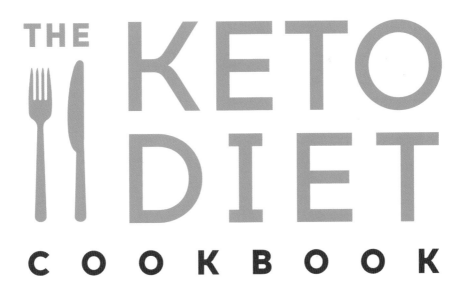

THE KETO DIET

COOKBOOK

140+ FLEXIBLE MEALS FOR EVERY DAY

LEANNE VOGEL

VICTORY BELT PUBLISHING INC.

Las Vegas

First published in 2019 by Victory Belt Publishing Inc.

ISBN-13: 978-1-628603-42-2

The author is not a licensed practitioner, physician, or medical professional and offers no medical diagnoses, treatments, suggestions, or counseling. The information presented herein has not been evaluated by the U.S. Food and Drug Administration, and it is not intended to diagnose, treat, cure, or prevent any disease. Full medical clearance from a licensed physician should be obtained before beginning or modifying any diet, exercise, or lifestyle program, and physicians should be informed of all nutritional changes.

The author claims no responsibility to any person or entity for any liability, loss, or damage caused or alleged to be caused directly or indirectly as a result of the use, application, or interpretation of the information presented herein.

Front and back cover photography and photos of author by Leanne Vogel and Nathan Elson

Food photography by Tatiana Briceag

Cover design by Justin-Aaron Velasco

Interior design by Yordan Terziev, Boryana Yordanova, and Justin-Aaron Velasco

Printed in Canada

TC 0119

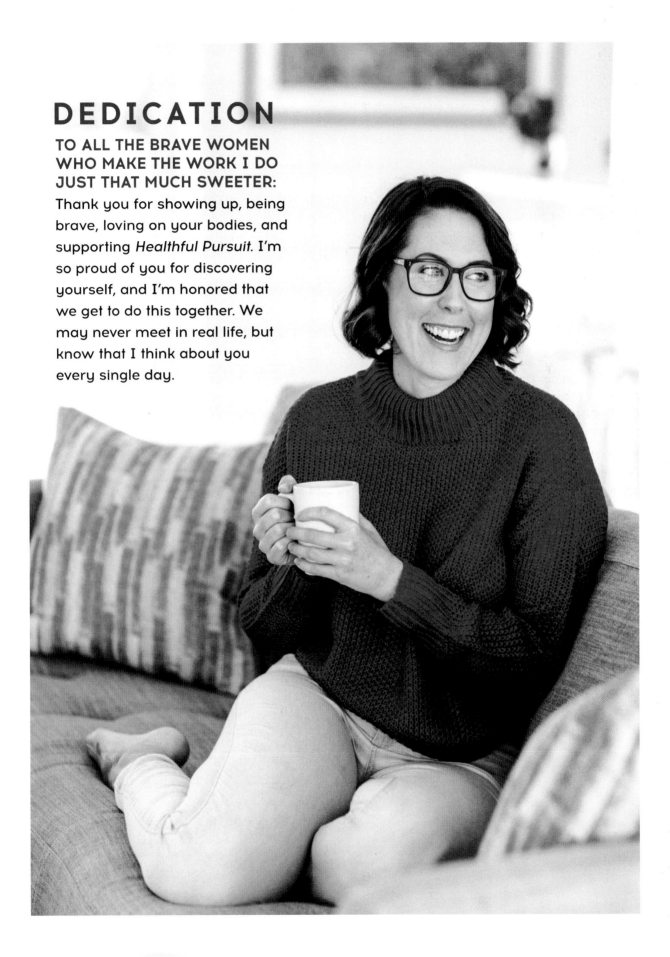

DEDICATION

TO ALL THE BRAVE WOMEN WHO MAKE THE WORK I DO JUST THAT MUCH SWEETER: Thank you for showing up, being brave, loving on your bodies, and supporting *Healthful Pursuit*. I'm so proud of you for discovering yourself, and I'm honored that we get to do this together. We may never meet in real life, but know that I think about you every single day.

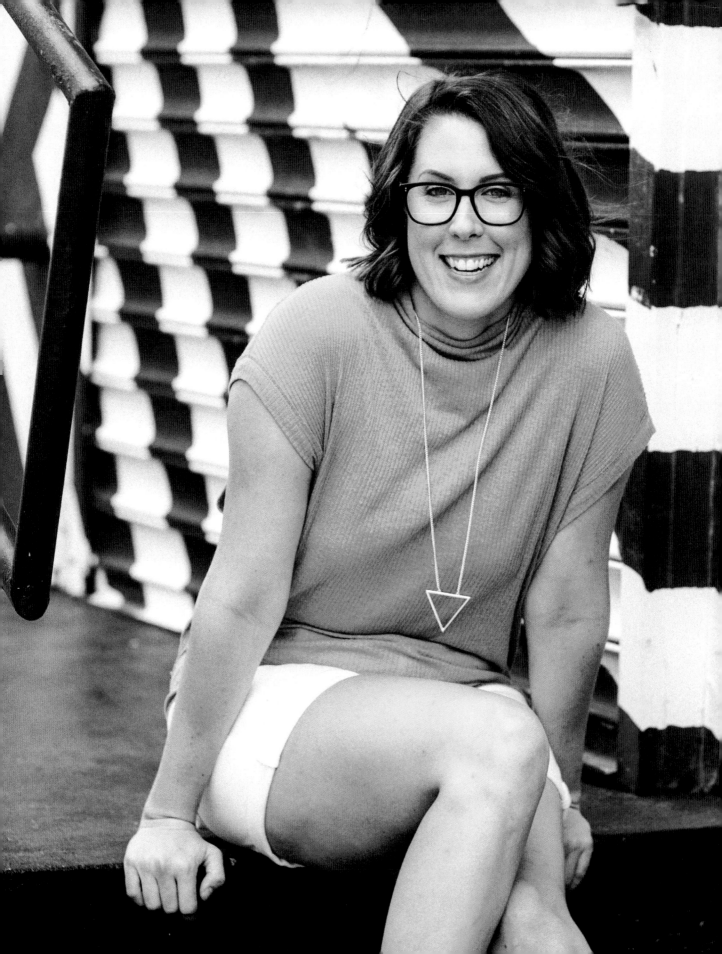

CONTENTS

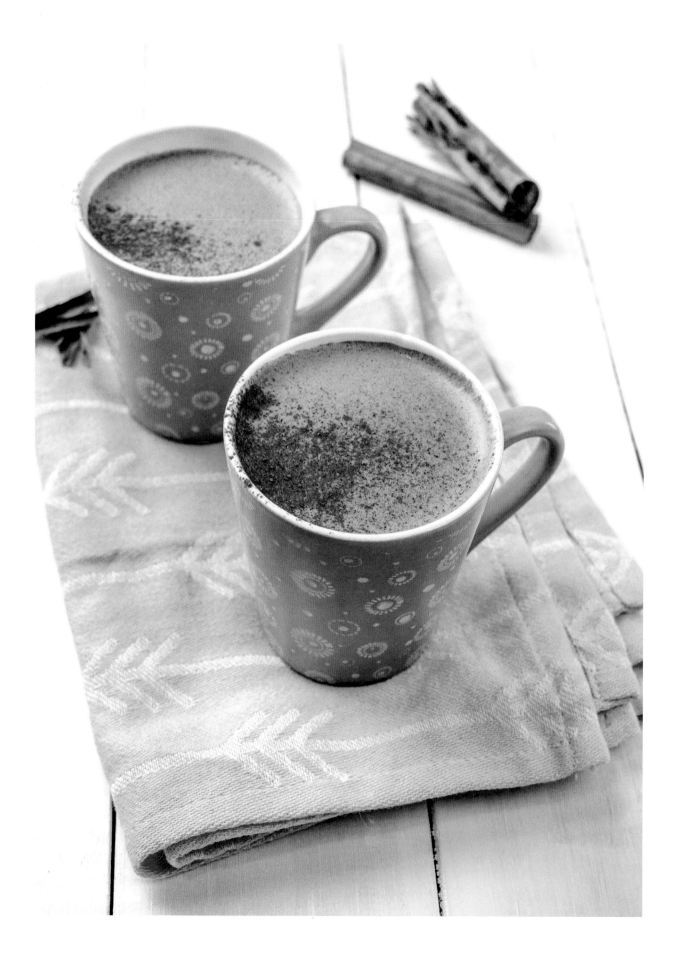

SPECIAL **THANK-YOU**

There are many of you who make doing this work so, so sweet. I've enjoyed getting to know you, gifting you various little goodies throughout the year, and relying on your feedback. This book, my podcast, blog posts, videos, recipes, and just about everything I do on *Healthful Pursuit* would not be possible without your support.

A very special thank-you to the following lovely humans:

Amber	Deanna F.	Jazmin J.	Kristi S.	Nanette S.	Stacey B.
Ann G.	Debbie W.	Jennifer E.	Kristie P.	Nicole B.	Stephanie J.
Anne M.	Deborah C.	Jennifer L.	Kristina S.	Nicole S.	Susan H.
Annie U.	Denise D.	Jennifer S.	Kristy F.	Pamela J.	Susan N.
Ashley C.	DiAnn W.	Jerri A.	Lacy L.	Pamela P.	Susan S.
Barbara I.	Elizabeth G.	Jessica D.	Laura L.	Pascale H.	Tamara R.
Beth G.	Erica S.	Jessica H.	Lindsay K.	Patti W.	Tanya S.
Brandy	Erin T.	Jocelyne B.	Lindsey W.	Paula F.	Teresa B.
Caitlin M.	Eva R.	Josephine B.	Lisa H.	Rachael P.	Terri F.
Cara F.	Francine M.	Judy H.	Lisa L.	Robbin K.	Theresa D.
Carol W.	Genevie	Kaitlin J.	M. J.	Roxana C.	Todd M.
Carolina L.	Gina R.	Kallie T.	Maggie B.	Samantha K.	Toni C.
Carrie H.	Hannah B.	Karen L.	Marci B.	Sandy	Victoria O.
Christin H.	Heather R.	Kate S.	Marisa S.	Sarah E.	Victoria S.
Christine C.	Holly K.	Katie W.	Marnie F.	Sarah K.	Wendi M.
Christine K.	Jamie G.	Kellie I.	Maureen W.	Sarah S.	Yvonne
Cindy B.	Jana G.	Kelly R.	Melody R.	Shaye W.	Yvonne A.
Colleen H.	Janet K.	Kelly S.	Michelle A.	Sheila G.	
Connie A.	Janine B.	Kerry I.	Michelle P.	Sherri S.	
Corie M.	Jared G.	Kim B.	Michelle R.	Shirley J.	

Thank you for cheering me on.

XO,
Leanne

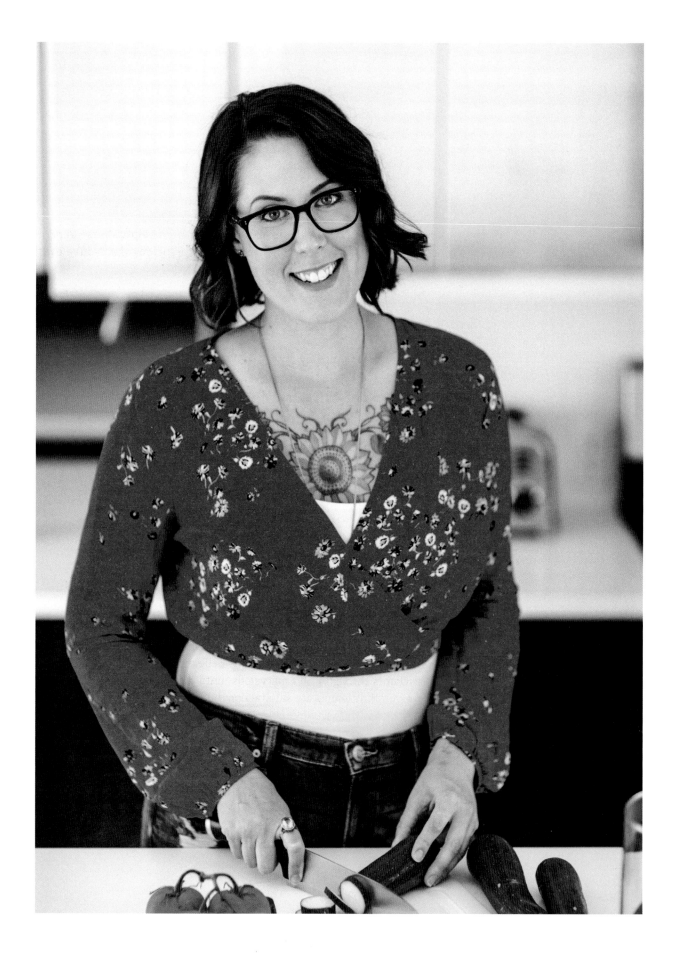

INTRODUCTION

Hi, friend. Before I share a bunch of the recipes that have been helpful to me in my five-plus years of eating keto, laid out in a completely different way than you've ever seen before, I want to set the tone for our time together.

You may have picked up this book because you're feeling fed up with the way your life is going, and you believe that changing the way you look, losing a little (or a lot of) weight, and finally getting in control of your body will change everything for you. You imagine a life filled with yeses, where you have the confidence to do the things you want to do when you want to do them. Perhaps this new life will include having better sex with your partner, completing a marathon, or finally wearing that cute (and currently way too tight) pair of jeans that you've kept in your closet as a motivator for the last four diets you've tried.

If this is you, I'm here to tell you to stop.

STOP!

Yup, you read that right. I'm suggesting that you stop. Why? Because I know that this chase never, ever works out in the long run. When all that was important to me was how I looked, I was never happy, was always miserable, and constantly felt like I was failing. That's not a pleasant way to live.

Why chasing after a perfect body doesn't work: You're different. And that's OK.

It's true that you can use the keto diet to lose a bunch of weight and feel hot in your bod, but that feeling of hotness lasts only so long. Believe me, I've done it, and I've walked countless clients through it. It's marvelous—until it isn't anymore. Of course, this book can give you that temporary satisfaction, but it can give you so much more if you let it. It all starts with the relationship you have with keto and with your body on keto.

Now, I can't speak for you. Maybe you want a hot bod no matter the cost. And hey, you can do that with keto! But maybe there's a small voice inside you that's seeking a bit more sustenance. Maybe that little voice is saying…

I want to live in a balanced body with loads of confidence.

I don't want to have to deal with horrible headaches anymore.

I want to choose joy.

I want to stop feeling like I need to drown myself in ice cream because "Who cares anyway?"

LEANNE, I WANT A BETTER LIFE; TELL ME YOUR SECRETS!

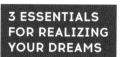
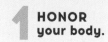
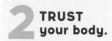
I feel you, and I invite you to join me in looking at your adjustment to keto or your life on keto a little differently. Making this adjustment will lead you to more success, less perceived failure, and ultimately more happiness.

Since 2007, I've been working hand in hand with people just like you, wanting to make a change in their life—workout goals, nutrition goals, education goals, you name it. And I think we often overlook the fact that changes come easiest when we side with our bodies. When we honor, trust, and nourish our bodies, we start to feel good, we make better decisions for ourselves, and we naturally progress toward our goals.

It's the relationship we have with ourselves that dictates the success we achieve…or don't achieve.

So, whether your goal is to be able to touch your toes again, boost your energy enough that you can chase your kids around the yard, finally live without an itchy scalp, or simply appreciate yourself a little, you got this.

What I'm proposing is that you

- Stop thinking you need to change your body before you can achieve happiness.
- Stop believing that you are only a body.
- Stop thinking you're weak.
- Start believing that your body wants to be healthy.
- Start trusting that your body wants what's best for you.
- Start appreciating all the wonderful things your body allows you to experience.

With this book and the recipes, meal planning system, and other resources in it, as well as all the free resources available on my blog, *Healthful Pursuit* (healthfulpursuit. com), we will work together to heal your body with a ketogenic diet. And as your body works its way toward healing, magical things will occur.

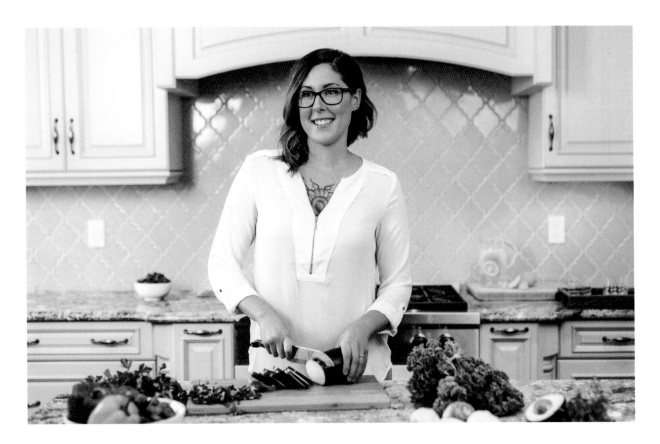

MY STORY

I guess I should formally introduce myself. My name's Leanne Vogel. I'm a Canadian who travels the world full-time, I'm a trained holistic nutritionist with more than eleven years in the field, and I used to be vegan.

I started *Healthful Pursuit* in 2010 after I realized that I couldn't reach many people working one-on-one day in and day out. Back then, *Healthful Pursuit* was a vegan blog where I shared plant-based recipes, meal plans, and my marathon training programs.

Right around 2013, I had gone six years without a menstrual period, and I decided that the path I was on wasn't working for me. Going six years without a period sounds great, but there comes a point when it's just not so great anymore. The lack of estrogen begins to affect bone density, the lack of cortisol affects muscle development, the lack of DHEA (another hormone) makes staying focused and happy next to impossible, and it all just gets to be a bit much.

Several doctors told me over the years that I wouldn't be able to have a natural period—ever. I went on hormone replacement therapy, and I gained weight very, very quickly. After about six months of being on hormone replacement therapy, I'd gained a whopping 40 pounds. I felt crazy every day of the week (the hormones made me so unstable), and I'd more than doubled my dose of ADHD medications to keep up with the demand.

This is when I found keto. July 2014 will forever be the month when my life took a 180-degree turn.

As I transitioned to a ketogenic diet, I made all the classic mistakes right out of the gate: not supplementing properly with electrolytes, working out too strenuously, not eating enough food, fasting too much, eating way too much dairy, and making macro-counting my number-one priority.

While the classic approach to a ketogenic diet—80 percent fat, 15 percent protein, and 5 percent carbohydrates, forever and ever amen—works for a lot of women, it didn't work for me. But I pushed my body into that paradigm for months because I thought I just needed to try harder until it finally worked.

Fast-forward one year and, although I'd been able to go off my ADHD medications (yay!), lose the hormone-related weight gain, get six-pack abs, and help others achieve similar results, I still wasn't happy. I had become so obsessed with food, my body, macros, calories, counting, tracking, and manipulating that I had distanced myself from…my *life*.

It wasn't until I took a step back and realized that I'd gone too far in the other direction (and still hadn't gotten my period back) that I accepted that the classic ketogenic protocol just wasn't for me.

Over the course of the next nine months, I researched, tested, and created focus groups on what I now call the Fat Fueled Protocol (find more details at healthfulpursuit.com/fatfueled), where women focus on three fundamental principles:

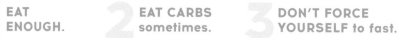

1 EAT ENOUGH. **2 EAT CARBS** sometimes. **3 DON'T FORCE YOURSELF** to fast.

After following this protocol for nine months, I got my period back. That was in 2015, and I've been ovulating, menstruating, and all the other –atings ever since. Take that, doctors who said I couldn't!

The moral of the story: You *can* heal your body, but you need patience, trust, and maybe a little chocolate. Wait, I ate *a lot* of chocolate, so let's say, "a healthy dose of chocolate."

Since getting my period back, I've gone on to work with women in regaining their health with a ketogenic diet: with the book *The Keto Diet* (ketodietbook.com) in 2017; with my twelve-week video training series, *Happy Keto Body* (happyketobody.com) in 2018; and now with this cookbook you hold in your hands.

My main point is that defining keto on *my* terms changed everything, and I'm confident that it can work for you, too. Consequently, you'll notice that a lot is going on with the recipes in this book. I delve deeper into the details in Chapter 3, but for now, you should know that I really wanted to make these recipes as accessible as I could for all sorts of people. If you respond best to incorporating dairy into your keto diet, I have you covered. If you can't do dairy (like I can't), every single recipe in this book can be made dairy-free. If you're sensitive to FODMAPs or nightshades or you aren't in the mood for a big meal, I have you covered, too.

WHY I MADE THIS

As a consumer, nothing irks me more than purchasing a book and discovering that it has all the same things in it as another book by the same author; the only difference is the cover. In other words, the same information is packaged a little differently, but I have to pay as much or more than I paid for the first book. Seriously, it's happened to me more times than I'd like to admit. (I really need to start looking *inside* books before I buy them.)

My first book, *The Keto Beginning*, delivers thirty days of keto instruction for keto newbies. My second book, *Fat Fueled*, delivers information on how to heal your body with a ketogenic diet. My third book, *The Keto Diet*, is…well, people call it their "keto bible." It's a 448-page, 2-pound beast of a book that emphasizes how to make keto work for you, no matter what your situation.

Honesty time: It's really hard to top *The Keto Diet*. I left nothing out. I put so much into that book that it took me nearly two years to find inspiration to write this one.

Instead of re-creating that same book, my vision for *The Keto Diet Cookbook* is to teach you how to eat keto with foods you have in your kitchen, introduce new ingredients to you, and show you how you can make keto work with the resources you have available right now.

If you're looking for more instruction on how to do keto—how to overcome hurdles, how to create an eating style that works best for your body, or how to change your relationship with your body—I have those answers for you, too! Head over to healthfulpursuit.com/shop to check out all the resources I've created and figure out what your logical next step would be.

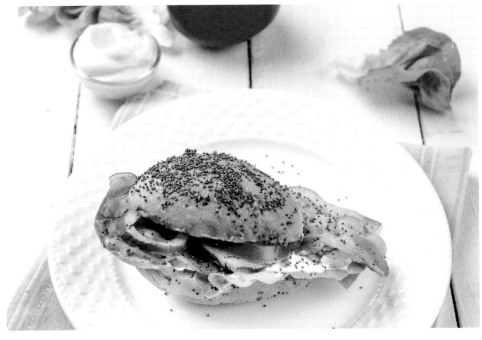

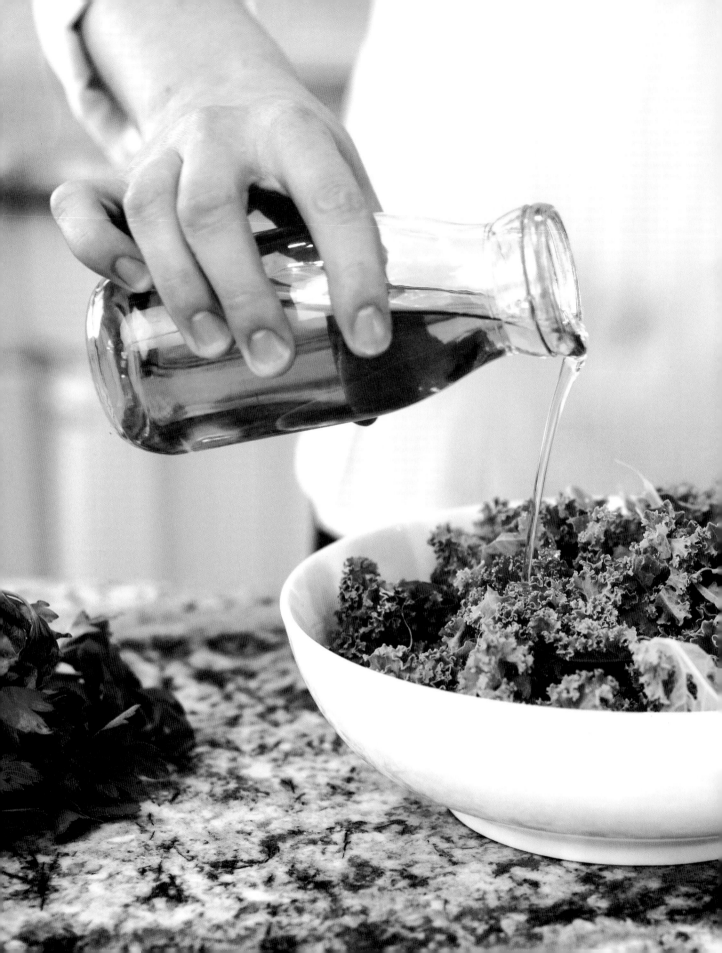

1.

THE KETO LOWDOWN

Ask anyone to define what keto is, why it's helpful, and what it can do for someone's health, and everyone will say something a little different. When you truly understand what the eating style you've chosen can do for your body, you sit in the driver's seat of your own health, wellness, and overall success. So, in this chapter, we'll cover:

1. **HOW TO KNOW WHETHER YOUR BODY NEEDS HEALING**

2. **HOW KETO DOES THE JOB**

3. **SETTING UP YOUR MACROS RIGHT...THE FIRST TIME**

4. **ADJUSTING KETO TO SUIT YOUR BODY**

WHAT KETO IS

Okay, time for ye ol' elevator pitch. You know—someone asks me what I do for work, I tell them that I create books and podcasts focused on the keto diet, and they instantly ask, "What's a keto?" To which I reply...

Keto is a low-carb, high-fat eating style whereby we reduce our carbohydrate intake so that we can burn fat for energy. The fat we use as energy comes from body fat or from the fats we consume. And, when we're using fat for fuel, we generate ketones, a by-product of fat breakdown that's used therapeutically by the whole body. When we're in this state, it is referred to as being "in ketosis."

Right now, you're burning glucose as energy. Glucose comes from carbohydrates like bread, potatoes, pasta, and sugary things. The problem with using glucose as energy is that it's really inefficient. You have to eat often, which leads to cravings, and you'll generally feel sluggish if the quality of the foods you've chosen doesn't align well with your body.

So, by eating keto, we eliminate the need to run primarily on glucose and instead run on fat! Fat is very efficient because we have so much on our bodies to use. All you have to do to access the fat on your body and burn it as fuel is to eat more fat and fewer carbs.

Seriously, I've said this so many times that I have it memorized. But it does such a great job of introducing keto that I just can't stop using it.

SIGNS IT'S TIME TO HEAL YOUR BODY

You may be thinking, "I don't have anything to heal. I just want to lose weight, and my body isn't cooperating." You'd be amazed at how many signs, symptoms, and imbalances cause our bodies to shut down and not do what we want them to do. Here are some signs that your body is in need of healing:

ITCHY SCALP
MOODINESS
DIZZINESS
ACNE

ANXIETY
HEADACHES
NASAL CONGESTION

BLOOD SUGAR HIGHS AND LOWS
SUGAR CRAVINGS

LACK OF INTEREST IN FOOD
FOOD ADDICTION
UNCONTROLLABLE HUNGER

CONSTIPATION
DIARRHEA

JOINT PAIN
PAINFUL PERIODS
LOW SEX DRIVE
SEVERE PMS

HOW KETO HEALS

When we reduce our consumption of carbohydrates and increase our intake of healthy fats, we see the following improvements:

 Inflammation goes down, which allows us to physically move more and be free from inflammatory conditions such as psoriasis, acne, and arthritis.

 Triglycerides decrease, which lowers cardiovascular disease risk.

 We naturally drink more water, which helps balance energy levels and relieve constipation.

 Quality of sleep improves, which leaves us feeling rested throughout the day.

 Our exposure to nutrients increases because we're pairing fat with fat-soluble vitamins.

 Endurance improves and muscle is spared, which leads to more gains at the gym.

 Our metabolism is regulated as blood sugar balances, which means we don't crave foods as often, and mood stabilizes.

 Hormones are better managed, which increases fertility and leads to more enjoyable periods, pregnancies, and menopause experiences.

No other diet heals the body like keto. As you satisfy yourself by consuming all the fats (I get to which fats are best on page 29), snacking on nut butter, and actually enjoying vegetables, your body is upregulating, balancing, and healing itself to a new normal. It's not uncommon for the body to change so drastically in such a short time that following a strict ketogenic protocol becomes unnecessary—or rather, what worked for you as you were healing your body becomes less of a concern in later months of eating keto.

Unlike other "diets," when you follow a ketogenic diet, your weight regulates itself without immense effort. Your anxiety subsides, your hair grows quickly and becomes strong, your appetite regulates itself without appetite suppression products, and all you have to worry about is ensuring that you eat enough fatty foods to keep yourself satiated. No self-loathing, guilt, or calorie counting required.

Your main takeaway from this chapter is that keto shouldn't be hard and doesn't have to be complex. I hope I make that point very, very clear in what's to come in the rest of this book.

BENEFITS OF KETOSIS

BLOOD SUGAR REGULATION

As you lower your carbohydrate intake, your elevated blood sugar level goes down and balances out, meaning that you have less need for insulin, the hormone that regulates blood sugar. When you start using fat as fuel, you become more and more insulin sensitive, whereby your body responds properly to carbohydrate intake, effectively releasing insulin when it should, with cells reacting to insulin as they should.

Once ketosis takes hold, you can say goodbye to eating every three to four hours in order to regulate your blood sugar. No more hangry feelings and no more pre-meal shakiness. You'll be riding the wave of blood sugar balance and enjoying the benefits after only days of following a ketogenic diet.

CLEARER SKIN

Carbohydrates might be the main dietary culprit for acne because of how they negatively affect hormone regulation. So, when you lower your carbohydrate intake via a ketogenic diet, you are effectively reducing your intake of the macronutrient that could be contributing to your hormone imbalances. In turn, you're balancing hormones that, when unbalanced, can result in acne.

It's incredible how much clearer my skin has become as a result of this eating style. I'm much more in tune with how my body responds to eating certain foods, and I've been able to determine that eggs, nightshades, and nuts affect my skin negatively.

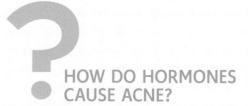

HOW DO HORMONES CAUSE ACNE?

Androgens, such as testosterone, cause increased sebum production, which leads to oily skin. When sebum production increases, cell production ramps up, and dead skin cells aren't shed in the normal fashion. The extra cells combine with the excess sebum, which causes blockages or plugs in the skin.

SUPPRESSED APPETITE

The keto diet is naturally satiating because fats are satiating. When you're in fat-burning mode, fat is a constant fuel source that your body can access on demand.

When I dieted in the past, food ruled my world. I always felt hungry and had to play mind games with myself to resist chowing down. With keto, I don't need to make an effort to avoid food the way I did before. I just...don't want to eat. With this shift comes great freedom—I can hop on a flight without snacks, I can go the whole morning without getting hungry, and I generally am not the least bit concerned about food.

BALANCED BLOOD WORK

Your biomarkers change as the way you fuel your body is flipped upside down with keto. Cholesterol, the precursor to all sex hormones, aids in balancing your endocrine system, HDL increases due to a higher saturated fat intake, HsCRP (a marker of overall inflammation) is reduced as you eat fewer inflammatory foods, and so much more.

As a vegan, and even when I was Paleo, I could never get a handle on my numbers. My total cholesterol, HDL, LDL, triglycerides, estrogen, progesterone, insulin, cortisol—everything was all over the place. But, after I had been in ketosis for six months, my blood panel looked marvelous, and it still does! My HDL is higher, my triglycerides are low, and my cortisol has balanced out.

ENHANCED BRAIN FUNCTION

Ketones are a powerful source of fuel for the brain. Fueling a brain with only glucose results in blood sugar highs and lows, which affect brain function and cause fluctuations in energy, focus, and ability to complete tasks efficiently, or at all.

After two months of eating this way, I was able to work with my doctor to stop taking all the ADHD medications I'd been on since I was eleven years old. I felt as if a veil had been lifted, and I was able to think clearly for the first time.

MOOD STABILIZATION

As your blood sugar levels off, so does your mood. Also, many of the foods you may have had negative reactions to—such as those containing artificial colors, flavors, and preservatives—are no longer part of your eating style, which contributes to further mood stabilization and healing through a focus on whole, unprocessed foods.

My moods have stabilized dramatically. Now, when I do eat a touch more carbohydrate than I'm used to, I'm reminded of just how crazy I used to feel all the time! These days, I can clearly identify my emotions and make levelheaded choices based on how I'm feeling instead of having the erratic and involuntary emotional reactions that so often controlled me in the past.

ACCESS TO FAT STORES FOR ENERGY

In a state of nutritional ketosis, our cell walls can stay wide open, which makes them ready to release fats into the energy chain through lipolysis. When you're fueled by glucose, insulin is out partying in your bloodstream and causes your cell walls to stay closed, which makes lipolysis much more difficult.

When you go keto, you activate your body fat as fuel for nearly every one of your body's daily processes. This fat energy is available at any time, so you have a steady stream of energy rather than suffering the peaks and valleys you experience when you're fueled by glucose.

IMPROVED MENTAL FOCUS

Think of ketones as rocket fuel for the brain. When your brain is receiving ketones, either in the form of exogenous (external to the body) ketones or endogenous (internal to the body) ketones, your brain lights up!

Regardless of the time of day, when you're fueled by fat, your brain has the ability to fire on all cylinders. You can expect improved focus and concentration the whole day through.

MEET THE KETONE: YOUR NEW BEST BUD

Ketones, also known as "ketone bodies," are by-products created when the body breaks down fat for energy. There are three types of ketone bodies: acetoacetate (AcAc), beta-hydroxybutyric acid (BHB), and acetone.

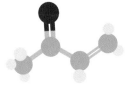

KETONES

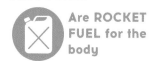 Are ROCKET FUEL for the body

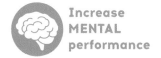 Increase MENTAL performance

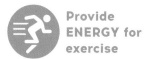 Provide ENERGY for exercise

How do you get this wonder drug? All you have to do is eat a ketogenic diet!

If you want to boost your body's natural ketone levels, you can supplement with MCT oil, which boosts ketones indirectly, or exogenous ketones, which are a pure ketone supplement that delivers ready-to-use ketones to the systems in your body that need them the most.

Exogenous ketones are not an absolute fix-everything supplement, and not everyone needs them. Also, using them improperly can lead to some serious drawbacks. For example, you should not use exogenous ketones to "erase" poor eating choices, such as consuming excess carbohydrates. You also shouldn't use them to extend fasting beyond what your body is comfortable with, or think that if you supplement with them, you don't have to focus on food quality and eat a well-rounded keto diet. Most importantly, it is possible to rely too heavily on exogenous ketones, so keep that in mind if you decide to try them out. However, if you use them responsibly and purposefully, then they can be an awesome keto game-changer!

THE BASICS OF THE KETOGENIC DIET

IT'S IMPORTANT THAT YOU UNDERSTAND THE FOLLOWING DEFINITIONS:

MACROS (short for MACRONUTRIENTS) are fats, proteins, and carbohydrates.

When someone asks, "What are your keto macros?" what they're asking is, how much of each macronutrient do you consume?

Macros can be displayed as percentages, such as 80% fat, 15% protein, and 5% carbohydrate, or as gram amounts, such as 178 grams of fat, 75 grams of protein, and 25 grams of carbohydrate. The carbohydrate amount refers to *total* carbohydrates consumed, not net carbohydrates.

TOTAL CARBOHYDRATES include all carbohydrates consumed.

NET CARBOHYDRATES are total carbohydrates minus any fiber and sugar alcohol consumed.

The premise of the ketogenic diet is to eat a lot of fat, moderate protein, and limited carbohydrates, like this:

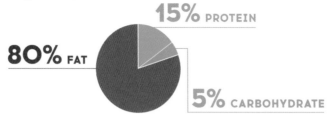

15% PROTEIN

80% FAT

5% CARBOHYDRATE

Think of these percentages as the amounts of food you eat in a day. All the food you eat equals 100 percent, with fats, proteins, and carbohydrates being the three pieces of the pie.

Here's an example to bring it all together for you:

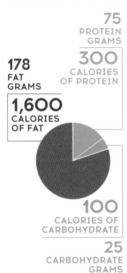

2,000
CALORIES IN A DAY

75
PROTEIN
GRAMS

300
CALORIES
OF PROTEIN

178
FAT
GRAMS

1,600
CALORIES
OF FAT

100
CALORIES OF
CARBOHYDRATE

25
CARBOHYDRATE
GRAMS

Your goal is to eat 2,000 calories in a day, and you want your macros to be 80 percent fat, 15 percent protein, and 5 percent carbohydrate. To figure out how much of each macronutrient to eat, you need to know that 1 gram of carbohydrate or protein equals 4 calories, while 1 gram of fat equals 9 calories. With that information in hand, you can translate the percentages to caloric equivalencies:

Calories of fat in a day = 2,000 x 80% = 1,600

Calories of protein in a day = 2,000 x 15% = 300

Calories of carbohydrate in a day = 2,000 x 5% = 100

Now, you can calculate how many grams make up each of these groups of calories by doing the following calculations:

Grams of fat in a day = 1,600 calories / 9 calories per gram = 178

Grams of protein in a day = 300 calories / 4 calories per gram = 75

Grams of carbohydrate in a day = 100 calories / 4 calories per gram = 25

The grams in these calculations represent the grams of actual fat, protein, and carbohydrate found in a food item rather than the physical weight of that food item. For example, 100 grams of chicken breast as weighed with a food scale does not contain 100 grams of protein; it has 31 grams of protein. So remember that these calculations don't refer to the physical weight of the food, but to the fat, protein, or carbohydrate the food contains.

To give you an idea of what 178 grams of fat looks like, it is about 1¼ cups (315 grams of physical weight) of almond butter. (Remember that almond butter also contributes carbohydrates and protein to the equation.) Here are two other examples:

· 75 grams of protein equates to about 2½ chicken thighs cooked with the skin on.

· 25 grams of carbohydrate equates to a small head of broccoli.

Understanding these concepts is super helpful when you're looking at the portions on your plate. It helps to know that fat contains more than double the energy (that is, calories) of protein or carbohydrate.

ADJUSTING KETO FOR YOUR BODY

You don't necessarily have to commit to specific macronutrient ratios in order to reach keto success. I've formulated the recipes in this book in such a way that if you make use of the recipes and meal planning strategies (see Chapter 3), you'll be quite close to the standard ketogenic ratios.

Once you get the hang of combining small, medium, large, and huge meals to create a meal plan that suits you best, you can start to tweak things here and there as you learn more about your body, your needs, and how adjusting the macro percentages affects your progress toward your goals.

You might be thinking, "Great! I know the keto macros; I'm set!" However, figuring out which macro percentages work best for you depends on what your body needs at any given time; the numbers might be different for someone else.

Many people (including me) respond best to keto when they adjust their macronutrients to their current circumstances. Perhaps you'll have days when you eat more protein than usual as you reduce your carbohydrates to nearly zero. On other days, you might consume less fat than normal so you can incorporate more leafy greens or load up on animal protein.

Let's run through some of the most common adjustments people can make to their macros based on their health imbalances or overall goals.

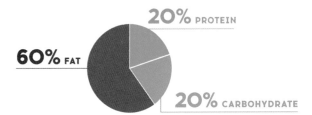

NO GALLBLADDER OR FATTY ACID DIGESTIVE ISSUES

Best for: People who know that they don't digest fat well or who do not have a gallbladder.

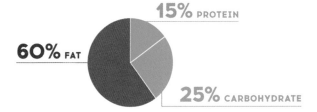

THYROID IMBALANCE, ADRENAL DYSFUNCTION, OR DIFFICULTY SLEEPING*

Best for: People with thyroid imbalance, adrenal dysfunction, or difficulty sleeping.

Eating low-carb, high-fat all day and then incorporating a touch more carbohydrates in the evening in the form of fruits (like apples and berries) and grain-free starches (like parsnips, squash, and sweet potatoes) might feel best.

Don't worry too much about whether the boost in carbohydrates will affect your ketone level. The amount of carbs you consume is so minimal that you'll be back to burning fat in the morning, and having that touch of carbs will go a long way toward balancing out the body systems that need it most.

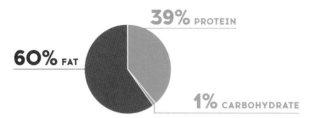

39% PROTEIN

60% FAT

1% CARBOHYDRATE

REACTING TO PLANTS OR WANTING TO LOSE FAT

Best for: People who are working on healing their digestive system, react to plant foods (such as vegetables, fruits, or nuts), or want to shed excess fat and develop muscle definition.

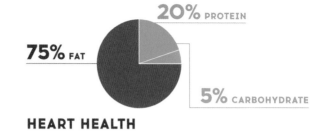

20% PROTEIN

75% FAT

5% CARBOHYDRATE

HEART HEALTH

Best for: Those concerned with the health of their heart.

If you find that when you eat keto, your cholesterol increases and you gain weight quickly, try reducing your intake of saturated fats and focus on monounsaturated fats such as olive oil and avocado oil.

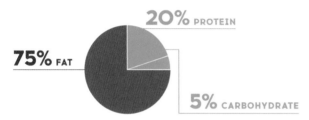

20% PROTEIN

75% FAT

5% CARBOHYDRATE

INFLAMMATION, AUTOIMMUNE CONDITIONS, OR PCOS

Best for: Those who have an autoimmune condition, struggle with inflammation, or have been diagnosed with polycystic ovary syndrome (PCOS).

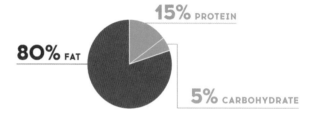

15% PROTEIN

80% FAT

5% CARBOHYDRATE

NEUROLOGICAL IMBALANCES

Best for: People who have imbalances of the nervous system, including biochemical, electrical, or structural abnormalities in the brain, nerves, or spinal cord—for example, struggling with poor coordination, loss of sensation, confusion, muscle weakness, or paralysis. Conditions that can cause these imbalances include ADHD, Alzheimer's disease, dementia, dyslexia, and restless leg syndrome.

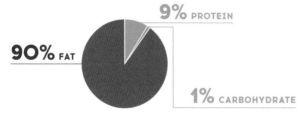

9% PROTEIN

90% FAT

1% CARBOHYDRATE

POST-SURGERY OR FEELING UNDER THE WEATHER

Best for: People whose immune systems have taken a hit, either with an oncoming flu bug, during a stressful period in life, or following a surgery where the body needs to do a bunch of healing and resting.

LADIES! SYNCING HORMONES WITH YOUR KETO PROTOCOL

If you're experiencing a monthly menstrual cycle, or you're at an age where a monthly cycle is expected of your body, understanding the hormones that influence your cycle is key to understanding hormone imbalance and how a ketogenic diet can help correct this imbalance. With just a slight tweak to your macronutrient ratios, you can support the ebb and flow of the two main hormones responsible for a balanced menstrual cycle: estrogen and progesterone.

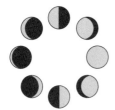

If you do not have a cycle due to a condition called amenorrhea, this information applies to you as well. Your body still might go through the hormonal ebb and flow, but that ebb and flow is not strong enough to produce menstruation. If you're unsure of where you are in your cycle, use the phases of the moon as a guide. A full moon can signify ovulation. When is the next full moon? Count backward 14 days from that date and pick that as day 1 of your next cycle.

A menstrual cycle results from hormonal changes between the ovaries and the pituitary gland (located in the brain). A typical cycle is between 24 and 35 days.

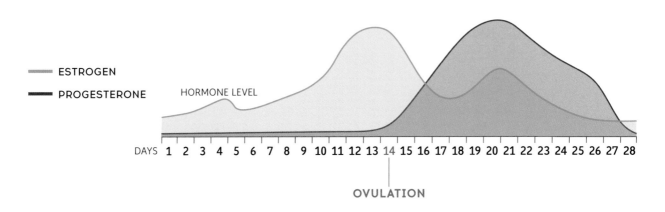

ESTROGEN matures an egg before ovulation. This is why you see an estrogen increase just before ovulation. Additionally, it matures the uterine lining that is shed when a period takes place, which is why the level increases again in the luteal phase.

Signs of excess estrogen: bloating, decreased sex drive, mood swings, headaches, acne, PMS

Signs of decreased estrogen: painful intercourse, depression, hot flashes, mood swings, irregular periods, increased instances of UTIs

PROGESTERONE works to balance out the effects of estrogen during the maturation of the uterine lining in the luteal phase. This is why it increases during the estrogen increase.

Signs of excess progesterone: bloating, decreased sex drive, swelling and tenderness of the breasts in the luteal phase

Signs of decreased progesterone: low sex drive, thyroid dysfunction (primarily hypothyroidism), weight gain, irregular menstrual cycle

Changing Your Macros with Your Cycle

The following macro adjustments assume that your period lasts for five days, you ovulate on the fourteenth day of your cycle, and your full menstrual cycle is 28 days. If your body is different, you will need to adjust the following to suit your pattern.

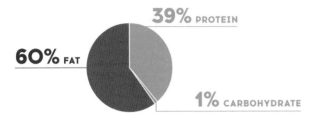

CYCLE DAYS 1 TO 5

During your period, your body may respond best to a higher protein intake.

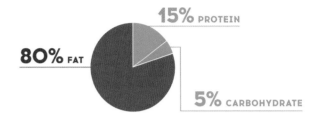

CYCLE DAYS 6 TO 11

The first day after your period until two days before ovulation. This is when women are most responsive to the ketogenic diet, able to eat severely low-carb or no-carb with boundless energy.

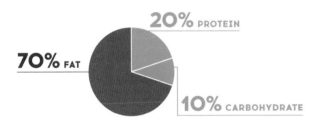

CYCLE DAYS 12 TO 16*

Two days before ovulation, ovulation itself, and two days after ovulation. A woman's body still responds well to eating low-carb during this phase, but you may benefit from a boost in glutathione, specifically in the evening. Food sources of glutathione include apples, avocados, broccoli, garlic, grapefruit, oranges, parsley, and tomatoes.

You could also benefit from maintaining your usual keto macros for breakfast and lunch and then increasing your carbohydrate intake after 5 p.m., preferably with fruit. Do this each evening during these days of your cycle.

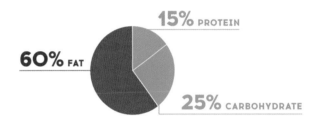

CYCLE DAYS 17 TO 28*

The third day following ovulation through the day before you get your period. Your body will likely begin to crave carbohydrates as you approach the end of your cycle.

You could benefit from maintaining your usual keto macros for breakfast and lunch and then increasing your carbohydrate intake after 5 p.m., preferably with starchy vegetables like cassava, plantains, potatoes, and sweet potatoes. Do this each evening during these days of your cycle.

Don't worry too much about whether you register ketones during this phase. The amount of carbohydrates you consume is so minimal that you'll be back to burning fat in the morning, and you will feel much better through the remainder of your cycle.

Menopause

Women who are currently experiencing menopause or are post-menopausal can typically follow standard 80/15/5 ketogenic ratios.

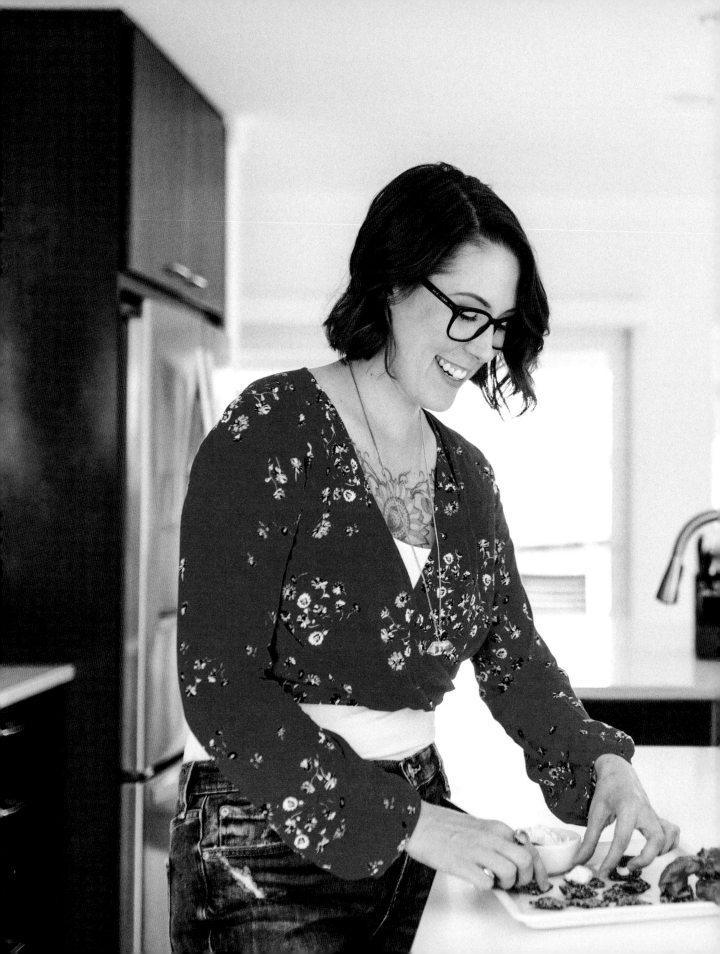

2.

4 STEPS TO KETO ✓ SUCCESS

Regardless of what brought you here or what your goals are, you can achieve a ketogenic state. The process goes like this:

1. SET YOUR MACROS AND EAT GOOD FOOD.

2. GET YOUR BODY INTO KETOSIS.

3. BECOME FAT-ADAPTED.

4. FIGURE OUT WHICH FOODS MAKE YOU FEEL GOOD AND HELP YOU HIT YOUR GOALS.

Let me break down each of these steps into bite-sized pieces for you.

SET YOUR MACROS

The way I see it, there are two ways of looking at macronutrient consumption:

- **PERCENTAGE INTAKE:** You would say, "My macronutrient consumption today was 73 percent fat, 15 percent protein, and 12 percent carbs." This approach is great when you're just getting started and you're trying to understand how the components relate to one another.

- **GRAM INTAKE:** You would say, "My macronutrient consumption today was 150 grams of fat, 70 grams of protein, and 55 grams of carbs." This approach is best once you have determined the exact ratios of macronutrients that work best for you. Then it's just a matter of hitting the target number of grams of each macronutrient every day.

The two approaches convey the same information; they just come from different viewpoints.

A good place to start is 75 to 80 percent fat, 15 percent protein, and 5 to 10 percent carbohydrate. In *The Keto Diet* (ketodietbook.com), I call this the Classic Keto Fat Fueled Profile. For more macro options, flip back to pages 22 to 25.

Maybe you're wondering WHICH FOODS TO EAT in order to hit these macros? I thought you'd never ask!

The health-promoting foods in the following lists are classic parts of a whole food–based ketogenic lifestyle. Where quality is a concern for a specific item, I've listed what to look for directly after the name of the item or at the top of the list.

Some people react to perfectly healthful foods in the form of inflammation, allergy symptoms, and/or a reduction in ketones. This isn't to say the food is bad for keto, but rather unhelpful for the individual. So, in this list, I've marked some of the potentially problematic food items that may be standing in the way of your living a fully healthy life. Don't get me wrong, there's nothing wrong with these foods, but if you're having issues on your keto diet and think that food items could be a culprit, here's where to look.

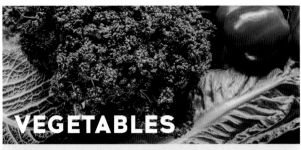

VEGETABLES

Alfalfa

Artichoke hearts ⚠️

Arugula

Asparagus ⚠️

Bok choy

Broccoli

Brussels sprouts ⚠️

Cabbage

Capers

Cauliflower ⚠️

Celeriac

Celery, *organic* ⚠️

Chard

Chives

Collards

Cucumbers, *organic*

Daikon

Eggplant ⚠️

Endive/Escarole

Fennel

Garlic ⚠️

Ginger ⚠️

Jicama

Kale

Kimchi ⚠️

Kohlrabi

Lettuce, *organic*

Mushrooms ⚠️

Okra ⚠️

Olives

Onions ⚠️

Peppers, sweet and hot ⚠️

Radishes

Rhubarb

Sauerkraut

Shallots ⚠️

Spinach, *organic*

Swiss chard

Tomatoes ⚠️

Turnips

Water chestnuts

Zucchini, *non-GMO*

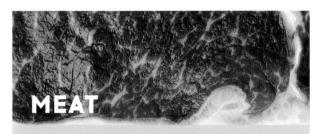

MEAT

All animal-based proteins are safe. Opt for grass-fed/pasture-raised when possible.

Bacon

Beef muscle meat and organ meat

Chicken muscle meat and organ meat

Cold cuts ⚠️

Lamb muscle meat

Pork muscle meat

Turkey muscle meat and organ meat

Wild game muscle meat and organ meat

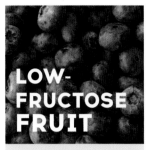

LOW-FRUCTOSE FRUIT

Avocados ⚠️

Blackberries ⚠️

Blueberries

Cranberries

Grapefruit ⚠️

Lemons ⚠️

Limes ⚠️

Raspberries

Strawberries

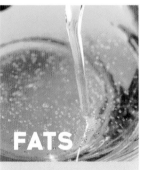

FATS

Avocado oil

Cacao/Cocoa butter ⚠️

Chicken fat (schmaltz), *free-range*

Chocolate, unsweetened ⚠️

Coconut

Coconut oil

Duck fat, *free-range*

Goose fat, *free-range*

Hazelnut oil ⚠️

Lard, *pasture-raised*

Macadamia nut oil ⚠️

MCT oil

MCT oil powder

Olive oil

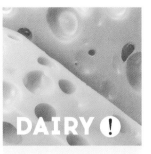

DAIRY ⚠️

Opt for high-fat, grass-fed/pasture-raised when possible.

Butter

Cheese

Cottage cheese

Cream cheese

Ghee

Heavy whipping cream

Milk

Sour cream

Whey

Yogurt

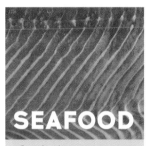

SEAFOOD

Opt for low-mercury fish as often as possible.

Anchovies

Mackerel

Oysters

Salmon, *wild-caught*

Sardines

Scallops

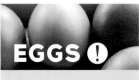

EGGS ⚠️

Chicken eggs

Duck eggs

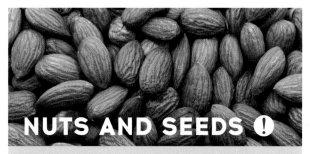

NUTS AND SEEDS ❗

Including nut and seed butters and flours.

Almonds	Pili nuts
Brazil nuts	Pine nuts
Cashews	Pistachios
Chia seeds	Poppy seeds
Flax seeds	Pumpkin seeds
Hazelnuts	Sesame seeds
Hemp seeds	Sunflower seeds
Macadamia nuts	Walnuts
Pecans	

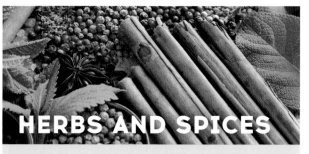

HERBS AND SPICES

Basil	Garlic powder ⓘ
Bay leaves	Ginger powder ⓘ
Black pepper ⓘ	Mint
Cardamom ⓘ	Mustard seed ⓘ
Carob powder	Nutmeg ⓘ
Cayenne pepper ⓘ	Onion powder ⓘ
Chili powder ⓘ	Oregano
Chipotle powder ⓘ	Paprika ⓘ
Cinnamon	Parsley
Cocoa powder	Rosemary
Cumin ⓘ	Sage
Curry powder ⓘ	Taco seasoning ⓘ
Dill	Thyme
Fennel seed ⓘ	Turmeric powder

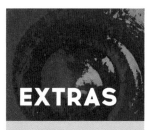
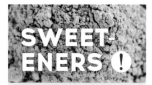

SWEET-ENERS ❗

Erythritol

Monk fruit

Stevia

Xylitol

EXTRAS

Apple cider vinegar

Balsamic vinegar

Bone broth

Coconut aminos

Coconut butter

Coconut vinegar

Collagen peptides

Gelatin

Hot sauce ⓘ

Ketchup, *unsweetened* ⓘ

Mayonnaise, *made with avocado oil*

Mustard ⓘ

Nutritional yeast

Salad dressings, *unsweetened* ⓘ

Salsa ⓘ

Vanilla extract, *alcohol-free*

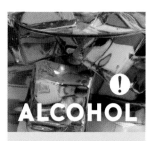

❗ ALCOHOL

Brandy

Champagne

Gin

Red wine, *dry farmed*

Tequila

Vodka

Whiskey

White wine, *dry farmed*

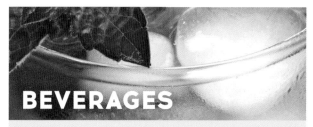

BEVERAGES

Coconut water	Herbal tea	Water kefir
Green tea	Kombucha ⓘ	

IS ALCOHOL ACTUALLY OKAY?

Alcohols like brandy, champagne, gin, dry-farmed white or red wine, tequila, vodka, and whiskey are pretty safe to have on a ketogenic diet; just understand that if you're struggling with health imbalances, drinking alcohol is not going to help the situation. However, if you are out with friends, at a function, or need a stiff drink, these are the best alcohols to opt for! Just know that your ketone levels will dip a bit before returning to normal. And alcohol is best avoided during the first couple of weeks of eating a ketogenic diet.

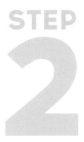

STEP 2
GET YOUR BODY INTO KETOSIS

Following a ketogenic eating style using the macros outlined in Step 1 will eventually put you into a state of ketosis. When you're in a state of ketosis, your body breaks down your body fat, using it as energy and developing ketones that are released into your bloodstream. Being "in ketosis" is a normal metabolic state that you achieve either by fasting or with the support of a high-fat, moderate-protein, low-carb eating style.

The process of getting into a ketogenic state, where you're generating ketones, can take anywhere from two weeks to a couple of months. How slow or fast your body gets there is dependent on many factors, but the most common is the state of your metabolism when you start.

STEP 3
BECOME FAT-ADAPTED

One of the goals of the ketogenic eating style is to become "fat-adapted." Being fat-adapted means that your body is primed for functioning optimally on very little glucose. This is where the healing happens.

When you first enter ketosis, the fat you will be using for energy will be in limited supply. The reason is that breaking down fat requires different enzymes than the ones needed to break down glucose, and your body won't have had sufficient time to produce many fat-converting enzymes.

Up until now, your body has focused on breaking down excess glucose rather than breaking down fats, so when you get started on a ketogenic lifestyle, your body needs a bit of time to "catch up" and build a store of fat-converting enzymes. This is one of the main reasons why many people feel tired when they begin altering their eating habits.

Once the fat-focused enzymes have built up, your cells miraculously change their preferred way of acquiring energy, and you become fully fat-adapted. The process of becoming fully fat-adapted can take anywhere from a month to a couple of months.

Once you've become fat-adapted, fatty acids and their substrates, ketone bodies, become your body's preferred fuel, and this is when all kinds of good things begin to happen. Your hormone levels balance out, levels of glycogen (the form in which glucose is stored in the liver and muscles) are depleted, your body carries around less water, and your energy is restored to normal levels. I strongly recommend that you stick with a keto plan for at least 30 days, and sometimes even longer, to allow your body ample time to become fully fat-adapted.

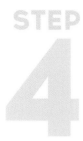
FIGURE OUT WHICH FOODS MAKE YOU FEEL GOOD

When I first started eating keto, I had it in my head that there were *good* and *bad* foods. You know: eat a lot of coconut and avocado, but don't eat fruit or starches of any kind, and stay far, far, far away from sugar.

Although there are foods that will benefit you far more than others when you follow a ketogenic diet, approaching keto—or any eating style, for that matter—with the "good versus bad" mentality will likely end in binges, going off plan, and feeling miserable about yourself.

So, what should you do instead? I go by one keto motto with almost everything I choose to eat. (I say "almost" only because I do indulge in a little popcorn here and there because I'm human, and popcorn is essential on epic movie nights.) Here's the motto:

I eat whole food, try to stay away from the artificial stuff, and if it's hard to pronounce, it's probably not best.

In keto, there's less debate about good versus bad than there is debate about what's whole versus not-so-whole. (Think "unprocessed versus processed.") There's also a focus on asking yourself, "How does my body feel with that certain food?"

For example, let's chat about dairy. I can't do dairy. I just *cannot*. Whenever I eat it, I get horrible acne, painful periods, constipation, diarrhea, brain fog—bad symptoms of a food that doesn't agree with me. Dairy is keto, for sure. But it doesn't work for me.

Next up, sweeteners. My opinion on keto-safe sweeteners has changed over time, and it continues to evolve. When I first started keto, I was metabolically damaged, which means I couldn't handle much sweetness without experiencing cravings, glucose spikes, and sleepiness. Now, five-plus years later, I can sweeten recipes with whole-food sweeteners like overripe banana, applesauce, or Medjool dates without seeing any effect on my ketones. Erythritol, xylitol, allulose, and stevia are all considered safe in keto. They likely won't spike your blood sugar as drastically as white sugar would (although some individuals experience some blood sugar spiking), and they're great options if you're metabolically damaged, you want a treat, and your body isn't responding well to whole-food sweeteners like fruit.

Nuts and seeds are other foods that work with a ketogenic lifestyle in some cases. Some people respond well to them; others do not.

So you see, there are keto foods that even many keto people can't eat. And we can adjust our eating styles to better support our bodies with the foods that make us feel our best, even if those foods aren't completely "keto." When you eat the best foods for your body, inflammation goes down, healing ramps up, and you're better able to stay in a ketogenic state.

Filling your life with the right foods will fuel you with energy, positivity, and rockin' good times. The wrong foods will give you headaches, bloating, cramps, and irritability.

Now, you might be thinking, "How the heck am I supposed to know which foods work well for me and which do not?" Let me tell you a particularly effective approach.

Food Journaling

Using a food journal is a great way to track the foods you eat and how you feel after eating them. I've provided a journal template that will help you make sense of the subtle cues your body sends you. You'll learn to listen to your body, understand yourself, and get healthy with every winning decision you make!

Here's how it works:

1 Photocopy the template and fill in your answers, writing notes on your phone, or creating your own template in a paper journal.

2 Take 15 minutes each day to record what you ate and how you felt before and after eating your meals.

3 Keep an open mind and a forgiving heart. Just write it all down!

You don't have to carry your food journal everywhere with you. Keep it at the office, at home, in the car—whatever works best for you. Set aside a little time each day to enter your foods in your journal and keep track of how you feel after you eat. How you feel after a meal is the most important part, and that information will tell you far more than you realize.

FOOD JOURNALING TIPS:

Begin with the date. I highly recommend that you keep track of the days of the week instead of listing just numbers. This information will come in handy when you start to link together your eating patterns.

Fill out the chart with details: the time you ate, the quantity (roughly) of food, the type of food (fruit, vegetable, protein, fat, etc.), and the symptoms you experienced after your meal.

At the end of the day, jot down how many hours you slept, how much water you drank, and what physical activity you did that day. Also sum up your total intake of veggies, fruit, and so on.

At the end of the week, answer the Weekly Reflection questions to document what you've learned about yourself.

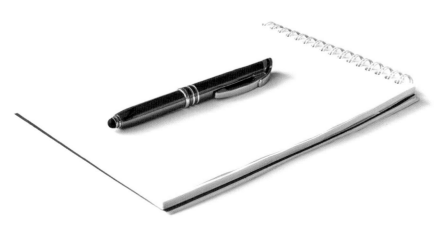

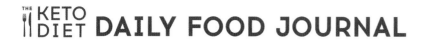

DAILY FOOD JOURNAL

Date: ....

TIME	FOOD/BEVERAGE & QUANTITY	SYMPTOMS

Hours of sleep last night: .... Glasses of water drunk today:..............................

Physical activity today:..

Summary of my day (cravings, situations, timing of meals, etc.):...

....

....

WEEKLY REFLECTION

Date: ....

Which foods do I gravitate to?..

....

Do I eat at the same time every day? What impacts my eating patterns?...

....

Do my portion sizes vary? If so, why?..

....

Where do I generally enjoy my meals? Do I feel better when I eat in certain places or environments?

....

....

Do I prefer eating alone or with a group?...

....

What emotional state am I usually in while I eat?..

....

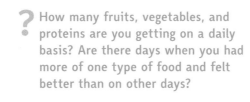

Here are some patterns to look for as you're journaling:

? How many fruits, vegetables, and proteins are you getting on a daily basis? Are there days when you had more of one type of food and felt better than on other days?

? Are you skipping meals and subsequently overeating later in the day?

? Are your meals balanced? Are you eating all of your starchy foods in the morning and packing in the protein in the afternoon?

? Are there long spans of time between meals?

? Do you notice any food groups that are completely missing?

? Do you notice that you overeat if you wait too long between meals?

? Do you notice your eating pattern changes when you fast in the morning versus in the evening?

? What is the perfect amount of time between your meals? What is too long, and what is too short?

? Do you experience a particular symptom after eating a certain type of food?

? What is the ideal day for you? What patterns were you following that day? Why do you think you felt so good?

? Is there a specific food that you ate consistently, perhaps too often?

? When you consider the day as a whole, is most of what you consume whole, unprocessed food, or is it primarily packaged?

Write answers to these questions in your food journal or, better yet, in a page of your journal or on sticky notes in your kitchen so that you have reminders of what works for you and what doesn't.

If you observe that you had a negative reaction on a particular day and you aren't sure how to pinpoint what specific thing caused that reaction, you could repeat the day in its entirety. You mirror your food choices, actions, and sleep patterns as much as possible except you adjust one thing. If you have the same negative reaction that you experienced previously, repeat the day again but adjust a different thing. Continue repeating the day and adjusting one thing at a time until you pinpoint what it is causing the reaction.

You can continue to food journal as long as you wish. When you come to a point where you feel you know what works for you and what doesn't, feel free to stop journaling for a while. Your journal will be available to you if you need it down the road.

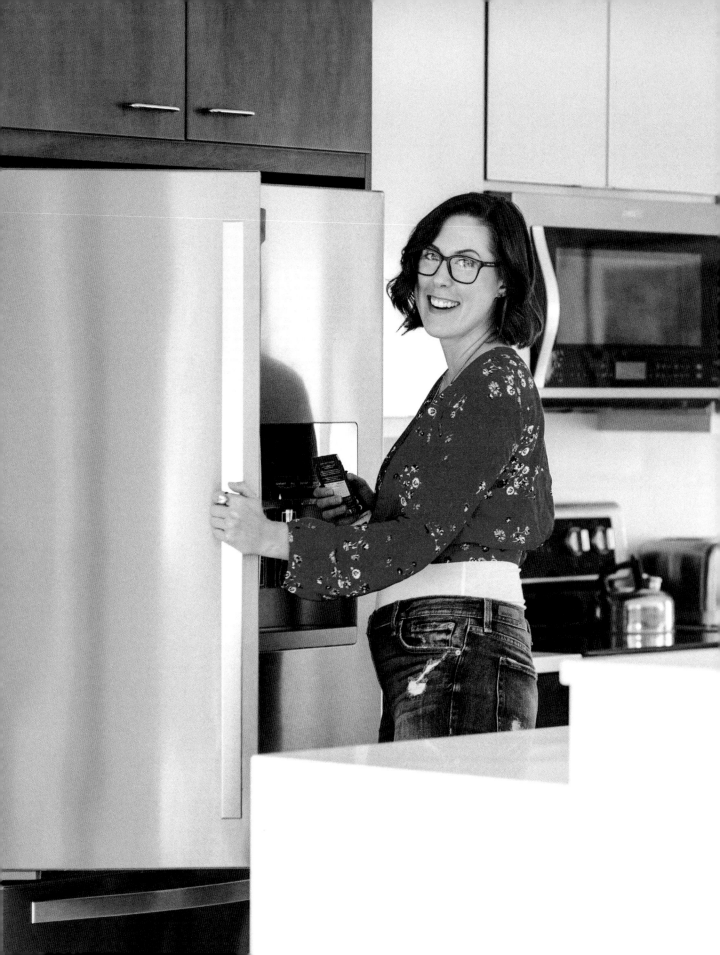

3.

THE KETO DIET MEAL PLANNING SYSTEM

Wanna know a secret? The key to keto success isn't found in a calorie counting app or somewhere on the internet. It's inside you! In this chapter, I'm going to share the unique meal planning system that'll help you get in touch with your hunger and eat what's right for you. All you gotta do is follow this clear template and slide in your choice of the all-inclusive recipes, and you'll be meal planning in moments! You're going to develop a meal plan using the following techniques:

1. **DEFINE YOUR MEAL PLANS BASED ON HUNGER AND GOALS.**

2. **CREATE MEALS BASED ON YOUR NEEDS.**

3. **USE THE INGREDIENTS YOU HAVE ON HAND.**

MEAL PLANNING

Whether you're planning each and every meal on your keto diet or you need some strategies to make dinnertime a little easier, these resources will get you on your way!

The way I see it, there are three ways to meal plan:

1 **YOUR CALORIE INTAKE GOALS OR HUNGER LEVEL.** There's nothing worse than following a meal plan designed for someone with a huge appetite or, on the flip side, having to over-prep because the plan outlined in your favorite cookbook gives you 1,400 calories to work with in a day when you actually need 2,000 calories. By basing your meal plan on your personal calorie target or overall hunger level, you can build a plan that's more unique to you.

2 **WHAT YOU NEED WHEN YOU NEED IT.** You know how much time you have to devote to prepping your meals, how many people are going to be enjoying those meals, and which kitchen appliances you have and don't have. For instance, you wouldn't add blender-based recipes to your meal plan if you don't own a blender!

Following a cookie-cutter meal plan could have you spending more time than you want to spend preparing meals, leave you with too many leftovers, or call for using kitchen appliances you don't own.

3 **THE INGREDIENTS YOU HAVE ON HAND.** If there's a bunch of chicken in your freezer, you probably want to include a couple of recipes in this week's meal plan that use chicken. Likewise, if there's a kale sale (try saying that ten times fast!), you'll probably be looking for recipes that use up the 5 pounds of kale you just purchased. Meal planning with the ingredients already in your home will save you time, energy, and money.

Let's go through these strategies individually, and I'll show you how to make the most of each one.

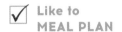

Your calorie intake goals or hunger level

Whether your calorie requirement is 1,500 or 2,500, having calorie variance in your plan is important. With calorie variance, you aim close to your calorie goal but often come in either below or above that goal. Some days you hit it spot on, other days you fall below it, and other days you come in above it. Calorie variance mimics natural eating, allowing for metabolic maintenance. People report easier weight loss, better energy, and an easier time sticking to a diet when calorie variance is in play.

If you've ever intermittent fasted for a couple of days, you know all about calorie variance! On days when you fast, you eat less. On days when you don't fast, you eat a little more.

CALORIE VARIANCE is especially helpful if you:

☑ Like to
MEAL PLAN

☑ Have been at the
SAME CALORIE LEVEL
for a long time

☑ Like to
FAST

I practice calorie variance by categorizing my meals into small, medium, large, and huge, mixing and matching meal sizes based on my hunger level and my overall goals.

Since all the recipes have similar keto macro percentages, you shouldn't see grave differences in your macro intake from day to day.

If you're already thinking, "But Leanne, so many keto coaches recommend that I not pay attention to calories, and you've even said it yourself...what gives?" That's a fair question. Remember, this is one of three meal planning strategies. If calories aren't the thing for you, pick another strategy.

However, if you're willing to give it a shot, I think you'll be pleasantly surprised. With the recipes being categorized as small, medium, large, and huge, you can use calorie variance to your advantage, choosing the meal size that meets your needs at that particular time. And, when all these meals are keto to start, it really comes down to your hunger levels/how much you want to eat per day to realize your goals.

SMALL
less than 300 calories
per serving

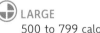MEDIUM
300 to 499 calories
per serving

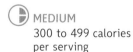LARGE
500 to 799 calories
per serving

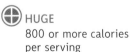HUGE
800 or more calories
per serving

This isn't an exact science, but it may be just the strategy you need to design your own meal plans using the recipes in this book.

The chart on the next page provides twelve combinations of small, medium, large, and huge meals to make up a day of eating.

Start by locating your daily calorie goal. Then view the meal size combination you'll use to build your daily meal plan.

For example, if your daily goal is 1,800 calories, you would have:

MEDIUM + LARGE + HUGE

Or, if your daily goal is 2,100 calories, you would have:

LARGE + LARGE + LARGE + SMALL

You could choose to have all your meals at one time, or you could eat two meals a day, three meals a day, or even four meals a day.

Also, note that there's more than one way to combine meal sizes to hit your daily goal. For example, if your goal is 1,800 calories, you could choose to eat four medium-sized meals rather than one medium, one large, and one huge meal. It's up to you!

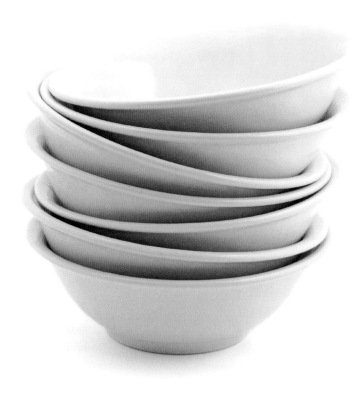

MEAL PLANNING COMBINATIONS

Here's how calorie variance comes into play with this method: Because each meal size category has a minimum and a maximum number of calories to it, combining your meals means that on one day, you could be at the low end of the combination (represented as min calorie intake), and on another day, you could be at the high end (represented as max calorie intake). If you add up your daily caloric intake for the week and divide that number by 7, you should be close to your daily calorie goal.

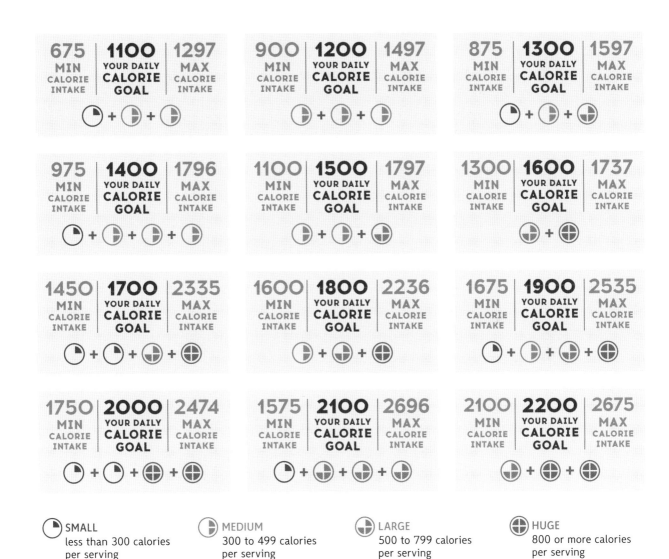

675 MIN CALORIE INTAKE	1100 YOUR DAILY CALORIE GOAL	1297 MAX CALORIE INTAKE
900 MIN CALORIE INTAKE	1200 YOUR DAILY CALORIE GOAL	1497 MAX CALORIE INTAKE
875 MIN CALORIE INTAKE	1300 YOUR DAILY CALORIE GOAL	1597 MAX CALORIE INTAKE

975 MIN CALORIE INTAKE	1400 YOUR DAILY CALORIE GOAL	1796 MAX CALORIE INTAKE
1100 MIN CALORIE INTAKE	1500 YOUR DAILY CALORIE GOAL	1797 MAX CALORIE INTAKE
1300 MIN CALORIE INTAKE	1600 YOUR DAILY CALORIE GOAL	1737 MAX CALORIE INTAKE

1450 MIN CALORIE INTAKE	1700 YOUR DAILY CALORIE GOAL	2335 MAX CALORIE INTAKE
1600 MIN CALORIE INTAKE	1800 YOUR DAILY CALORIE GOAL	2236 MAX CALORIE INTAKE
1675 MIN CALORIE INTAKE	1900 YOUR DAILY CALORIE GOAL	2535 MAX CALORIE INTAKE

1750 MIN CALORIE INTAKE	2000 YOUR DAILY CALORIE GOAL	2474 MAX CALORIE INTAKE
1575 MIN CALORIE INTAKE	2100 YOUR DAILY CALORIE GOAL	2696 MAX CALORIE INTAKE
2100 MIN CALORIE INTAKE	2200 YOUR DAILY CALORIE GOAL	2675 MAX CALORIE INTAKE

SMALL less than 300 calories per serving

MEDIUM 300 to 499 calories per serving

LARGE 500 to 799 calories per serving

HUGE 800 or more calories per serving

Once you have a combination in mind, use the meal size chart on the following pages to prep your plan!

◐ SMALL fewer than 300
CALORIES PER SERVING

RECIPE NAME	PAGE	SERVES	FREEZER-SAFE	AIP	COCONUT-FREE	DAIRY-FREE	EGG-FREE	LOW-FODMAP	NIGHTSHADE-FREE	NUT-FREE	VEGAN	VEGETARIAN
BREAKFAST												
AVOCADO BREAKFAST MUFFINS	110	6			○	✓				✓		✓
BUFFALO CHICKEN BREAKFAST MUFFINS	114	6			○	○		○	○	✓		
CHOCOHOLIC GRANOLA	108	14	❄		○	✓	✓	○	✓	✓	✓	✓
HERB CHICKEN SAUSAGES WITH BRAISED BOK CHOY	112	5	❄	○	○	○	✓	○	○	✓		
PROSCIUTTO BISCUITS	116	6	❄			✓		✓	✓	✓		
LUNCH												
CHILI LIME CHICKEN BOWLS	154	4	❄		✓	✓	✓			✓		
GERMAN NO-TATO SALAD	156	5			✓	✓	○	○	✓	✓		
SNACKS: SAVORY												
CAULIFLOWER PATTIES	270	5	❄		○	○			✓		○	✓
CRUNCHY JICAMA FRIES	260	4		○	✓	✓	○		○	✓	○	✓
FRIED CABBAGE WEDGES	276	6		✓	○	✓	✓	○	✓	✓	○	✓
HUMMUS CELERY BOATS	274	10			✓	✓	✓	○	○		✓	✓
LIVER BITES	264	24	❄	○	✓	✓	✓		✓	✓		
MAC FATTIES	268	20	❄			✓	✓	○	○		✓	✓
SALAMI CHIPS WITH BUFFALO CHICKEN DIP	278	6		○		✓	✓	○	○	✓		
SAUTÉED ASPARAGUS WITH LEMON-TAHINI SAUCE	262	4			✓	✓	✓		✓	✓	✓	✓
TAPENADE	272	6			✓	✓	✓			✓	○	○
WEDGE DIPPERS	266	4		○					✓	✓	○	
SNACKS: SWEET												
BROWNIE CAKE	322	8	❄		○	○			✓			✓
CHEESECAKE BALLS	312	12	❄		○	○	✓	✓	✓		○	✓
CINNAMON BOMBS	314	8	❄	○	○	○	✓	✓	✓	○	○	✓
CINNAMON SUGAR MUFFINS	324	12	❄		○	○		○	✓			✓
FUDGE BOMBS	320	8	❄		○	○	✓	✓	✓	○	○	✓
GRANDMA'S MERINGUES	308	6			○	✓		✓	✓	✓		✓
HAYSTACK COOKIES	310	10	❄		○	✓	✓	✓	✓	✓	○	✓
JELLY CUPS	318	16		○	○	○	✓	✓	✓	○		
KETONE GUMMIES	304	8		✓	✓	✓	✓	✓	✓	✓		
STRAWBERRY SHORTCAKE COCONUT ICE	306	4		○	○	✓	✓	✓	✓	✓	✓	✓
SUPERPOWER FAT BOMBS	316	8	❄		○	○	✓	✓	✓	✓	○	○
DRINKS												
CHILLED CHAI	360	1		○	○	○	✓	✓	✓	○	○	○
EGG CREAM	340	1			○	○	✓	✓	✓	○	○	○
FROZEN MARGARITAS!	350	4		○	✓	✓	✓	○	✓	✓	✓	✓
KETO ARNOLD PALMER	336	2		○	✓	✓	✓	✓	✓	✓	✓	✓
KETO FIZZ	352	1		✓		✓	✓	✓	✓	✓	✓	✓
MATCHA MILKSHAKE	356	1	❄		○	○	✓		✓	○	○	✓
STRAWBERRY MILKSHAKE	354	2	❄	✓	○	✓	✓	✓	✓	✓	✓	✓
THE ULTRA GREEN	358	2	❄	✓	○	✓	✓		✓	✓	○	○
TURMERIC KETO LEMONADE	338	2		○	✓	✓	✓	✓	✓	✓	✓	✓
VANILLA SHAKE	362	1	❄		○	○		✓	✓	○		○
WATERMELON COOLER	348	4		○	✓	✓	✓	✓	✓	✓	✓	✓

RECIPE NAME	PAGE	SERVES	FREEZER-SAFE	AIP	COCONUT-FREE	DAIRY-FREE	EGG-FREE	LOW-FODMAP	NIGHTSHADE-FREE	NUT-FREE	VEGAN	VEGETARIAN
BREAKFAST												
CROSS-COUNTRY SCRAMBLER	130	2			✓	✓		✓		✓		
EGGS BENEDICT	132	4			O	O		✓	✓	O		
FULL MEAL DEAL	126	4			O		O	✓				✓
HEY GIRL	120	1		O	O	✓	O	✓	✓	✓	O	O
INDIAN MASALA OMELET	140	2			✓	O				✓		✓
KETO BREAKFAST PUDDING	136	3			✓	✓	✓	O	✓	✓	O	O
LIVER SAUSAGES & ONIONS	128	6	❄	O	✓	O	✓			✓		
MUG BISCUIT	134	1	❄			O		✓	✓	✓		✓
PEPPER SAUSAGE FRY	138	4	❄	O	O	✓	✓	O	O	✓		
PUMPKIN SPICE LATTE OVERNIGHT "OATS"	122	2			O	O	✓	✓	✓	O	O	✓
ROCKET FUEL HOT CHOCOLATE	124	2		O	O	✓	✓	✓	✓	✓	O	O
SALMON BACON ROLLS WITH DIPPING SAUCE	118	4		O	✓	✓	O	O	O	O		
STICKY WRAPPED EGGS	142	6			O	✓		✓	O	✓		
LUNCH												
ANTIPASTO SALAD	164	4			✓	✓	✓			✓		
BROCCOLI GINGER SOUP	162	4	❄	O		✓	✓			✓		
CAJUN SHRIMP SALAD	170	4			✓	✓	✓			✓		
EASY CHOPPED SALAD	168	1		O	✓	✓	✓		O	✓	✓	✓
SALMON SALAD CUPS	158	4		O	✓	✓	O	✓	✓	✓		
SAUERKRAUT SOUP	166	4	❄	O	✓	✓	✓		✓	✓		
SPECKLED SALAD	172	1		O	✓	✓	✓	O	✓	✓	✓	✓
STEAK FRY CUPS	160	6	❄		O	✓	✓			✓		
DINNER												
BBQ BEEF & SLAW	204	4	❄	O	✓	✓	✓		O	✓		
CHICKEN LAKSA	218	4	❄		O	✓	✓		O	✓		
CREAM OF MUSHROOM-STUFFED CHICKEN	206	4	❄	O	O	O	✓		✓	✓		
CREAMY SPINACH ZUCCHINI BOATS	214	4			✓	O			O	✓		
CRISPY PORK WITH LEMON-THYME CAULI RICE	208	4	❄	O	O	O	✓		✓	✓		
CRISPY THIGHS & MASH	198	6	❄	O	O	O	✓		✓	✓		
EPIC CAULIFLOWER NACHO PLATE	222	4			O	O	O			✓		
MY FAVORITE CREAMY PESTO CHICKEN	216	4	❄		O	✓	✓	O	O	O		
NOODLES & GLAZED SALMON	200	4	❄	O	O	✓	✓	O	O	O		
ONE-POT PORKY KALE	210	4	❄	O	O	O	✓		O	O		
SALMON & KALE	212	4	❄	O	✓	✓	✓		O	✓		
SCALLOPS & MOZZA BROCCOLI MASH	202	4	❄	O	O	O	✓		✓	✓		
SHHH SLIDERS	224	4	❄		✓	✓		O	O	✓		
SHRIMP CURRY	226	4	❄		O	✓	✓			✓		
SUPER CHEESY SALMON ZOODLES	220	4	❄	O	O	O	✓	O	O	✓		
SNACKS: SAVORY												
BLT DIP	292	10			✓	✓	O					
BREADED MUSHROOM NUGGETS	286	4			✓	✓			O			✓
CHIMICHURRI	284	6		O	✓	✓	✓	O		✓	O	O
CUCUMBER SALMON COINS	288	2			✓	✓	O	O	✓	✓		
DAIRY-FREE (BUT JUST AS GOOD) QUESO	280	5			O	✓	✓				O	O
RADISH CHIPS & PESTO	290	2			✓	✓	✓			✓	✓	✓
TOASTED ROSEMARY NUTS	282	5	❄		O	O	✓	✓	O		O	✓
SNACKS: SWEET												
BLUEBERRY CRUMBLE WITH CREAM TOPPING	330	6	❄		O	✓			✓		O	✓
CHOCOLATE SOFT-SERVE ICE CREAM	332	4		O	✓	✓		✓	✓		O	O
EDANA'S MACADAMIA CRACK BARS	326	12	❄		O	O		✓	✓			✓
N'OATMEAL BARS	328	16	❄			✓	✓	✓	✓	✓	✓	✓

⊕ LARGE 500 to 799
CALORIES PER SERVING

RECIPE NAME	PAGE	SERVES	FREEZER-SAFE	AIP	COCONUT-FREE	DAIRY-FREE	EGG-FREE	LOW-FODMAP	NIGHTSHADE-FREE	NUT-FREE	VEGAN	VEGETARIAN
BREAKFAST												
ALL DAY ANY DAY HASH	144	4	❄		○	○	✓			✓		
COFFEE SHAKE	150	1			○	○	✓	✓	✓	✓	○	✓
SOMETHING DIFFERENT BREAKFAST SAMMY	146	1			✓	✓	○		○	✓	○	○
SUPER BREAKFAST COMBO	148	1	❄	○	○	✓	✓	○	✓	○	○	○
LUNCH												
BLT-STUFFED AVOCADOS	190	4		○	✓	✓	✓		○	✓		
BROCCOLI TABBOULEH WITH GREEK CHICKEN THIGHS	192	6	❄	○	✓	✓	✓		○	✓		
CHIMICHURRI STEAK BUNWICHES	182	4	❄		✓	✓			○	✓		
COCONUT RED CURRY SOUP	180	4	❄	○		✓	✓			✓		
CREAM CHEESE MEAT BAGELS	188	6	❄		○	○		○	○	✓		
KALE SALAD WITH SPICY LIME-TAHINI DRESSING	176	4			✓	✓	✓			✓	✓	✓
KETO LASAGNA CASSEROLE	174	6	❄		○	○				○		
MEXICAN CHICKEN SOUP	184	4	❄		○	○	✓			✓		
SAMMIES WITH BASIL MAYO	186	2			✓	✓	○		✓	✓		
ZUCCHINI PASTA SALAD	178	4			✓	✓	○	✓		○	○	✓
DINNER												
BACON-WRAPPED STUFFED CHICKEN	244	4	❄	○	✓	✓	✓		✓	✓		
CABBAGE & SAUSAGE WITH BACON	228	4	❄	○	✓	✓	✓		○	✓		
CHEESY MEATBALLS & NOODLES	236	6	❄	○	○	○	✓			✓		
MEXICAN MEATZZA	240	4			○	○	✓			○		
NOODLE BAKE	242	6		○	○	○	✓		○	✓		
ONE-POT STUFFIN'	246	4	❄	○	✓	✓	✓		✓	○		
ROASTED BROCCOLI & MEAT SAUCE	234	4	❄		✓	✓	✓	○		✓		
SECRET STUFFED PEPPERS	230	4	❄	○	✓	○	✓	○	○	✓		
SHRIMP FRY	232	4	❄	○	○	✓	✓	○	○	✓		
SOUTHERN PULLED PORK "SPAGHETTI"	248	6	❄		✓	✓	✓			✓		
SWEET BEEF CURRY	250	4	❄		○	✓	✓		○	✓		
ZUCCHINI LASAGNA	238	6	❄		○	○				✓		
SNACKS: SAVORY												
BACON-WRAPPED AVOCADO FRIES	300	4		✓	✓	✓	✓		✓	✓		
KETO DIET SNACK PLATE	298	1			✓	✓				✓		
TUNA CUCUMBER BOATS	294	1			✓	✓	○	○	✓	✓		
ZUCCHINI CAKES WITH LEMON AIOLI	296	2				✓			✓	✓		

⊕ HUGE 800 or more
CALORIES PER SERVING

RECIPE NAME	PAGE	SERVES	FREEZER-FRIENDLY	AIP	COCONUT-FREE	DAIRY-FREE	EGG-FREE	LOW-FODMAP	NIGHTSHADE-FREE	NUT-FREE	VEGAN	VEGETARIAN
LUNCH												
PAPRIKA CHICKEN SANDWICHES	194	4			○	✓	○		○	✓		
DINNER												
BREADED SHRIMP SALAD	254	4			○	✓						
OPEN-FACED TACOS	252	4	❄		○	○	✓	○		✓		
SHREDDED MOJO PORK WITH AVOCADO SALAD	256	4	❄		✓	✓	✓			✓		

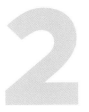

2 What you need when you need it

When meal prepping, it's important to find what you want when you know you'll need it. From quick meals, single-serving recipes when you're eating solo, and fast snacks to meals made in a pressure cooker, the recipes highlighted below will make your meal planning that much easier.

In addition, remember that every recipe is equipped with a guide showing you whether it is safe for your lunch kit, which allergens it is free of, whether it's family-friendly, or if it can be stored in the freezer for later use. All these features will make meal planning a breeze. See pages 52 and 53 for an outline of these features and pages 364 to 366 for a table of these features, which makes it super easy to find the kinds of recipes you're looking for.

UNDER 25 MINUTES

Breakfast

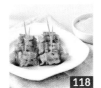 118
Salmon Bacon Rolls with Dipping Sauce

 122
Pumpkin Spice Latte Overnight "Oats"*

 124
Rocket Fuel Hot Chocolate*

 126
Full Meal Deal

 136
Keto Breakfast Pudding*

Lunch

 158
Salmon Salad Cups*

 164
Antipasto Salad*

 172
Speckled Salad*

 186
Sammies with Basil Mayo*

 190
BLT-Stuffed Avocados

Dinner

 200
Noodles & Glazed Salmon

 224
Shhh Sliders

 232
Shrimp Fry

 254
Breaded Shrimp Salad

also no-bake/cook

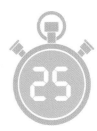

FAST SNACKS

Toasted Rosemary Nuts — 282

Tuna Cucumber Boats* — 294

Tapenade* — 272

Keto Diet Snack Plate* — 298

Cinnamon Bombs* — 314

Fudge Bombs* — 320

Strawberry Shortcake Coconut Ice* — 306

Chilled Chai* — 360

Keto Fizz* — 352

The Ultra Green* — 358

also no-bake/cook

SOLO MEALS AND SNACKS

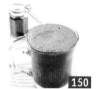
Coffee Shake — 150

Hey Girl — 120

Mug Biscuit⁺ — 134

Something Different Breakfast Sammy — 146

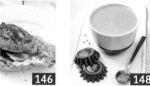
Super Breakfast Combo — 148

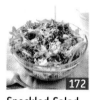
Speckled Salad — 172

Easy Chopped Salad — 168

Tuna Cucumber Boats — 294

Keto Diet Snack Plate — 298

Egg Cream — 340

⁺*Serve with leftover meat, roasted vegetables, or avocado with sesame seeds.*

LUNCH KIT-FRIENDLY

Pumpkin Spice Latte Overnight "Oats" — 122

Liver Sausages & Onions — 128

Cross-Country Scrambler — 130

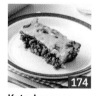
Keto Lasagna Casserole — 174

Broccoli Ginger Soup — 162

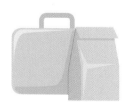

Speckled Salad — 172

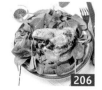
Kale Salad with Spicy Lime-Tahini Dressing — 176

Cream of Mushroom–Stuffed Chicken — 206

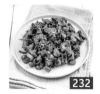
Salmon & Kale — 212

Shrimp Fry — 232

QUICK COOKING WITH A PRESSURE COOKER

While having a pressure cooker isn't a requirement for preparing any of the recipes in this book, if you do have one, here are a couple of days' worth of meals you can make to cut down on prep time.

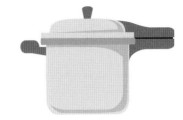

Breakfast

144

All Day Any Day Hash

138

Pepper Sausage Fry

Lunch

184

Mexican Chicken Soup

174

Keto Lasagna Casserole

180

Coconut Red Curry Soup

166

Sauerkraut Soup

Dinner

228

Cabbage & Sausage with Bacon

234

Roasted Broccoli & Meat Sauce

250

Sweet Beef Curry

246

One-Pot Stuffin'

3

The ingredients you have on hand

There are two ways to find what you need in this book based on the ingredients you have on hand:

1. The book's index (beginning on page 372) lists key ingredients and which recipes include those ingredients. If you have kale, it'll tell you which recipes use kale. If you have almonds, it'll tell you that, too!

2. The table on the following pages outlines which key protein(s) are used in the meals and snacks throughout the book that are awesome choices for prepping your meal plan.

PROTEIN USED	RECIPE NAME	PAGE	TYPE	MEAL SIZE
BACON	CROSS-COUNTRY SCRAMBLER	130	Breakfast	MEDIUM
	SALMON BACON ROLLS WITH DIPPING SAUCE	118	Breakfast	MEDIUM
	STICKY WRAPPED EGGS	142	Breakfast	MEDIUM
	SOMETHING DIFFERENT BREAKFAST SAMMY	146	Breakfast	LARGE
	BLT-STUFFED AVOCADOS	190	Lunch	LARGE
	BACON-WRAPPED STUFFED CHICKEN	244	Dinner	LARGE
	CABBAGE & SAUSAGE WITH BACON	228	Dinner	LARGE
	BLT DIP	292	Snack: Savory	MEDIUM
	BACON-WRAPPED AVOCADO FRIES	300	Snack: Savory	LARGE
BEEF CHUCK	BBQ BEEF & SLAW	204	Dinner	MEDIUM
	SWEET BEEF CURRY	250	Dinner	LARGE
CHICKEN BREASTS	MEXICAN CHICKEN SOUP	184	Lunch	LARGE
	CREAM OF MUSHROOM-STUFFED CHICKEN	206	Dinner	MEDIUM
	MY FAVORITE CREAMY PESTO CHICKEN	216	Dinner	MEDIUM
CHICKEN THIGHS	CHILI LIME CHICKEN BOWLS	154	Lunch	SMALL
	BROCCOLI TABBOULEH WITH GREEK CHICKEN THIGHS	192	Lunch	LARGE
	COCONUT RED CURRY SOUP	180	Lunch	LARGE
	PAPRIKA CHICKEN SANDWICHES	194	Lunch	HUGE
	CHICKEN LAKSA	218	Dinner	MEDIUM
	CRISPY THIGHS & MASH	198	Dinner	MEDIUM
	BACON-WRAPPED STUFFED CHICKEN	244	Dinner	LARGE
	OPEN-FACED TACOS	252	Dinner	HUGE
COLLAGEN	BROCCOLI GINGER SOUP	162	Lunch	MEDIUM
	CREAMY SPINACH ZUCCHINI BOATS	214	Dinner	MEDIUM
COLLAGEN/ PROTEIN POWDER	HEY GIRL	120	Breakfast	MEDIUM
	KETO BREAKFAST PUDDING	136	Breakfast	MEDIUM
	ROCKET FUEL HOT CHOCOLATE	124	Breakfast	MEDIUM
	SUPER BREAKFAST COMBO	148	Breakfast	LARGE
	SUPERPOWER FAT BOMBS	316	Snack: Sweet	SMALL
	CHILLED CHAI	360	Drink	SMALL
	THE ULTRA GREEN	358	Drink	SMALL
	VANILLA SHAKE	362	Drink	SMALL
DELI MEAT	GERMAN NO-TATO SALAD	156	Lunch	SMALL
	CREAM CHEESE MEAT BAGELS	188	Lunch	LARGE
	SAMMIES WITH BASIL MAYO	186	Lunch	LARGE
EGGS	AVOCADO BREAKFAST MUFFINS	110	Breakfast	SMALL
	BUFFALO CHICKEN BREAKFAST MUFFINS	114	Breakfast	SMALL
	CROSS-COUNTRY SCRAMBLER	130	Breakfast	MEDIUM
	EGGS BENEDICT	132	Breakfast	MEDIUM
	INDIAN MASALA OMELET	140	Breakfast	MEDIUM
	STICKY WRAPPED EGGS	142	Breakfast	MEDIUM
	KETO DIET SNACK PLATE	298	Snack: Savory	LARGE
FISH, OTHER	SHHH SLIDERS	224	Dinner	MEDIUM
	TUNA CUCUMBER BOATS	294	Snack: Savory	LARGE
GELATIN	JELLY CUPS	318	Snack: Sweet	SMALL
	KETONE GUMMIES	304	Snack: Sweet	SMALL
GROUND BEEF	SAUERKRAUT SOUP	166	Lunch	MEDIUM
	KETO LASAGNA CASSEROLE	174	Lunch	LARGE
	MEXICAN MEATZZA	240	Dinner	LARGE
	OPEN-FACED TACOS	252	Dinner	HUGE

PROTEIN USED	RECIPE NAME	PAGE	TYPE	MEAL SIZE
GROUND CHICKEN	HERB CHICKEN SAUSAGES WITH BRAISED BOK CHOY	112	Breakfast	SMALL
GROUND PORK	CREAM CHEESE MEAT BAGELS	188	Lunch	LARGE
	EPIC CAULIFLOWER NACHO PLATE	222	Dinner	MEDIUM
	CHEESY MEATBALLS & NOODLES	236	Dinner	LARGE
GROUND TURKEY	CHEESY MEATBALLS & NOODLES	236	Dinner	LARGE
	ROASTED BROCCOLI & MEAT SAUCE	234	Dinner	LARGE
	ZUCCHINI LASAGNA	238	Dinner	LARGE
LEFTOVER CHICKEN	BUFFALO CHICKEN BREAKFAST MUFFINS	114	Breakfast	SMALL
	SALAMI CHIPS WITH BUFFALO CHICKEN DIP	278	Snack: Savory	SMALL
LIVERS, CHICKEN	LIVER SAUSAGES & ONIONS	128	Breakfast	MEDIUM
	SECRET STUFFED PEPPERS	230	Dinner	LARGE
	LIVER BITES	264	Snack: Savory	SMALL
NUTS	ZUCCHINI PASTA SALAD	178	Lunch	LARGE
	HUMMUS CELERY BOATS	274	Snack: Savory	SMALL
	MAC FATTIES	268	Snack: Savory	SMALL
	BLT DIP	292	Snack: Savory	MEDIUM
	DAIRY-FREE (BUT JUST AS GOOD) QUESO	280	Snack: Savory	MEDIUM
	RADISH CHIPS AND PESTO	290	Snack: Savory	MEDIUM
	TOASTED ROSEMARY NUTS	282	Snack: Savory	MEDIUM
PORK CHOPS	CRISPY PORK WITH LEMON-THYME CAULI RICE	208	Dinner	MEDIUM
	ONE-POT PORKY KALE	210	Dinner	MEDIUM
PORK SHOULDER	SOUTHERN PULLED PORK "SPAGHETTI"	248	Dinner	LARGE
	SHREDDED MOJO PORK WITH AVOCADO SALAD	256	Dinner	HUGE
PROSCIUTTO	PROSCIUTTO BISCUITS	116	Breakfast	SMALL
ROTISSERIE CHICKEN	BLT-STUFFED AVOCADOS	190	Lunch	LARGE
SALAMI	ANTIPASTO SALAD	164	Lunch	MEDIUM
	SALAMI CHIPS WITH BUFFALO CHICKEN DIP	278	Snack: Savory	SMALL
	KETO DIET SNACK PLATE	298	Snack: Savory	LARGE
SALMON	SALMON BACON ROLLS WITH DIPPING SAUCE	118	Breakfast	MEDIUM
	SALMON SALAD CUPS	158	Lunch	MEDIUM
	NOODLES & GLAZED SALMON	200	Dinner	MEDIUM
	SALMON & KALE	212	Dinner	MEDIUM
	SUPER CHEESY SALMON ZOODLES	220	Dinner	MEDIUM
	CUCUMBER SALMON COINS	288	Snack: Savory	MEDIUM
SAUSAGE	PEPPER SAUSAGE FRY	138	Breakfast	MEDIUM
	CABBAGE & SAUSAGE WITH BACON	228	Dinner	LARGE
	NOODLE BAKE	242	Dinner	LARGE
	ONE-POT STUFFIN'	246	Dinner	LARGE
	SHRIMP FRY	232	Dinner	LARGE
SEA SCALLOPS	SCALLOPS & MOZZA BROCCOLI MASH	202	Dinner	MEDIUM
SEEDS	SPECKLED SALAD	172	Lunch	MEDIUM
	KALE SALAD WITH SPICY LIME-TAHINI DRESSING	176	Lunch	LARGE
	N'OATMEAL BARS	328	Snack: Sweet	MEDIUM
SHRIMP	CAJUN SHRIMP SALAD	170	Lunch	MEDIUM
	SHRIMP CURRY	226	Dinner	MEDIUM
	SHRIMP FRY	232	Dinner	LARGE
	BREADED SHRIMP SALAD	254	Dinner	HUGE
STEAK	ALL DAY ANY DAY HASH	144	Breakfast	LARGE
	STEAK FRY CUPS	160	Lunch	MEDIUM
	CHIMICHURRI STEAK BUNWICHES	182	Lunch	LARGE

MEAL TYPES

Hurrah, we're to the part where the eating happens! The recipe chapters of this book are organized by meal type, with the recipes in each chapter ordered from smallest to largest. This will make planning your meals ahead of time—or picking out a recipe at the last minute—so much easier.

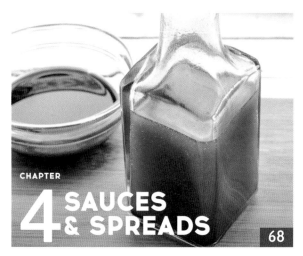

CHAPTER 4 SAUCES & SPREADS 68

These are the dressings and marinades called for throughout the book that'll make just about any keto dish delicious!

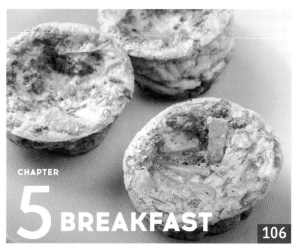

CHAPTER 5 BREAKFAST 106

As you adapt to keto, you'll be less and less interested in breakfast, but that isn't to say it'll never happen. And who doesn't love breakfast for dinner once in a while? This chapter also has a couple of fast-extending recipes like Hey Girl (page 120) that, if your goal is insulin regulation, can be enjoyed during your fast.

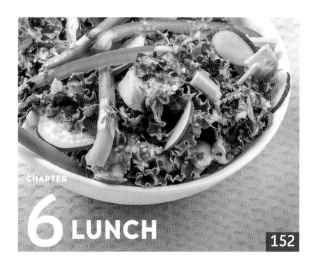

CHAPTER 6 LUNCH 152

Recipes that are quick to put together or fare well in a packed lunch. There's a good collection of sandwiches, salads, stews, and the like.

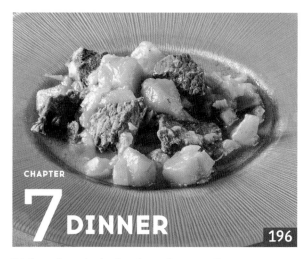

CHAPTER 7 DINNER 196

Dishes the whole family will enjoy. Every recipe makes at least four servings, and many make awesome leftovers for the next day or can be frozen for later.

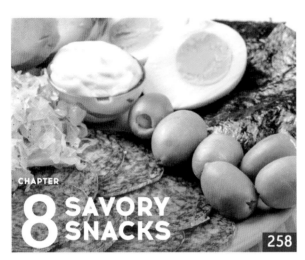

Act as snacks or quick mini meals that are lighter in volume but pack the same punch. You'll find snacking becomes less and less important to you as you become fat-adapted, but it's always better to be prepared with a couple of fat bombs in your freezer.

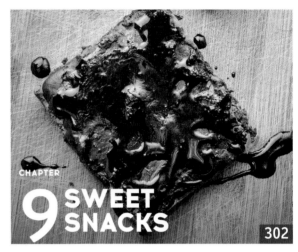

Act as snacks or quick sweet tooth satisfiers. All are family-friendly, and some are pretty enough to serve to guests (like Grandma's Meringues on page 308 or Brownie Cake on page 322).

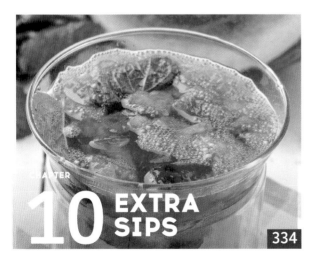

Treat the drinks in this chapter as snacks, bedtime sips, or accompaniments to your main meal.

RECIPE GUIDE

Here's how to interpret the recipe pages that follow.

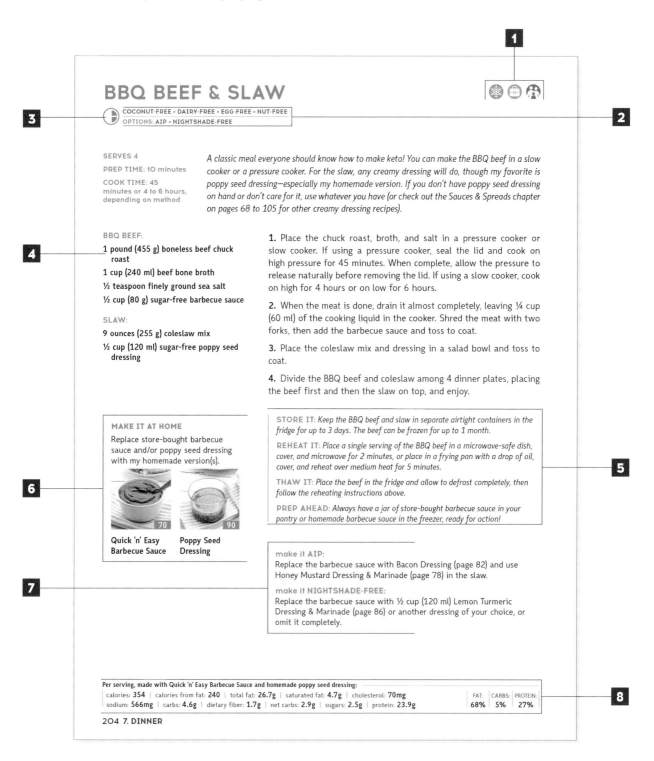

1

BBQ BEEF & SLAW

COCONUT-FREE • DAIRY-FREE • EGG-FREE • NUT-FREE
OPTIONS: AIP • NIGHTSHADE-FREE

3

2

SERVES 4

PREP TIME: 10 minutes

COOK TIME: 45 minutes or 4 to 6 hours, depending on method

A classic meal everyone should know how to make keto! You can make the BBQ beef in a slow cooker or a pressure cooker. For the slaw, any creamy dressing will do, though my favorite is poppy seed dressing—especially my homemade version. If you don't have poppy seed dressing on hand or don't care for it, use whatever you have (or check out the Sauces & Spreads chapter on pages 68 to 105 for other creamy dressing recipes).

BBQ BEEF:

1 pound (455 g) boneless beef chuck roast

1 cup (240 ml) beef bone broth

½ teaspoon finely ground sea salt

½ cup (80 g) sugar-free barbecue sauce

SLAW:

9 ounces (255 g) coleslaw mix

½ cup (120 ml) sugar-free poppy seed dressing

4

1. Place the chuck roast, broth, and salt in a pressure cooker or slow cooker. If using a pressure cooker, seal the lid and cook on high pressure for 45 minutes. When complete, allow the pressure to release naturally before removing the lid. If using a slow cooker, cook on high for 4 hours or on low for 6 hours.

2. When the meat is done, drain it almost completely, leaving ¼ cup (60 ml) of the cooking liquid in the cooker. Shred the meat with two forks, then add the barbecue sauce and toss to coat.

3. Place the coleslaw mix and dressing in a salad bowl and toss to coat.

4. Divide the BBQ beef and coleslaw among 4 dinner plates, placing the beef first and then the slaw on top, and enjoy.

MAKE IT AT HOME

Replace store-bought barbecue sauce and/or poppy seed dressing with my homemade version(s).

70 — Quick 'n' Easy Barbecue Sauce

90 — Poppy Seed Dressing

6

STORE IT: Keep the BBQ beef and slaw in separate airtight containers in the fridge for up to 3 days. The beef can be frozen for up to 1 month.

REHEAT IT: Place a single serving of the BBQ beef in a microwave-safe dish, cover, and microwave for 2 minutes, or place in a frying pan with a drop of oil, cover, and reheat over medium heat for 5 minutes.

THAW IT: Place the beef in the fridge and allow to defrost completely, then follow the reheating instructions above.

PREP AHEAD: Always have a jar of store-bought barbecue sauce in your pantry or homemade barbecue sauce in the freezer, ready for action!

5

make it AIP:
Replace the barbecue sauce with Bacon Dressing (page 82) and use Honey Mustard Dressing & Marinade (page 78) in the slaw.

make it NIGHTSHADE-FREE:
Replace the barbecue sauce with ½ cup (120 ml) Lemon Turmeric Dressing & Marinade (page 86) or another dressing of your choice, or omit it completely.

7

Per serving, made with Quick 'n' Easy Barbecue Sauce and homemade poppy seed dressing:
calories: **354** | calories from fat: **240** | total fat: **26.7g** | saturated fat: **4.7g** | cholesterol: **70mg**
sodium: **566mg** | carbs: **4.6g** | dietary fiber: **1.7g** | net carbs: **2.9g** | sugars: **2.5g** | protein: **23.9g**

FAT:	CARBS:	PROTEIN:
68%	5%	27%

8

204 7. DINNER

1 FEATURES

These icons point out key features of the recipes:

Freezer-safe recipes store well in the freezer. You'll find information about how best to store them at the ends of the recipes.

Lunch kit–friendly recipes won't melt on you or cause a mess in your packed lunch.

Family-friendly recipes make four servings or more.

Quickie recipes take 30 minutes or less to prepare from start to finish.

2&7 DIETARY GUIDELINES

For those of you who avoid certain foods or follow specific eating protocols, I've included some guidelines.

AIP: All the ingredients are compliant with the autoimmune protocol (AIP), or the recipe offers adjustments to make the dish compliant.

COCONUT-FREE: All the ingredients are coconut-free, or the recipe offers coconut-free modifications.

EGG-FREE: The recipe uses no eggs, or egg-free substitutions are listed.

LOW-FODMAP: The recipe is low in FODMAPs or offers suggestions to make the dish low-FODMAP.

NIGHTSHADE-FREE: The recipe has no nightshades or can be made nightshade-free with one or two simple swaps.

NUT-FREE: There are no nuts in the recipe, or it can easily be made nut-free.

VEGAN: The recipe does not contain animal products or can be modified for vegans.

VEGETARIAN: The recipe may contain eggs and/or give you the option to add dairy but does not contain any other animal protein, or vegetarian substitutions are given.

If a recipe as written is fully compliant with one of these designations, it appears in the first line below the recipe title. If adjustments can be made to make the recipe compliant with a particular designation, it appears in the line below that, next to the word *OPTION(S)*, with the necessary modifications outlined in a gray box.

3 MEAL SIZE

These icons, along with the accent color used on the page, help you decide which dishes to prepare based on your hunger level or calorie goals. On pages 39 to 44, I show you how to use this information when meal planning.

 SMALL   LARGE

 MEDIUM   HUGE

4 METRIC MEASUREMENTS

I have included metric equivalents throughout this book for all volume amounts of ¼ cup or greater, as well as for all temperatures, weights, and dimensions.

5 EXTRA INSTRUCTIONS

PREP AHEAD: Shares how to get a step ahead when preparing the recipe for guests or doing meal prep.

PRESSURE COOK IT: Describes how to prepare the recipe in your electric pressure cooker.

STORE IT: Provides storage instructions for the recipe.

THAW IT: Defrosting instructions accompany all recipes that can be stored in the freezer.

REHEAT IT: Outlines how to reheat leftovers that are best served warm on the stovetop, in the microwave, and/or in the oven, depending on the recipe.

6 RECIPE INTEGRATION

MAKE IT AT HOME You always have the option to use store-bought dressings and sauces for convenience, but if you'd like to make your own using the recipes in this book, look for the "Make It at Home" boxes.

USE IN THESE RECIPES For sauces and spreads that pair well with specific breakfast, lunch, dinner, and savory snack recipes throughout the book, I've included these handy boxes to highlight the different ways you can use them.

8 NUTRITION INFORMATION

For each recipe, I have provided the nutrition information per serving, clarifying which ingredients I used to arrive at those numbers if the recipe gives more than one ingredient option. I have also included macronutrient percentages for each recipe, along with the percentage of alcohol it contains, if applicable.

INGREDIENTS USED

The goal of *The Keto Diet Cookbook* is to give you recipes that are easy to prepare, with ingredients you are likely to have on hand. I've included various ingredient choices in each recipe so that you don't have to break the bank to stock your pantry in order to eat good food.

In this section, save for fresh produce, I've listed many of the ingredients I've used in this book so that you can plan your grocery shopping around it and also understand what's what.

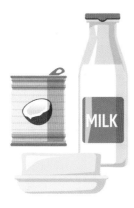

Dairy/Nondairy Options

Dairy doesn't work for a lot of people. It can lead to inflammation, a heavy reliance on dairy products (which limits variety in the diet), an increase in low-quality food consumption, and exposure to hormones and antibiotics. One of the main reasons I do not like promoting the consumption of dairy is that it means consuming the milk from another mammal—milk that's meant to grow a baby cow, goat, or sheep.

Think about it for a second: Would you drink pig milk? What about pigeon? How about cockroach? For serious. These animals do in fact make milk for their young.

My Fat Fueled Protocol, as outlined in my Fat Fueled Program (healthfulpursuit.com/fatfueled), my Happy Keto Body Program (happyketobody.com), and my previous book, *The Keto Diet* (ketodietbook.com), doesn't include dairy for these reasons. However, many of you told me that you wanted dairy options in my next book, so I've intertwined dairy and dairy-free options throughout this book so that the recipes meet you where you are, right at this moment. Dairy does work for some people, and for those people, being able to include dairy on keto can make all the difference. It provides a touch of flavor in recipes, and it can help you add variety to your diet and help you hit your fat macro that much more easily.

Dairy-free options trump dairy options throughout this book, meaning that all the recipes are dairy-free but can be made with dairy if you so choose.

DAIRY-FREE OR REGULAR CHEESE (shredded): If a recipe is better with a touch of shredded cheese, I called for either dairy-free or regular cheese.

Dairy-free cheese isn't a real food and should be viewed as a treat. If I can make my own cheese, like Walnut "Cheese" (page 241) or Melty "Cheese" (page 243), I do. But it's also important to show you how to use store-bought dairy-free options if convenience is important to you. My favorite dairy-free cheese brand is So Delicious.

By law, conventional American cheese has to be 51 percent cheese; the rest can be vegetable oil and fillers. It's important to look for cheese that's sourced from humanely raised cows, is Non-GMO Project Verified, and is made from pure, simple ingredients—never artificial. Artificial, you ask? Yes. Food coloring is often used in the making of cheese to give it its orange color. If you're looking for a reputable brand, Applegate Naturals is one of my favorites and is readily available.

Note that for ease of preparation, to save a bit of money, and because dairy-free cheese doesn't look as appetizing as the real thing, the recipe photos throughout this book picture real dairy cheese.

BUTTER (contains dairy): Butter is not called for in any of the recipes, but you're free to use butter anywhere I call for coconut oil or ghee. If food quality is important to you, opt for butter sourced from grass-fed and grass-finished cattle. My favorite brand is Vital Farms.

GHEE (contains dairy): Ghee is butter that's been cooked over low heat until the milk solids have started to brown lightly, creating a slightly nutty, caramelized flavor. It is shelf-stable, with a high smoke point and a deeply nutty flavor. Wherever ghee is a good option in a recipe, I've listed it. My favorite brand is Fourth and Heart.

NUTRITIONAL YEAST (dairy-free): Where a cheesy flavor is needed, nutritional yeast is a great option. It doesn't melt like cheese, but when combined with garlic powder, onion powder, and a little mustard, it has a similar taste! My favorite is made by Bob's Red Mill and is easy to find just about anywhere.

COCONUT CREAM (dairy-free): An alternative to heavy cream. It is thick like whipped cream directly from the can without needing to be chilled. It can be purchased in cans or Tetra Paks, although the canned versions are much easier to find. My favorite brands are Thai Kitchen and Native Forest. If you are following a low-FODMAP protocol, ⅓ cup (85 g) or less is safe. Any more than that and coconut cream becomes too high in FODMAPs.

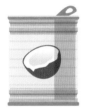

COCONUT MILK (dairy-free): There are many ways to incorporate coconut milk into your keto diet. I've compared coconut milk to various forms of dairy so that you understand how they perform when being cooked with.

If you are following a low-FODMAP protocol, ⅓ cup (80 ml) or less is safe. Any more than that and coconut milk of any kind becomes too high in FODMAPs.

Full-fat coconut milk is an alternative to homogenized milk or heavy cream. It is very dense directly from the can. When chilled, the cream will separate from the water, and you'll have thick coconut cream at the top of the can when you open it. My favorite brands are Thai Kitchen, Native Forest, and Thrive Market.

If you do not wish to use full-fat coconut milk, it can be replaced with an equal amount of full-fat dairy milk or heavy cream.

Lite coconut milk is an alternative to 1% or 2% milk. This type of coconut milk comes in cartons and is probably the more readily available option. You'll find it at the supermarket labeled as coconut milk. There are various options to choose from, many of them sweetened, so look for the unsweetened variety. Also, if you have gut issues, you may want to opt for a carrageenan-free coconut milk. My favorite brand is So Delicious.

If you do not wish to use lite coconut milk, you can use another nondairy milk or 1% or 2% dairy milk.

Coconut cream is the high-fat portion of full-fat coconut milk and is a great alternative to heavy whipping cream. You can purchase coconut cream on its own or chill a can of full-fat coconut milk and skim the fat from the top of the can once it's chilled.

MILK (dairy-free or regular): Whenever a recipe calls for just "milk," without specifying a particular type, I have used lite coconut milk, as outlined above. But you can use any type of milk you wish, from 1% dairy milk to cashew milk to hemp milk and beyond. As long as your choice is unsweetened, you're good to go!

OTHER NONDAIRY MILKS: There are dairy-free milk recipes on pages 342 to 347 if you would like to make your own. Alternatively, you can purchase all sorts of keto-friendly dairy-free milks at the supermarket, including almond milk, cashew milk, macadamia nut milk, and pea milk. Watch for carrageenan if you have a sensitive gut, and opt for the unsweetened variety.

If you're following an AIP protocol, your best option is coconut milk. If you're following a low-FODMAP protocol, your best options are almond, hemp, and macadamia nut milk.

| *Amp up the protein in your favorite nondairy milk by adding a scoop of collagen!*

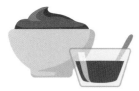

Homemade Versus Store-Bought Dressings and Sauces

I love dressings and marinades. They can mean the difference between getting excited for a home-cooked meal and opting for takeout. There's something so fun about dressing up a familiar dish with something new, learning how to prepare your own sauces, and saving money, too!

There's no shortage of store-bought keto-friendly dressings and sauces on the market today. Really, you're looking for options that are high-fat and unsweetened. You can find many of these at your local supermarket for a good price. If ingredient quality is important to you, one of my favorite brands for ketchup, dressings, marinades, and mayonnaise, all made with avocado oil, is Primal Kitchen.

Any recipe that calls for a dressing, marinade, or mayonnaise calls for the store-bought version of the ingredient. I did this because 75 percent of the *Healthful Pursuit* community asked for it. If you're among the 25 percent who would prefer to make your own high-fat/unsweetened keto versions at home, there are 18 recipes in this book to help you do just that! Each recipe that calls for a store-bought sauce of some sort has a feature labeled "Make It at Home," which shows you how to make that same sauce yourself, adjusting the ingredients to suit your needs.

Where applicable, I've outlined which homemade dressings and sauces are used in which recipes so that when you have a batch of, say, Green Speckled Dressing (page 80) primed and ready to go in the refrigerator, you know which recipes in the book use that dressing. No more waste! You can find this feature on each of the applicable dressing recipes in the "Use in These Recipes" box.

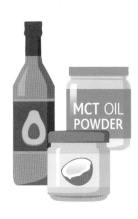

Fat and Oil Options

It's easy to go overboard on buying oils, but it doesn't need to be this way. All you really need is one oil that's safe for cooking and one that's best for cold uses, like salad dressings.

In the recipes, I sometimes list various options for fats. You'll see ingredient listings like:

3 tablespoons avocado oil, coconut oil, or ghee

None of them is the best option. Use whichever one you'd like.

In addition to butter and ghee, as outlined in the "Dairy/Nondairy Options" section on pages 54 to 56, there are a few fats that I use throughout the book that you may find helpful to have in your pantry. My favorites, listed from most readily available and versatile to least, are:

COCONUT OIL (for cooking and baking): Coconut oil is readily available, which is why it's my number-one recommended oil. You shouldn't have a problem finding it. You could use lard, tallow, butter, ghee, or cacao butter in its place.

BUTTER-FLAVORED COCONUT OIL (for cooking and baking): If you can't do butter but want the butter flavor, there are many coconut oils that are flavored with plant extracts to produce a buttery taste without the dairy. Anywhere where ghee or coconut oil is called for, you could use this butter-flavored coconut oil in its place. It's a fairly common item at supermarkets, and doesn't have the unhealthy processed oils like many of the butter substitutes on the market today. My favorite brand is Nutiva.

AVOCADO OIL (for cold uses, cooking, and baking): Avocado oil is the most versatile oil of all. It's awesome on salads and great for cooking because of its high smoke point. There are refined and nonrefined options. I prefer refined because it doesn't contribute an avocado flavor to recipes. My favorite brand is Chosen Foods. You could use olive oil in its place for the cold recipes only.

OLIVE OIL (for cold uses): Great for making your own mayonnaise and for adding to dressings, this oil is best used for recipes that are not cooked. I opt for extra-virgin olive oil, preferably organic. If I'm making mayonnaise, I like using a light olive oil with a minimal flavor. My favorite olive oil is the Kirkland brand from Costco.

CACAO BUTTER (for baking): Cacao butter, which is the fat from chocolate, is a little harder to find than the previous fats, and it's a bit more expensive than the other options. I purchase mine on Amazon. You're looking for a raw, unrefined, food-grade variety. You could use lard, tallow, ghee, coconut oil, or butter in its place.

MCT OIL POWDER (for cooking, baking, and drinks): MCT oil powder is made from spraying MCT oil on acacia fiber, a highly soluble fiber that's sourced from the sap of the acacia tree. It's different from MCT oil in that it fully incorporates into recipes without leaving a pool of fat behind. I don't particularly like MCT oil for this reason, and because it causes digestive distress in many people. But MCT oil powder doesn't have this effect. Considered more of a supplement, it's a great way to add fat to recipes, including baked goods and drinks; however, it's not essential to a keto diet.

See how unflavored MCT oil powder is used in these recipes:

    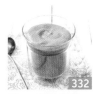

| 124 | 150 | 310 | 316 | 332 | 344 |

Rocket Fuel Hot Chocolate **Coffee Shake** **Haystack Cookies** **Superpower Fat Bombs** **Chocolate Soft-Serve Ice Cream** **Coconut Milk**

LARD (for cooking and baking): A suggested replacement item for coconut oil, ghee, or avocado oil in cooking, lard is best used in savory dishes or when baking cookies, muffins, or cakes. It's highly saturated, offering richness to the dish it's added to. Lard is easy to find online, or you can make your own by asking your butcher for unrendered fat, placing the fat pieces in your slow cooker, and cooking on high for 3 to 4 hours. Bits of protein will need to be strained afterward. The rendered fat will keep in the fridge for months and is quite cost-effective, too!

GARLIC-INFUSED OIL (for cold uses): Garlic-infused oil is just that—oil that's been infused with garlic, usually made with olive oil. If you're sensitive to garlic, as is the case for someone on a low-FODMAP diet, garlic-infused oil can add garlic flavor to a dish without causing digestive distress.

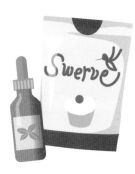

Sweeteners

There are many keto-friendly sweeteners to choose from, but I have opted to use the most common ones to keep you from running all over the city. My favorite sweeteners are:

ERYTHRITOL: This is my all-time favorite sweetener because of its versatility, ease of use (it replaces sugar one to one), and availability worldwide. My favorite brand is Swerve, which is a blend of erythritol, oligosaccharides, and natural flavors. Alternatively, you could use an equal amount of xylitol, monk fruit, or allulose; grind it finely in your blender or food processor if you need the powdered form. If you're following an AIP protocol, however, erythritol is not safe. Use stevia in its place, or enjoy dishes unsweetened.

Confectioners'-style erythritol (aka powdered erythritol) is the type I like to use because it becomes smooth in recipes without needing to be heated extensively. It's especially great when added to fat bombs, frostings, and drinks.

Granulated erythritol has a grainier texture and can be used in all recipes that call for granulated sugar.

In recipes where I simply call for erythritol, you can use either type. When I specify confectioners'-style or granulated, the type does matter to the end result of the recipe.

STEVIA (liquid): There are a bunch of liquid stevia brands on the market today that taste awful and have a horrible aftertaste. The only type of stevia I use is Now Foods stevia glycerite because it doesn't have that metallic aftertaste that many of us on keto have come to hate. Alternatively, you could use monk fruit drops.

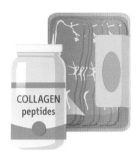

Protein

There are ample ways to hit your protein requirements on keto, and a lot of them are pretty straightforward—muscle meats, organ meats, seafood, eggs, and dairy (if you tolerate it). But I have used some other proteins in the recipes that may be unfamiliar to you, so it's worth a little introduction.

COLLAGEN PEPTIDES AND/OR PROTEIN POWDER: These two ingredients can be used interchangeably throughout the book. With either option, be cognizant of choosing unsweetened, unflavored varieties. If you use a flavored and/or sweetened variety, it will affect the end result of the recipe.

I use unsweetened, unflavored collagen peptides because they have no taste, incorporate seamlessly into recipes, and benefit the gut. Collagen peptides are widely accessible in many supermarkets, health food stores, and online. My favorite brands are Equip and Thrive Market.

See how collagen is used in these recipes:

   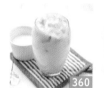

| 120 | 310 | 316 | 358 | 360 | 362 |

Hey Girl   Haystack Cookies   Superpower Fat Bombs   The Ultra Green   Chilled Chai   Vanilla Shake

Protein powder, on the other hand, can be a bit tricky. How well a protein powder integrates with other ingredients will rely on the type of protein it contains. Pea protein is notoriously more challenging to work with than something like egg white, beef, or whey protein due to its fiber content.

GELATIN: Think of gelatin as a sister to collagen. When collagen is added to hot or cold liquid, it integrates fully and does not alter the consistency, but when gelatin is mixed into something hot, it turns gelatinous as it cools, like a gummy.

CRUSHED PORK RINDS: A great replacement for panko breadcrumbs. You can make your own by purchasing pork rinds, placing them in a resealable bag, and crushing them on the counter, or you can purchase them already crushed. My favorite brand is Bacon's Heir.

BONE BROTH: There truly is a difference between cooking with stock and broth. While not necessary, because of its richness, broth sure does make meals taste better! You can make your own broth or purchase it from a store. My two favorite brands are Kettle & Fire and Bonafide Provisions.

BACON: There are all sorts of bacon choices out there, some better than others. If your budget allows, opt for uncured and nitrate-free bacon. My favorite brand is Pederson's Natural Farms.

A little tip: To make perfect crispy bacon, cook it in the microwave!

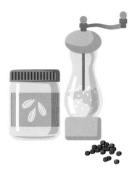

Pantry Goods and Refrigerated Items

HIMALAYAN SALT AND SEA SALT: Everywhere sea salt is called for, you can use Himalayan salt instead, but not the other way around. You'll notice that I use Himalayan salt in drinks, because drinking seawater is never a good time, no matter how much you love the ocean. But for real, sea salt in drinks tastes a little off to me, which is why you'll find two types of salt used in this book.

BLACK PEPPER: I love cooking with black pepper, but if you're following an AIP protocol, you probably know that black pepper is off-limits in some of the phases. This is why many of the recipes in this book include a warning about black pepper.

ALMOND BUTTER: I enjoy smooth unsweetened almond butter because it has fewer carbs than almond butter made with almonds with the skins still on, and it's more versatile for baking. The key is to find an almond butter without added sugar or processed oils.

COCONUT BUTTER (COCONUT MANNA): Coconut butter is to coconuts as peanut butter is to peanuts. Basically, coconut butter is ground coconut. My favorite brand of coconut butter is Artisana, and for coconut butter treats, I like Synchro.

SEED BUTTER: An awesome replacement for coconut butter or any nut butter, seed butter could be made from sunflower seeds, hemp seeds, or pumpkin seeds. I also call for tahini (ground sesame seeds) in a couple of the recipes.

CACAO, COCOA, AND CAROB POWDER: I bake exclusively with cacao powder. It tastes better, is better for you, and usually comes from more ethical sources. I call for cocoa powder in the recipes because it is more readily available and less costly, and the recipes will turn out fine if you use it. But if you can swing it, upgrade to cacao powder. You'll never go back to the other stuff.

Additionally, if you're AIP, cacao and cocoa are off-limits, but you can get away with eating a bit of carob. Carob is less bitter than chocolate and has a roasted, naturally sweet flavor. Just be mindful of the ingredients in carob products, as many of them come sweetened and use grain-based sweeteners like barley syrup. Your best bet is to use pure carob powder.

RICED CAULIFLOWER: Recipes like Chili Lime Chicken Bowls (page 154) and Cauliflower Patties (page 270) call for riced cauliflower. If you haven't been introduced to riced cauliflower yet, consider this your introduction! Riced cauliflower is finely chopped raw cauliflower that can be used in place of white or brown rice. It may not sound like much, but riced cauliflower will become a staple in your keto diet. To make riced cauliflower, cut the base off a head of cauliflower and remove the florets. Then transfer the florets to a food processor or blender and pulse three or four times to break them up into small (¼-inch/6-mm) pieces. And there you have it, riced cauliflower! Or you can purchase already riced cauliflower in the frozen section of most grocery stores.

INGREDIENT SUBSTITUTIONS

I've tried to make *The Keto Diet Cookbook* accessible to all sorts of people and their food preferences. Wherever possible, I provide various ingredient options so that you can make adjustments for your preferences.

That's the reason I've included dairy in this book, even though I don't consume it myself. Thanks go to my loving husband, Kevin, who chowed down on all the dairy-containing dishes featured here to ensure that you get what you need to succeed with your keto diet.

I've opted for two main sweeteners throughout the book: erythritol and stevia. If you respond better to a different type of sweetener, use that instead. If you respond better to a touch of overripe banana than to a sweetener, use it!

Each recipe is as holistic as I could make it, but as hard as I tried, I'm sure I didn't think of everything and everyone. So I'm providing some general adjustments here for people who require them. The following substitution lists will help you navigate keto should you need to remove specific foods, such as dairy, coconut, or nuts, from your diet.

What makes these lists unique is that all the foods included are keto-friendly. Online lists include all foods rather than just keto foods, which can be confusing. I've taken out the guesswork to provide you with keto-friendly dos and don'ts.

Let's get to it!

Dairy

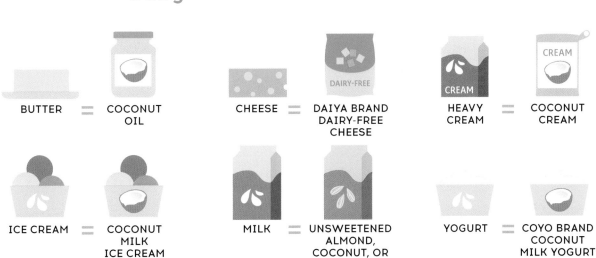

BUTTER = COCONUT OIL

CHEESE = DAIYA BRAND DAIRY-FREE CHEESE

HEAVY CREAM = COCONUT CREAM

ICE CREAM = COCONUT MILK ICE CREAM

MILK = UNSWEETENED ALMOND, COCONUT, OR HEMP MILK

YOGURT = COYO BRAND COCONUT MILK YOGURT

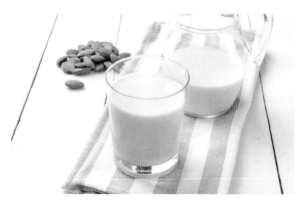

MILK SUBSTITUTES

Instead of relying heavily on dairy milk, try making your own nut or seed milk with just about any nut or seed you have lying around. All you have to do is soak, strain, rinse, and blend.

Yield: 4 cups (950 ml)

Soak 1 cup (115 to 175 g) of raw nuts or seeds in water for 12 to 24 hours, then strain with a fine-mesh sieve and rinse. Place the nuts or seeds in a blender with 4 cups (950 ml) fresh water. Blend, strain the mixture through cheesecloth, and enjoy. Store in an airtight container in the fridge for up to 5 days.

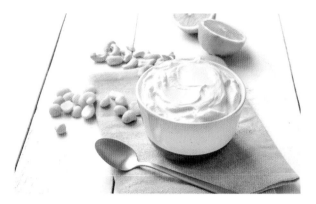

SOUR CREAM SUBSTITUTE

This recipe is essential if you're like me and refuse to spend $8 on a tiny tub of dairy-free sour cream. Also, the ingredients in the homemade version are far superior.

Yield: 1 cup (240 g)

Soak 1 cup (155 g) of raw cashews in water for 6 hours, then strain with a fine-mesh sieve and rinse. Place the cashews in a blender with ½ cup (120 ml) water, ⅓ cup (80 ml) lemon juice, ¼ cup (40 g) raw macadamia nuts, 1 tablespoon nutritional yeast, ¾ teaspoon finely ground sea salt, and ½ teaspoon ground white pepper. Blend until creamy. Store in a sealed jar in the fridge for up to 5 days.

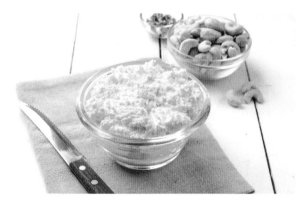

CREAM CHEESE SUBSTITUTE

Cream cheese doesn't have to be made with dairy to be delicious! Either make your own (see page 74 for my recipe; for plain cream cheese, just omit the onion powder, garlic powder, and chives), or purchase soy-based (not my favorite), nut-based, or even pea-based cream cheese products at the supermarket. While some of the options are pretty tasty, they are a bit pricey.

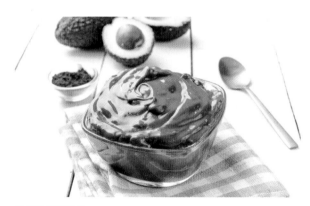

PUDDING

This pudding is awesome when you're craving a little sweetness but don't have time for an epic recipe. Creamy and delicious, it'll hit the spot every time!

Yield: 1 cup (280 g)

Place the flesh of 3 medium Hass avocados, ⅓ cup (80 ml) lemon juice OR ¼ cup (20 g) cocoa powder, ½ teaspoon vanilla extract, ⅛ teaspoon finely ground sea salt, and 4 drops liquid stevia in a blender or food processor and blend until smooth. Best enjoyed immediately.

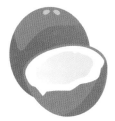

Coconut

The last time you ate something containing coconut—shredded coconut, coconut oil, or coconut butter—did you feel a slight tingling sensation in your mouth or throat? If so, what you experienced could very well be due to an allergy, but it also could be due to the way the coconut was processed, especially if your experience was with coconut oil. It turns out that the methods used to process many coconut oils can lead to the development of bacteria, which you might sense in your mouth as a tingly feeling.

You may have experienced this sensation and sworn off all coconut products because you assumed you had an allergy. In case bacteria is to blame, though, you should see if you experience the same reaction when you consume full-fat coconut milk from a freshly opened can. If that test goes okay, try Alpha Health DME Virgin Coconut Oil or Skinny Coconut Oil. (I know; I don't like the "Skinny" name either, but it's a fabulous product!) Using either of these products should eliminate any reaction that is the result of bacteria present in your coconut oil.

If you suspect you're sensitive to coconut itself (rather than being affected by the presence of bacteria), it's best to avoid it altogether and see how things go.

If it has become obvious that coconut itself is the culprit, what's a keto seeker to do? I have some suggestions for coconut substitutions you can use in your favorite keto dishes.

LITE COCONUT MILK

1 cup (240 ml) LITE COCONUT MILK = 1 cup (240 ml) NUT OR SEED MILK

COCONUT FLOUR

FOR SAVORY RECIPES:

 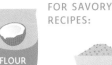

½ cup (50 g) COCONUT FLOUR = ¾ cup (55 g) ROUGHLY GROUND PORK RINDS

SHREDDED COCONUT

1 cup (100 g) UNSWEETENED SHREDDED COCONUT = ¾ cup (110 g) HULLED HEMP SEEDS

COCONUT CREAM OR FULL-FAT COCONUT MILK

    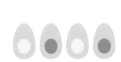

1 cup (250 g) COCONUT CREAM OR 1 cup (240 ml) FULL-FAT COCONUT MILK = ¾ cup (180 ml) NUT OR SEED MILK blended with ¼ cup (40 g) SOAKED RAW CASHEWS

1 cup (250 g) COCONUT CREAM = FLESH OF 2 MEDIUM HASS AVOCADOS (8 oz/220 g), blended

COCONUT OIL

FOR SAVORY RECIPES:

1 cup (210 g) COCONUT OIL = 1 cup (210 g) BEEF TALLOW OR LARD

FOR BAKED GOODS:

1 cup (210 g) COCONUT OIL = 1 cup (210 g) LARD OR 1 cup (240 g) CACAO BUTTER

FOR SWEET FAT BOMBS:

1 cup (210 g) COCONUT OIL = 1 cup (240 g) CACAO BUTTER

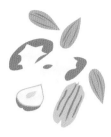

Nuts

Here are some of my tried-and-true suggestions for living without nuts:

- **For fat bombs:** Replace nut butters with sunflower seed butter or tahini.
- **For recipes that include ground nuts:** Use hulled hemp seeds.
- **For breading meat and fish:** Coat the meat or fish with crushed pork rinds.
- **For snacking:** Eat more nourishing veggies, fats, and meats. If you're on the go, try sugar-free jerky or coconut flakes for a quick snack.

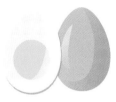

Eggs

If you're sensitive to egg white, try these substitutions:

- **For making mayonnaise:** Use only egg yolks (3 yolks = 1 whole large egg).
- **For baking and cooking:** Make egg white scrambles for your loved ones and save the yolks for yourself! Egg yolks work fabulously in almost every dish that calls for whole eggs.
- **For baking:** Use flax eggs. For the equivalent of 1 large egg, combine 1 tablespoon ground flaxseed (measure after grinding) with 3 tablespoons water. Stir well and place in the refrigerator for 15 minutes to set. After 15 minutes, you'll have a sticky egglike substitute.
- **For baking or general cooking:** Prepare a gelatin egg using the following instructions: Place ¼ cup (60 ml) of water in a small saucepan. Sprinkle the entire surface of the water with 1 tablespoon of unflavored gelatin powder. Let it sit untouched for 5 minutes. After 5 minutes, turn the burner on low and whisk for 1 minute, or until the texture is smooth. Use gelatin eggs as you would eggs in cakes, cookies, brownies, and more.

If you're sensitive to the whole egg, try these substitutions:

- **For making mayonnaise:** Use the egg-free mayo recipe on page 102.
- **For baking:** Use flax eggs as described above.
- **For baking or general cooking:** Prepare gelatin eggs as described above.
- **For breading meat and fish:** Dip the meat or fish in coconut milk to make the breading stick.

Foods that share a similar protein-to-fat ratio with eggs include smoked salmon, sardines, and crispy chicken skin. (Although you're free to substitute with omega-3 rich foods like salmon and sardines, I had to mention chicken skin in here somewhere!)

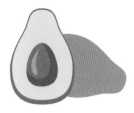

Avocados

Although avocado is one of the richest, most sought-after foods for high-fat living, it's not the end of the world if you can't eat avocado.

Replace avocado oil with

- MCT oil or olive oil for uncooked recipes
- Beef tallow, coconut oil, or red palm oil for recipes that involve cooking

Replace avocados with

- Full-fat coconut milk or soaked raw cashews in desserts where the avocado is used to thicken or add smoothness to the recipe. This works great for brownies, puddings, cookies, mousse, and other sweet recipes that call for mashed avocado.
- Soaked raw cashews, mayonnaise, or pureed zucchini in savory recipes where the avocado is used as a base. This works great in salad dressings and sauces.

If you can't do avocados, focus on consuming nutrient-rich greens throughout the day. My favorite way to do so is to chop up a bunch of greens (kale, mustard greens, chard, and the like) and sauté them in a health-promoting fat such as grass-fed tallow or coconut oil and some rich bone broth. Cook the greens for about a minute, then transfer them to an airtight container and chill them in the refrigerator overnight. The mixture will harden slightly, and you can add it to salads, eat it as a cold side dish, or reheat it. I love snacking on a bowl of chilled greens!

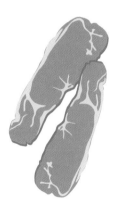

Pork Products

Other than good ol' bacon, there's not much you'll miss out on by omitting pork from your keto diet. Here are some suggested replacements:

- Instead of bacon, try turkey bacon or salmon bacon. Or embrace chicken skin! Sprinkle the skin with salt and pepper and roast in a 375°F (190°C) oven until crispy, about 25 minutes.
- Instead of ground pork, use ground beef.
- Instead of shredded pork, use shredded chuck roast.
- Instead of lard, use beef tallow or coconut oil.

KITCHEN APPLIANCES AND TOOLS

One can go a little crazy stocking the kitchen with all the (unnecessary) things. While I'll be the first to admit that there was a time when my food pantry served as storage for all of my kitchen appliances, I now see the value in having just a few good-quality tools and appliances as opposed to buying everything under the sun and rarely using it.

Sure, you can get the fancy things, or you can stock your kitchen with classics that'll work for just about every recipe! Here are my top tools and the items I've used throughout the book.

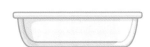

BAKING PANS: While there are many sizes to choose from, the most common sizes are the 8-inch (20-cm) square baking pan and the 13 by 9-inch (33 by 23-cm) baking pan. The most versatile materials are glass and silicone. If you choose silicone, you won't need to use as much parchment paper as you may need to use with glass or other materials.

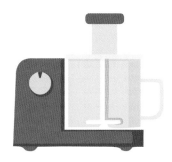

FOOD PROCESSOR: A food processor is similar to a blender in function; you don't need both appliances to prepare the recipes in this book. I call for either a blender or a food processor, but not both.

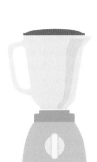

BLENDER: I used a Breville Fresh & Furious and a Vitamix blender to make the recipes in this book. When I call for a high-powered blender, I'm referring to a blender like a Vitamix. When a recipe simply says "blender," it truly means any blender you have access to.

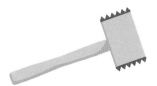

MEAT MALLET: An essential tool if you enjoy chicken thighs! I purchased my meat mallet from Amazon for $15 a couple of years ago and am impressed every time I use it. Though not required, it is super handy for recipes like the Paprika Chicken Sandwiches (page 194).

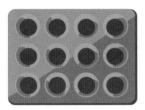

MUFFIN PAN: A 12-well silicone muffin pan will never steer you wrong. You can use it to make fat bombs, muffins, single-serve quiches, and so much more. I like using silicone more than other materials because it doesn't require muffin liners, which cuts down on cost and waste.

SILICONE MOLD: You'll be making a few fat bombs here and there, so getting a little silicone mold for them is never a bad thing. Now, if you opt for an 8-inch (20-cm) square silicone baking pan, you can kill two birds with one stone, using that baking pan whenever a silicone mold is called for. However, if you want a dedicated mold for fat bombs and other little treats, the most versatile option is a silicone mini muffin pan or silicone ice cube tray.

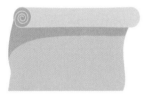

PARCHMENT PAPER OR SILICONE BAKING MAT: If you want to purchase only one or the other, go for parchment paper, which is more versatile. I use the If You Care brand of unbleached parchment paper.

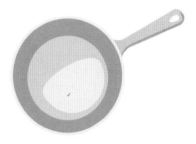

SAUCEPAN AND FRYING PAN: Medium to large is a safe bet. If they have lids, that's a plus!

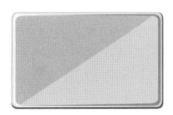

RIMMED BAKING SHEET: Similar to baking pans, there are many sizes of rimmed baking sheets to choose from, but the most common is an 18 by 13-inch (46 by 33-cm), which will fit most ovens comfortably.

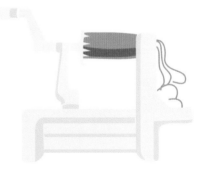

SPIRAL SLICER: Though not essential, I sure do love a good spiral slicer! If you don't want yet another tool taking up space in your kitchen, a vegetable peeler will work, too; just continuously peel the vegetable until there is nothing left. Alternatively, many supermarkets sell vegetables that are already spiral sliced (although you will pay quite a bit more for the convenience).

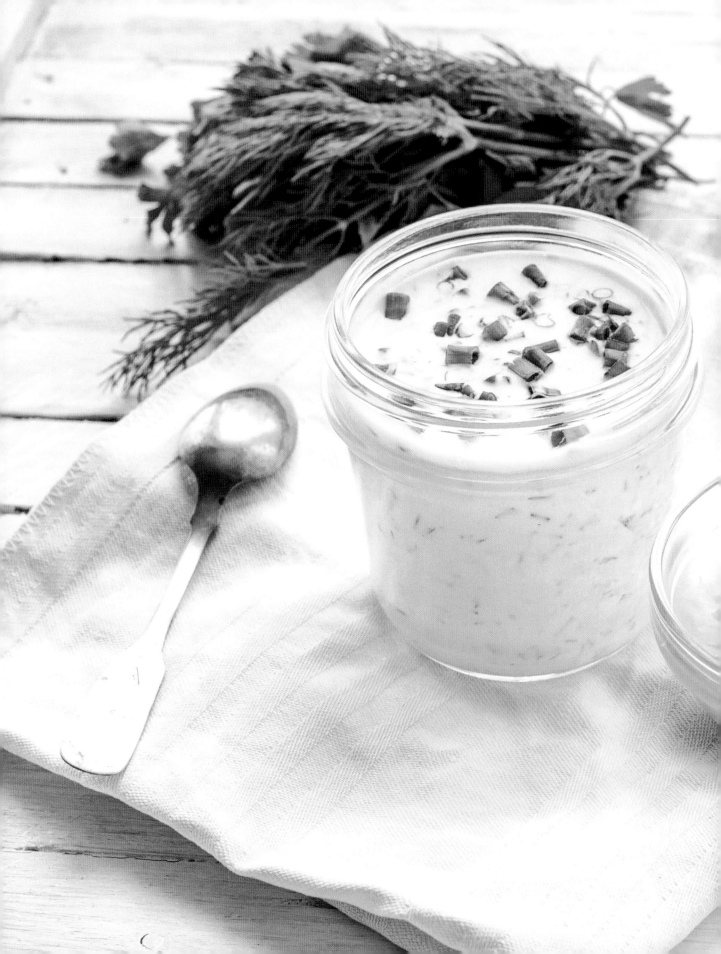

4.

SAUCES
& SPREADS

QUICK 'N' EASY BARBECUE SAUCE

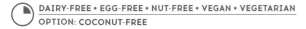

DAIRY-FREE • EGG-FREE • NUT-FREE • VEGAN • VEGETARIAN
OPTION: COCONUT-FREE

MAKES 1¼ cups (300 g)
PREP TIME: 5 minutes
COOK TIME: –

So many barbecue sauce recipes require you to cook down the ingredients and then cool the sauce before you can slather it on a burger. That's a lot of work, so I do it this way instead.

⅓ cup (80 ml) balsamic vinegar

⅓ cup (80 ml) water

1 (6-oz/170-g) can tomato paste

2 tablespoons coconut aminos

1 tablespoon Dijon mustard

½ teaspoon garlic powder

½ teaspoon onion powder

½ teaspoon paprika

½ teaspoon finely ground sea salt

¼ teaspoon ground black pepper

Place all the ingredients in a 16-ounce (475-ml) or larger airtight container. Cover and shake until incorporated.

STORE IT: *Keep in the fridge for up to 5 days or in the freezer for up to 1 month.*

THAW IT: *Set in the fridge to thaw completely before using.*

make it COCONUT-FREE:
Replace the coconut aminos with soy sauce, omit the salt, and add 1 tablespoon of confectioners'-style erythritol or 3 drops of liquid stevia.

USE IN THESE RECIPES

204
BBQ Beef & Slaw

248
Southern Pulled Pork "Spaghetti"

Per tablespoon:

| calories: **11** | calories from fat: **1** | total fat: **0.1g** | saturated fat: **0g** | cholesterol: **0mg** | FAT: | CARBS: | PROTEIN: |
| sodium: **66mg** | carbs: **2.1g** | dietary fiber: **0.4g** | net carbs: **1.7g** | sugars: **1.1g** | protein: **0.4g** | 8% | 76% | 16% |

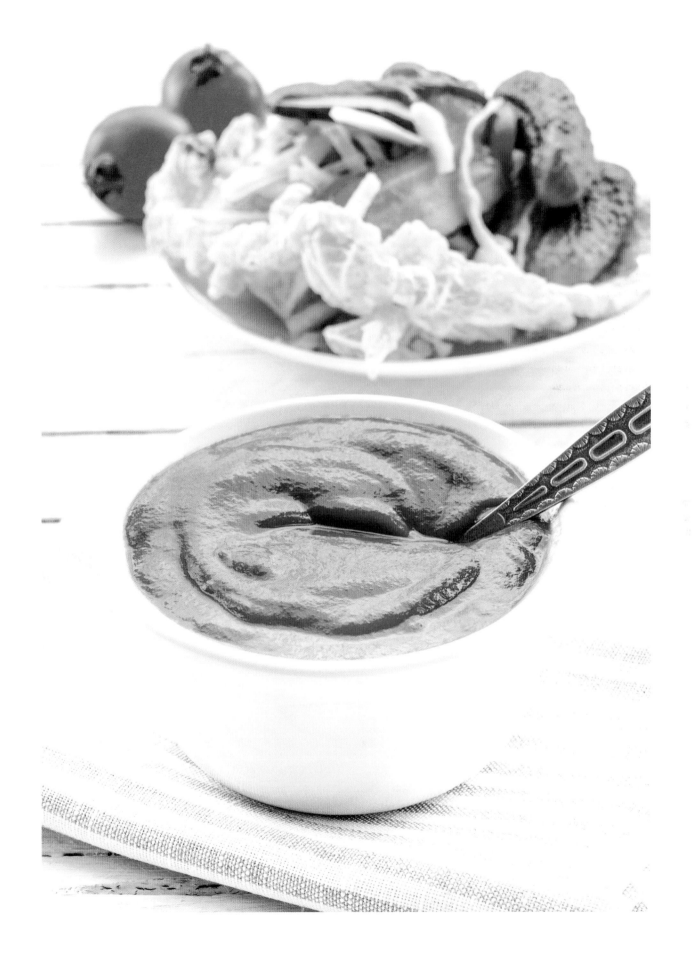

THAI DRESSING

DAIRY-FREE • EGG-FREE • VEGAN • VEGETARIAN
OPTIONS: NIGHTSHADE-FREE • NUT-FREE

MAKES 1 cup (240 ml)

PREP TIME: 5 minutes

COOK TIME: –

My favorite way to use this dressing is to drizzle it on fresh vegetables, broccoli especially. There are multiple ways to personalize this recipe, too. If you love dairy, replace the coconut milk with heavy cream. If you don't do toasted sesame oil or don't want to buy a bottle just for this recipe, replace it with avocado oil or olive oil.

If you don't have access to coconut aminos, you can replace it with an equal amount of soy sauce, omit the salt from the recipe, and add your favorite sweetener—either 10 drops of liquid stevia or 2 teaspoons of confectioners'-style erythritol should do the trick!

¼ cup (70 g) smooth unsweetened almond butter

¼ cup (60 ml) full-fat coconut milk

2 tablespoons apple cider vinegar

2 tablespoons coconut aminos

2 tablespoons toasted sesame oil

1 tablespoon lime juice

1 teaspoon garlic powder

½ teaspoon cayenne pepper

½ teaspoon finely ground sea salt

1. Place all the ingredients in a 12-ounce (350-ml) or larger airtight container. Cover and shake until incorporated.

2. When ready to serve, give the container a little shake and enjoy.

STORE IT: *Keep in the fridge for up to 5 days.*

make it NIGHTSHADE-FREE:
Omit the cayenne.

make it NUT-FREE:
Use sunflower seed butter in place of the almond butter.

USE IN THESE RECIPES

176

Kale Salad with Spicy Lime-Tahini Dressing

254

Breaded Shrimp Salad

266

Wedge Dippers

Per tablespoon:

calories: **22** | calories from fat: **18** | total fat: **2g** | saturated fat: **0.4g** | cholesterol: **0mg**
sodium: **61mg** | carbs: **0.7g** | dietary fiber: **0.1g** | net carbs: **0.6g** | sugars: **0.1g** | protein: **0.1g**

FAT:	CARBS:	PROTEIN:
86%	12%	2%

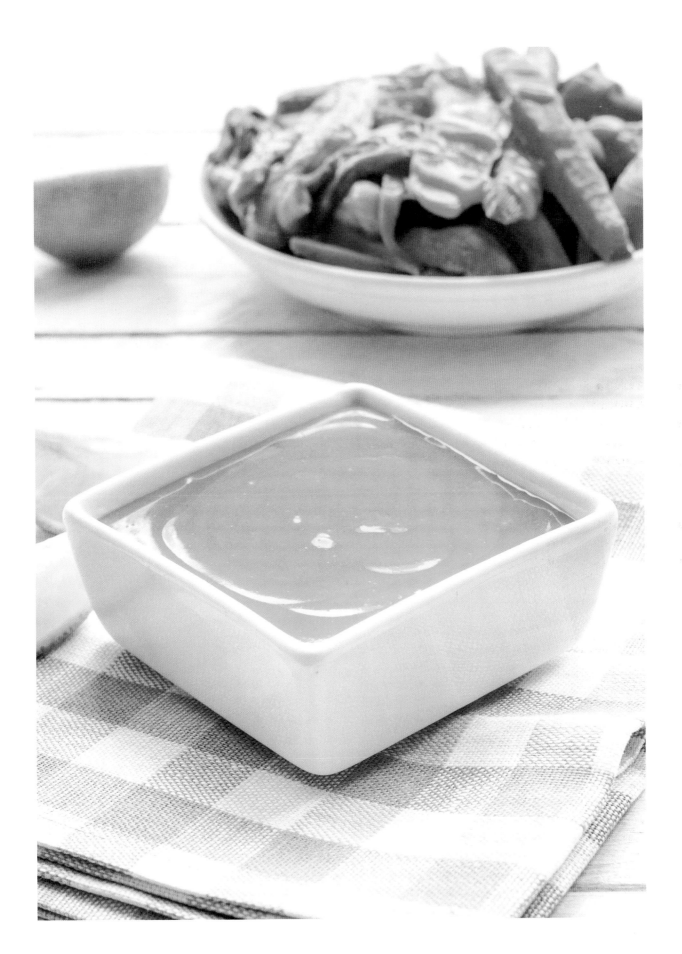

CHIVE & ONION CREAM CHEESE

DAIRY-FREE • EGG-FREE • NIGHTSHADE-FREE • VEGETARIAN • VEGAN

OPTION: COCONUT-FREE

MAKES 1 cup (270 g)

PREP TIME: 5 minutes, plus 12 hours to soak cashews

COOK TIME: –

If you can eat the real thing, I'm jealous. Sadly, for us "dairy-afflicted" folk, this is as close to real cream cheese as we'll ever get. But for real, this dairy-free version isn't a bad substitute at all. And of course, if dairy doesn't affect you, have at it!

1 cup (130 g) raw cashews

¼ cup (60 g) unsweetened plain dairy-free yogurt

2 tablespoons apple cider vinegar

2 teaspoons nutritional yeast

¾ teaspoon onion powder

½ teaspoon finely ground sea salt

¼ teaspoon garlic powder

2 tablespoons sliced fresh chives

1. Place the cashews in a 12-ounce (350-ml) or larger sealable container. Cover with water. Seal and place in the fridge to soak for 12 hours.

2. Once the cashews are ready, drain and rinse them, then place in a food processor or blender along with the remaining ingredients, except the chives. Blend on high until smooth.

3. Transfer to a 12-ounce (350-ml) or larger airtight container. Stir in the sliced chives. Set on the counter for an hour before serving to allow the flavors to meld.

STORE IT: *Keep in the fridge for up to 5 days.*

make it COCONUT-FREE:
Use a yogurt that is not coconut-based.

USE IN THIS RECIPE

188

Cream Cheese
Meat Bagels

Per tablespoon, made with coconut yogurt:

| calories: **55** | calories from fat: **37** | total fat: **4.1g** | saturated fat: **0.8g** | cholesterol: **0mg** | | FAT: | CARBS: | PROTEIN: |
| sodium: **62mg** | carbs: **3.2g** | dietary fiber: **0.5g** | net carbs: **2.7g** | sugars: **0.5g** | protein: **1.5g** | **67%** | **23%** | **10%** |

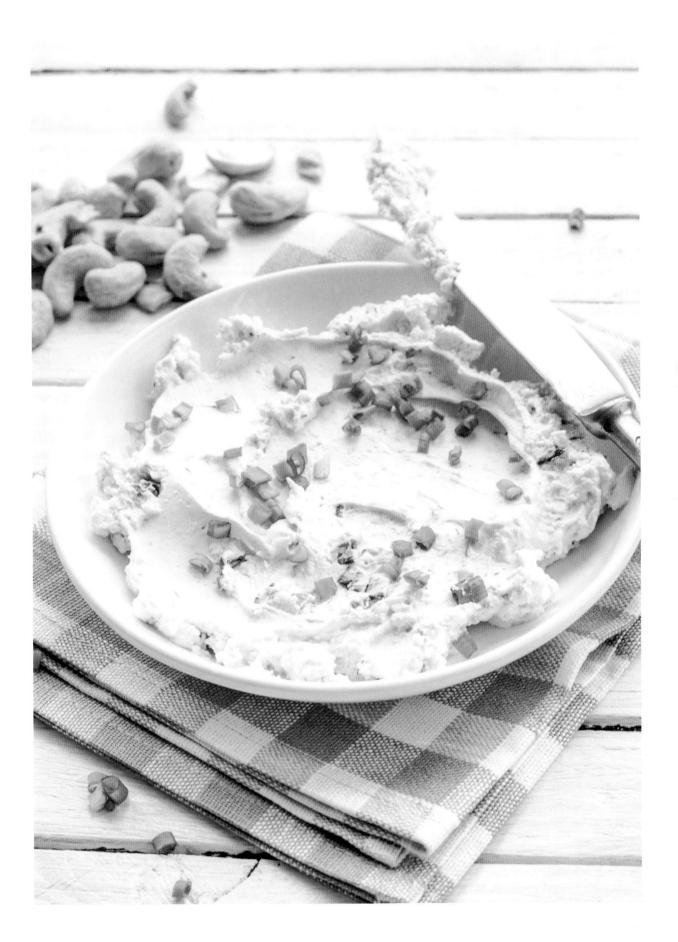

RANCH DRESSING

DAIRY-FREE · NIGHTSHADE-FREE · NUT-FREE · VEGETARIAN
OPTIONS: EGG-FREE · VEGAN

MAKES 2 cups (475 ml)

PREP TIME: 5 minutes

COOK TIME: –

Whether you can do eggs or not, this recipe is a dream. It tastes just like traditional ranch dressing and is good with just about anything you slather it on. My favorite is to double up on the garlic and drizzle it over roasted carrots.

1 cup (210 g) mayonnaise

½ cup (120 ml) full-fat coconut milk

3 tablespoons finely chopped fresh parsley

2 tablespoons sliced fresh chives

2 small cloves garlic, minced

1 tablespoon minced white onions

1 tablespoon finely chopped fresh dill

1 tablespoon apple cider vinegar

1 tablespoon lemon juice

¼ teaspoon finely ground sea salt

⅛ teaspoon ground black pepper

1. Place all the ingredients in a 20-ounce (600-ml) or larger airtight container. Cover and shake until incorporated.

2. When ready to serve, give the container a little shake and enjoy.

STORE IT: *Keep in an airtight container in the fridge for up to 5 days.*

make it EGG-FREE/VEGAN:
Use egg-free mayonnaise (see recipe on page 102).

MAKE IT AT HOME

Replace store-bought mayonnaise with my homemade version.

Mayonnaise

USE IN THESE RECIPES

Steak Fry Cups   Wedge Dippers   Bacon-Wrapped Avocado Fries

Per tablespoon, made with homemade mayonnaise:

calories: **57**	calories from fat: **55**	total fat: **6.1g**	saturated fat: **1.5g**	cholesterol: **7mg**	FAT:	CARBS:	PROTEIN:
sodium: **182mg**	carbs: **0.4g**	dietary fiber: **0.1g**	net carbs: **0.3g**	sugars: **0.1g**	protein: **0.1g**	**98%**	**1%**	**1%**

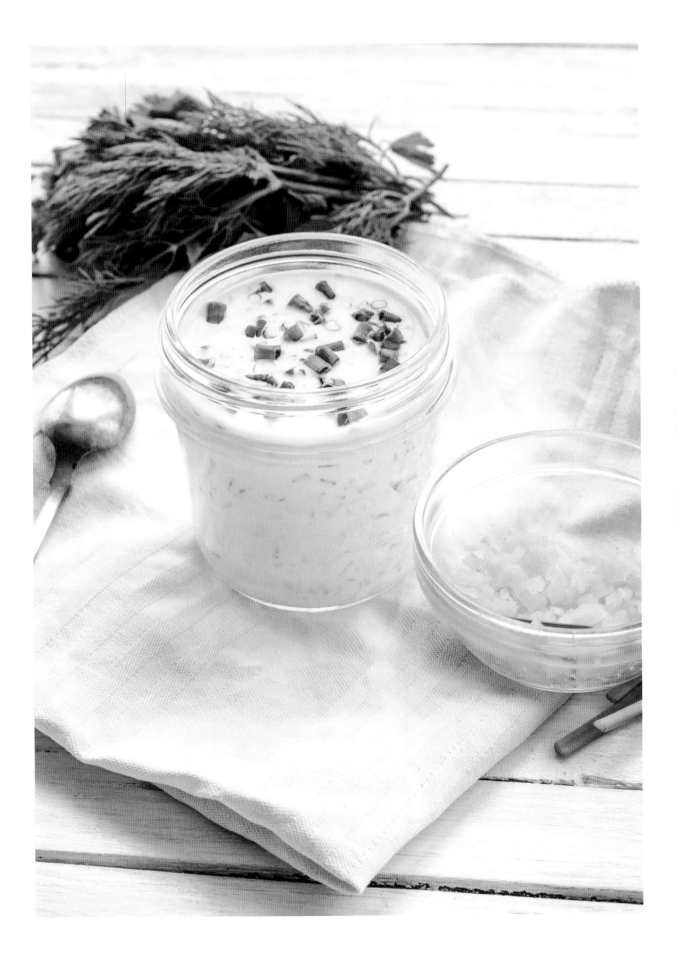

HONEY MUSTARD DRESSING & MARINADE

 AIP • COCONUT-FREE • DAIRY-FREE • EGG-FREE • NIGHTSHADE-FREE • NUT-FREE • VEGETARIAN

MAKES 1¾ cups (415 ml)
PREP TIME: 5 minutes
COOK TIME: –

This dressing is awesome on salads and fabulous as a marinade for chicken, and it triples as a wicked dip for homemade chicken fingers. Yes, there is honey in the recipe. And you're right, honey isn't a "keto food." But raw honey has some amazing health benefits, and, as you'll see in the nutrition information, it doesn't amp up the total carbohydrates in the dressing at all. If you're concerned, though, feel free to replace the honey with 2 teaspoons of confectioners'-style erythritol. The dressing just won't have that awesome honey taste!

Since the marinades in this book are likely to be heated, I've given avocado oil as an option in all the marinade recipes so you don't have to be concerned about the smoke point of the oil.

1 cup (240 ml) light-tasting oil, such as avocado oil or light olive oil

¼ cup (60 ml) apple cider vinegar

¼ cup (52 g) Dijon mustard

2 tablespoons lemon juice

1 tablespoon plus 1 teaspoon honey

½ teaspoon finely ground sea salt

1. Place all the ingredients in an 18-ounce (530-ml) or larger airtight container. Cover and shake until incorporated.

2. When ready to serve, give the container a little shake and enjoy.

STORE IT: *Keep in the fridge for up to 5 days or in the freezer for up to 1 month.*

THAW IT: *Set in the fridge to thaw completely before using.*

USE IN THESE RECIPES

 260
Crunchy Jicama Fries

 286
Breaded Mushroom Nuggets

 296
Zucchini Cakes with Lemon Aioli

Per tablespoon, made with avocado oil:

calories: **74** | calories from fat: **71** | total fat: **7.9g** | saturated fat: **0.9g** | cholesterol: **0mg**
sodium: **61mg** | carbs: **1g** | dietary fiber: **0.1g** | net carbs: **0.9g** | sugars: **0.9g** | protein: **0.1g**

FAT:	CARBS:	PROTEIN:
95%	**5%**	**0%**

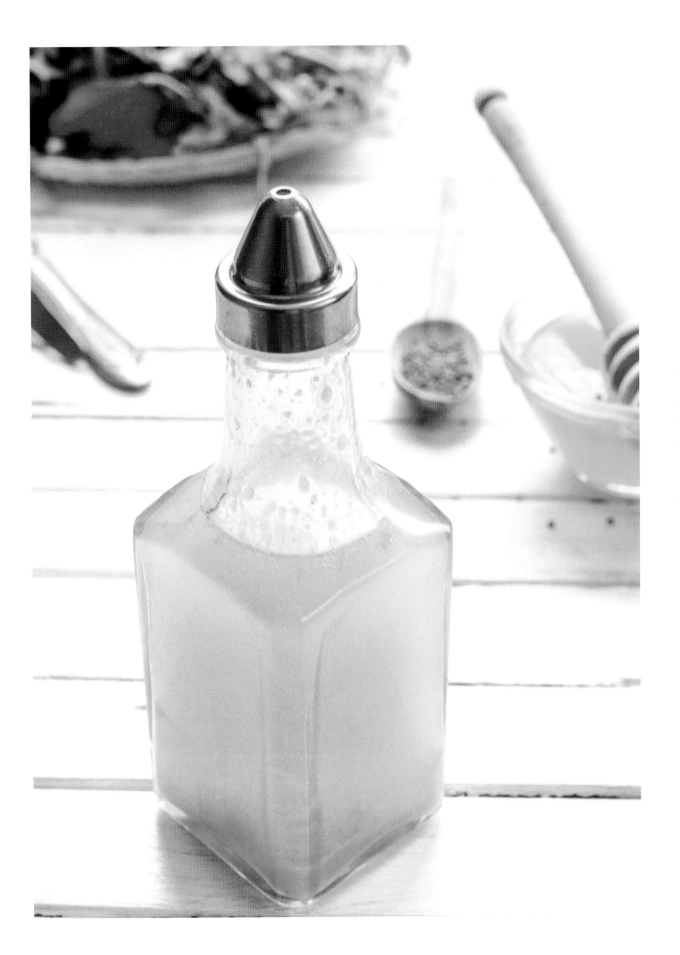

GREEN SPECKLED DRESSING

DAIRY-FREE • NIGHTSHADE-FREE • NUT-FREE • VEGETARIAN

OPTIONS: COCONUT-FREE • EGG-FREE • LOW-FODMAP • VEGAN

MAKES 1½ cups (350 ml)

PREP TIME: 5 minutes

COOK TIME: –

Inspired by green goddess dressing, but punchier. Make up a batch and you'll see what I mean!

½ cup (120 ml) light-tasting oil, such as avocado oil or light olive oil

½ cup (105 g) mayonnaise

3 tablespoons apple cider vinegar

2 tablespoons dried chives

2 teaspoons coconut aminos

2 teaspoons Dijon mustard

2 teaspoons dried parsley

1 teaspoon distilled vinegar

1 teaspoon garlic powder

½ teaspoon dried tarragon leaves

¼ teaspoon finely ground sea salt

1. Place all the ingredients in a 16-ounce (475-ml) or larger airtight container. Cover and shake until incorporated.

2. When ready to serve, give the container a little shake and enjoy.

STORE IT: *Keep in the fridge for up to 5 days.*

make it **COCONUT-FREE:**
Replace the coconut aminos with soy sauce and omit the salt.

make it **EGG-FREE/VEGAN:**
Use egg-free mayonnaise (see recipe on page 102).

make it **LOW-FODMAP:**
Omit the garlic powder.

USE IN THESE RECIPES

146
Something Different Breakfast Sammy

194
Paprika Chicken Sandwiches

276
Fried Cabbage Wedges

MAKE IT AT HOME

Replace store-bought mayonnaise with my homemade version.

104
Mayonnaise

Per tablespoon, made with avocado oil and homemade mayonnaise:

calories: **75** | calories from fat: **74** | total fat: **8.2g** | saturated fat: **1g** | cholesterol: **2mg**
sodium: **45mg** | carbs: **0.2g** | dietary fiber: **0g** | net carbs: **0.2g** | sugars: **0g** | protein: **0.1g**

FAT:	CARBS:	PROTEIN:
98%	1%	1%

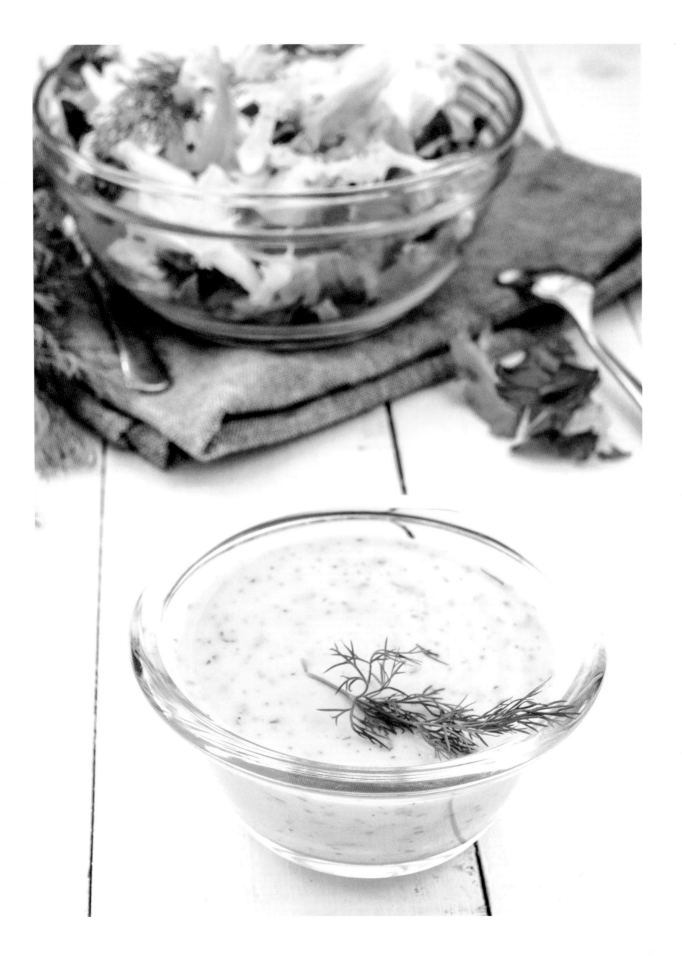

BACON DRESSING

COCONUT-FREE • DAIRY-FREE • EGG-FREE • LOW-FODMAP • NIGHTSHADE-FREE • NUT-FREE
OPTION: AIP

MAKES ½ cup (120 ml)

PREP TIME: 2 minutes

COOK TIME: –

I'm always trying to come up with unique uses for bacon grease, and this dressing is one of my favorites! It's a great way to use up leftover grease and boost your overall fat intake. Be forewarned, though, that this doesn't act like your everyday dressing. Bacon grease is so saturated that it hardens when it touches cold things. That's why this dressing is best on warm foods like roasted vegetables, warmed kale salad, or a pile of cooked meats and veggies.

If you don't have the amount of bacon grease needed for this recipe, you'll need to cook about 9 ounces (255 g) of bacon to get ⅓ cup (80 ml) of grease.

⅓ cup (80 ml) melted bacon grease

3 tablespoons lemon juice

¼ teaspoon finely ground sea salt

¼ teaspoon ground black pepper

make it AIP:
Omit the black pepper.

1. Place all the ingredients in a 7-ounce (210-ml) or larger airtight container. Cover and shake until incorporated.

2. Before serving, set the container on the counter for a couple of hours to soften, then give the container a little shake and enjoy.

STORE IT: *Keep in the fridge for up to 5 days or in the freezer for up to 1 month.*

THAW IT: *Set in the fridge to thaw completely before using.*

USE IN THESE RECIPES

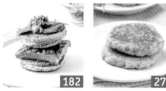

Chimichurri Steak Bunwiches 182

Cauliflower Patties 270

Per tablespoon:

calories: **79** | calories from fat: **77** | total fat: **8.6g** | saturated fat: **3.4g** | cholesterol: **8mg**
sodium: **60mg** | carbs: **0.2g** | dietary fiber: **0g** | net carbs: **0.2g** | sugars: **0.1g** | protein: **0.1g**

FAT:	CARBS:	PROTEIN:
99%	1%	0%

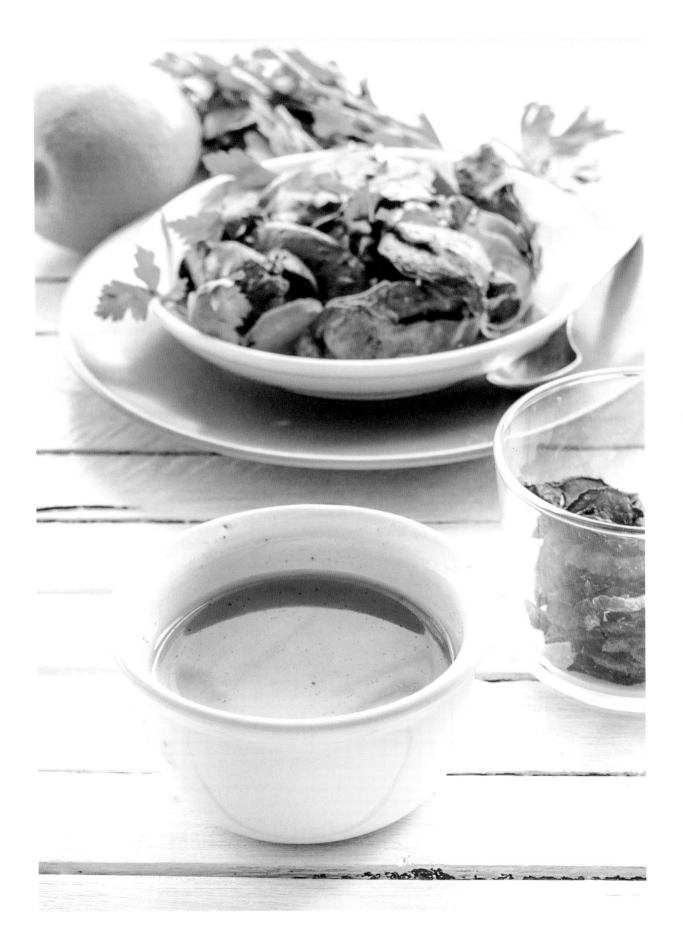

AVOCADO LIME DRESSING

 AIP • COCONUT-FREE • DAIRY-FREE • EGG-FREE • NIGHTSHADE-FREE • NUT-FREE • VEGAN • VEGETARIAN

MAKES 1¹⁄₃ cups (315 ml)
PREP TIME: 5 minutes
COOK TIME: –

The thing about avocados is that when they're ready to eat, they need to be eaten, and finding creative ways to enjoy them without getting avocado fatigue is a struggle. This dressing is awesome with celery and crazy good tossed with romaine lettuce. To keep it from turning brown, store it in an airtight container with a leftover avocado pit inside, and try to gobble it up as quickly as possible.

2 medium Hass avocados, peeled and pitted (about 8 oz/220 g of flesh)

²⁄₃ cup (160 ml) light-tasting oil, such as avocado oil or light olive oil

½ cup (115 g) roughly chopped white onions

½ packed cup (35 g) fresh cilantro leaves and stems

2 tablespoons lime juice

2 cloves garlic

½ teaspoon finely ground sea salt

1. Place all the ingredients in a blender or food processor. Blend until completely smooth.

2. Transfer the dressing to a 14-ounce (415-ml) or larger airtight container for storage.

STORE IT: *Keep in the fridge, with a piece of plastic wrap over the top to keep the dressing from browning, for up to 3 days.*

Per tablespoon, made with avocado oil:

calories: **84**	calories from fat: **76**	total fat: **8.5g**	saturated fat: **1.3g**	cholesterol: **0mg**
sodium: **45mg**	carbs: **1.6g**	dietary fiber: **0.9g**	net carbs: **0.7g**	sugars: **0.3g**	protein: **0.3g**

FAT:	CARBS:	PROTEIN:
91%	**8%**	**1%**

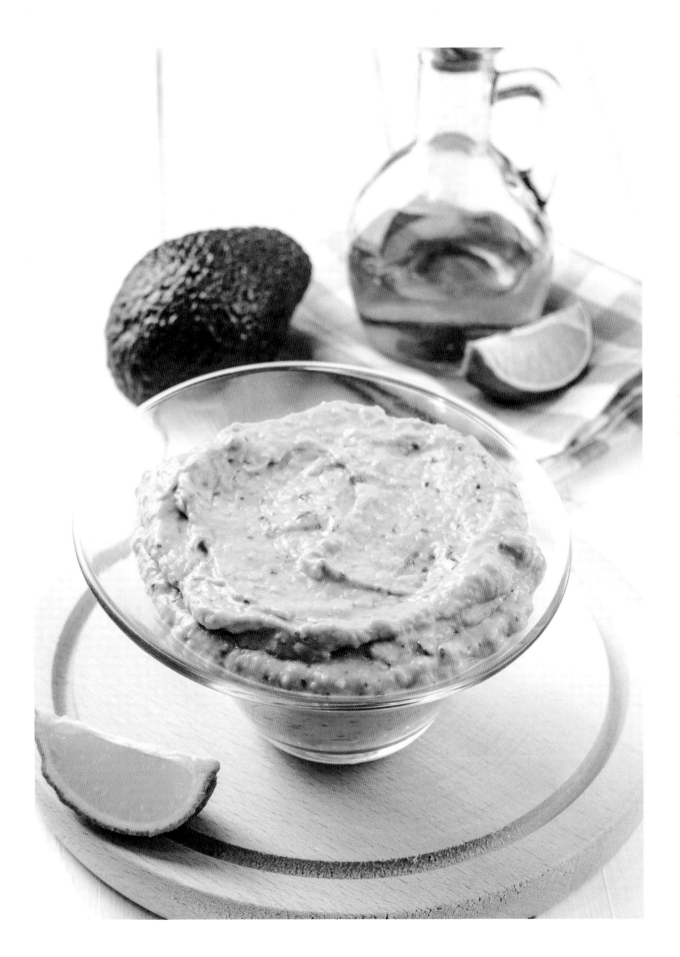

LEMON TURMERIC DRESSING & MARINADE

 AIP • COCONUT-FREE • DAIRY-FREE • EGG-FREE • NIGHTSHADE-FREE • NUT-FREE • VEGAN • VEGETARIAN

MAKES 1½ cups (350 ml)
PREP TIME: 5 minutes
COOK TIME: –

This dressing takes coleslaw to greater heights, adds a kick to browned ground beef, and is awesome in a stir-fry.

1 cup (240 ml) light-tasting oil, such as avocado oil or light olive oil

¼ cup (60 ml) apple cider vinegar

1 tablespoon plus 1 teaspoon lemon juice

2 teaspoons garlic powder

1½ teaspoons turmeric powder

1 teaspoon onion powder

½ teaspoon finely ground sea salt

1. Place all the ingredients in a 16-ounce (475-ml) or larger airtight container. Cover and shake until incorporated.

2. When ready to serve, give the container a little shake and enjoy.

STORE IT: *Keep in the fridge for up to 5 days or in the freezer for up to 1 month.*

THAW IT: *Set in the fridge to thaw completely before using.*

USE IN THESE RECIPES

144
All Day Any Day Hash

172
Speckled Salad

208
Crispy Pork with Lemon-Thyme Cauli Rice

Per tablespoon, made with avocado oil:

| calories: **84** | calories from fat: **81** | total fat: **9.1g** | saturated fat: **1.1g** | cholesterol: **0mg** | FAT: | CARBS: | PROTEIN: |
| sodium: **39mg** | carbs: **0.4g** | dietary fiber: **0.1g** | net carbs: **0.3g** | sugars: **0.1g** | protein: **0.1g** | **98%** | **2%** | **0%** |

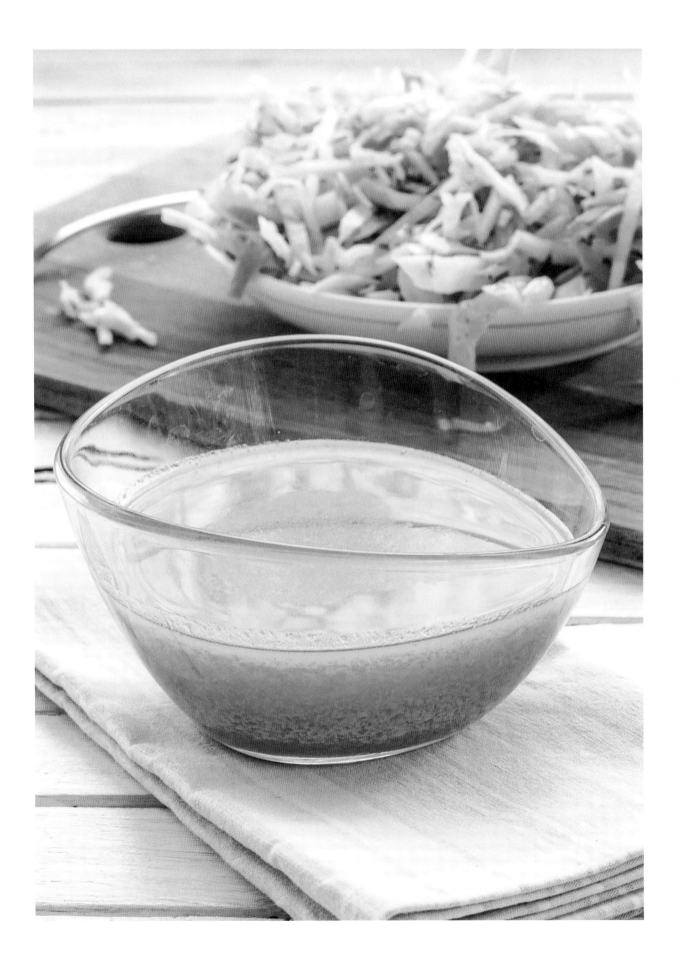

BASIL VINAIGRETTE & MARINADE

 COCONUT-FREE • DAIRY-FREE • EGG-FREE • NIGHTSHADE-FREE • NUT-FREE • VEGETARIAN
OPTIONS: AIP • LOW-FODMAP • VEGAN

MAKES 1½ cups (350 ml)
PREP TIME: 5 minutes
COOK TIME: –

There's this pâté recipe on my blog, Healthful Pursuit *(healthfulpursuit.com), that I created in 2012 and continues to be one of my favorite recipes to this day. Now, there's only so much almond-based pâté a girl can eat, so I decided to take all the flavors from the pâté and make a dressing version!*

2 cups (60 g) fresh basil leaves

1 cup (240 ml) light-tasting oil, such as avocado oil or light olive oil

½ cup (120 ml) lemon juice

2 cloves garlic

2 teaspoons honey, 1 teaspoon erythritol, or 3 drops liquid stevia

Grated zest of 1 lemon

½ teaspoon finely ground sea salt

1. Place all the ingredients in a blender or food processor. Blend until the basil leaves are ¼-inch (6-mm) specks.

2. Transfer the dressing to a 14-ounce (415-ml) or larger airtight container.

3. When ready to serve, give the container a little shake and enjoy.

STORE IT: *Keep in the fridge for up to 4 days.*

make it AIP:
Do not use erythritol.

make it LOW-FODMAP:
Omit the garlic and replace ¼ cup (60 ml) of the oil with garlic-infused oil. Use stevia.

make it VEGAN:
Do not use honey.

USE IN THESE RECIPES

130
Cross-Country Scrambler

168
Easy Chopped Salad

212
Salmon & Kale

Per tablespoon, made with avocado oil and honey:

calories: **85**	calories from fat: **82**	total fat: **9.1g**	saturated fat: **1.1g**	cholesterol: **0mg**
sodium: **40mg**	carbs: **0.7g**	dietary fiber: **0.1g**	net carbs: **0.6g**	sugars: **0.6g**	protein: **0.1g**

FAT:	CARBS:	PROTEIN:
96%	3%	0%

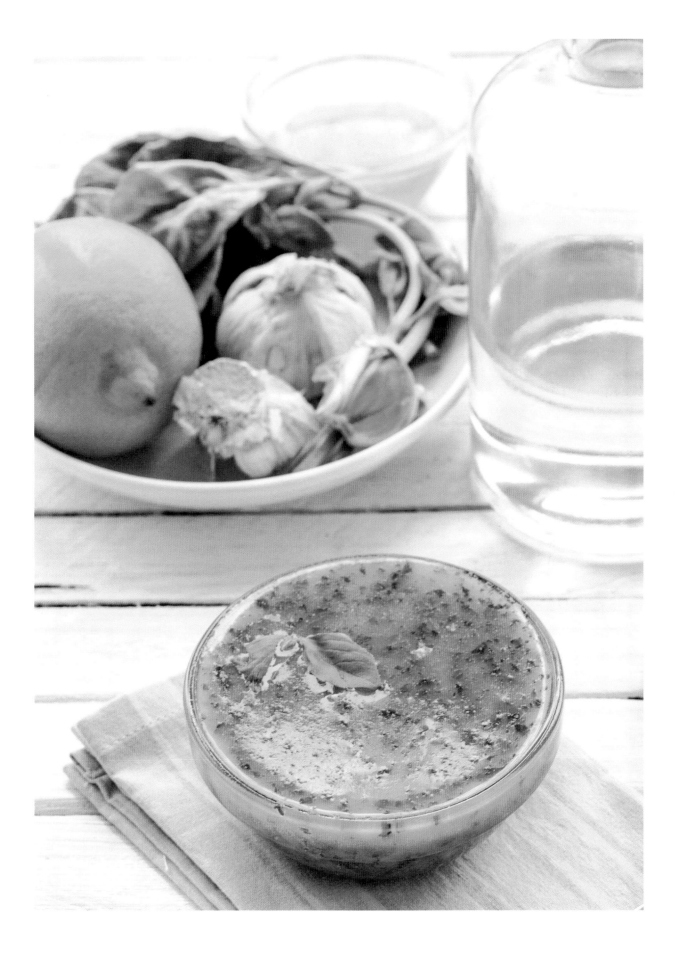

POPPY SEED DRESSING

COCONUT-FREE • DAIRY-FREE • EGG-FREE • NIGHTSHADE-FREE • NUT-FREE • VEGAN • VEGETARIAN
OPTION: LOW-FODMAP

MAKES 1½ cups (350 ml)
PREP TIME: 5 minutes
COOK TIME: –

Why use confectioners'-style erythritol for this dressing? Well, you could use granulated, but then you'd have to heat the mixture to dissolve the sweetener, and that seems like an awful lot of work. I always keep a bag of confectioners'-style erythritol on hand for recipes like this one where I don't want to spend added time in the kitchen. It tastes the same as granulated, without all the extra work. If you can't get your hands on confectioners', get a bag of granulated, blend it to a fine powder, and store it in your pantry. It'll be way, way easier to work with!

1 cup (240 ml) light-tasting oil, such as avocado oil or light olive oil

¼ cup (60 ml) distilled vinegar

2 tablespoons confectioners'-style erythritol, or 10 drops liquid stevia

1 tablespoon plus 1 teaspoon poppy seeds

2 teaspoons onion powder

1 teaspoon Dijon mustard

½ teaspoon finely ground sea salt

1. Place all the ingredients in a 16-ounce (475-ml) or larger airtight container. Cover and shake until incorporated.

2. When ready to serve, give the container a little shake and enjoy.

STORE IT: *Keep in the fridge for up to 5 days or in the freezer for up to 1 month.*

THAW IT: *Set in the fridge to thaw completely before using.*

make it **LOW-FODMAP:**
Omit the onion powder.

USE IN THIS RECIPE

BBQ Beef & Slaw

204

Per tablespoon, made with avocado oil:

calories: **85** | calories from fat: **83** | total fat: **9.3g** | saturated fat: **1.1g** | cholesterol: **0mg**
sodium: **42mg** | carbs: **0.3g** | dietary fiber: **0.1g** | net carbs: **0.2g** | sugars: **0.1g** | protein: **0.1g**

FAT:	CARBS:	PROTEIN:
98%	1%	1%

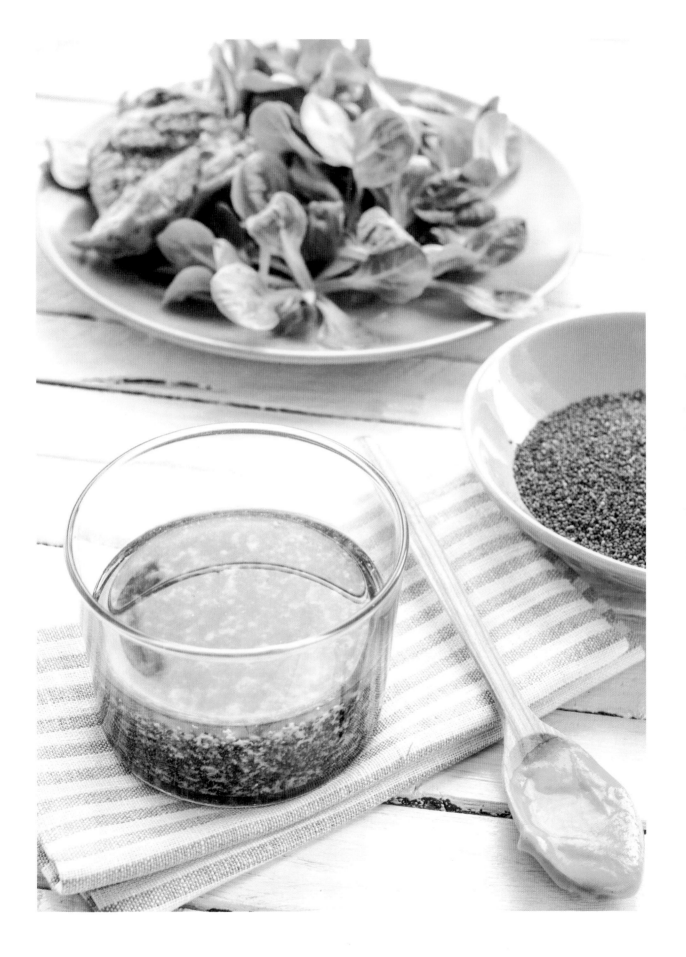

TERIYAKI SAUCE & MARINADE

DAIRY-FREE • EGG-FREE • NIGHTSHADE-FREE • NUT-FREE • VEGAN • VEGETARIAN

OPTION: COCONUT-FREE

MAKES 1½ cups (350 ml)

PREP TIME: 5 minutes

COOK TIME: –

Awesome as a marinade for pork or fresh-cut vegetables (especially broccoli or bok choy) and in a stir-fry. Try not to overthink your keto cooking! Chop up a couple of random vegetables, add some meat and this sauce, and you're well on your way to a keto meal.

1 cup (240 ml) light-tasting oil, such as avocado oil or light olive oil

¼ cup (60 ml) coconut aminos

2 tablespoons confectioners'-style erythritol

1 tablespoon apple cider vinegar

1 teaspoon garlic powder

1 teaspoon ginger powder

1 teaspoon finely ground sea salt

1. Place all the ingredients in a 16-ounce (475-ml) or larger airtight container. Cover and shake until incorporated.

2. When ready to serve, give the container a little shake and enjoy.

make it COCONUT-FREE:
Replace the coconut aminos with soy sauce and omit the salt.

STORE IT: *Keep in the fridge for up to 5 days or in the freezer for up to 1 month.*

THAW IT: *Set in the fridge to thaw completely before using.*

USE IN THIS RECIPE

Wedge Dippers

266

Per tablespoon, made with avocado oil:

calories: **85**	calories from fat: **82**	total fat: **9.1g**	saturated fat: **1.1g**	cholesterol: **0mg**	
sodium: **81mg**	carbs: **0.7g**	dietary fiber: **0g**	net carbs: **0.7g**	sugars: **0g**	protein: **0g**

FAT:	CARBS:	PROTEIN:
96%	**3%**	**1%**

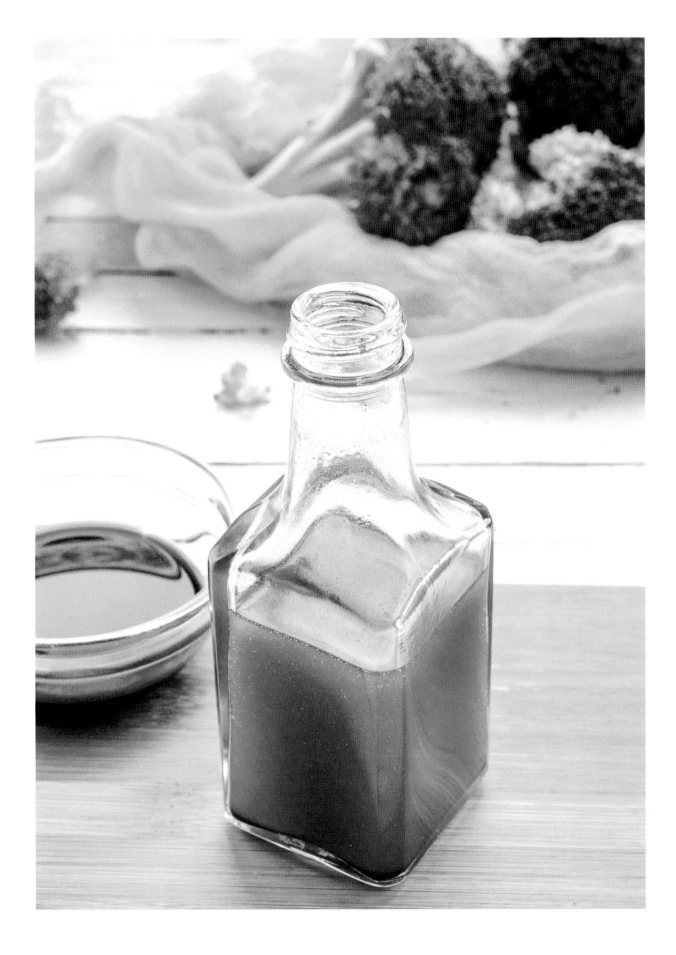

CREAMY ITALIAN DRESSING

COCONUT-FREE • DAIRY-FREE • NUT-FREE • VEGETARIAN
OPTIONS: EGG-FREE • LOW-FODMAP • NIGHTSHADE-FREE • VEGAN

MAKES 1½ cups (350 ml)
PREP TIME: 5 minutes
COOK TIME: –

Yes, you could make this dressing with fresh ingredients like crushed garlic, fresh thyme, and/or fresh basil, but that would take a lot of time and cost more. My vote? Double the recipe—or heck, even triple it—and spend less money eating more fat.

¾ cup (180 ml) light-tasting oil, such as avocado oil or light olive oil

¼ cup plus 2 tablespoons (80 g) mayonnaise

3 tablespoons red wine vinegar

1 tablespoon distilled vinegar

1 tablespoon lemon juice

1 tablespoon onion powder

1½ teaspoons dried basil

1½ teaspoons ground black pepper

¾ teaspoon garlic powder

¾ teaspoon dried oregano leaves

¾ teaspoon dried thyme leaves

½ teaspoon red pepper flakes

¼ teaspoon finely ground sea salt

1. Place all the ingredients in a 16-ounce (475-ml) or larger airtight container. Cover and shake until incorporated.

2. When ready to serve, give the container a little shake and enjoy.

STORE IT: *Keep in the fridge for up to 5 days.*

make it EGG-FREE/VEGAN:
Use egg-free mayonnaise (see recipe on page 102).

make it LOW-FODMAP:
Omit the onion and garlic powder.

make it NIGHTSHADE-FREE:
Omit the red pepper flakes.

USE IN THESE RECIPES

144

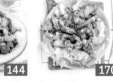
170

210

All Day Any Day Hash

Cajun Shrimp Salad

One-Pot Porky Kale

MAKE IT AT HOME

Replace store-bought mayonnaise with my homemade version.

104

Mayonnaise

Per tablespoon, made with avocado oil and homemade mayonnaise:

| calories: **86** | calories from fat: **83** | total fat: **9.3g** | saturated fat: **1.2g** | cholesterol: **1mg** | FAT: **97%** | CARBS: **2%** | PROTEIN: **0%** |
| sodium: **45mg** | carbs: **0.5g** | dietary fiber: **0.1g** | net carbs: **0.4g** | sugars: **0.1g** | protein: **0.1g** | | | |

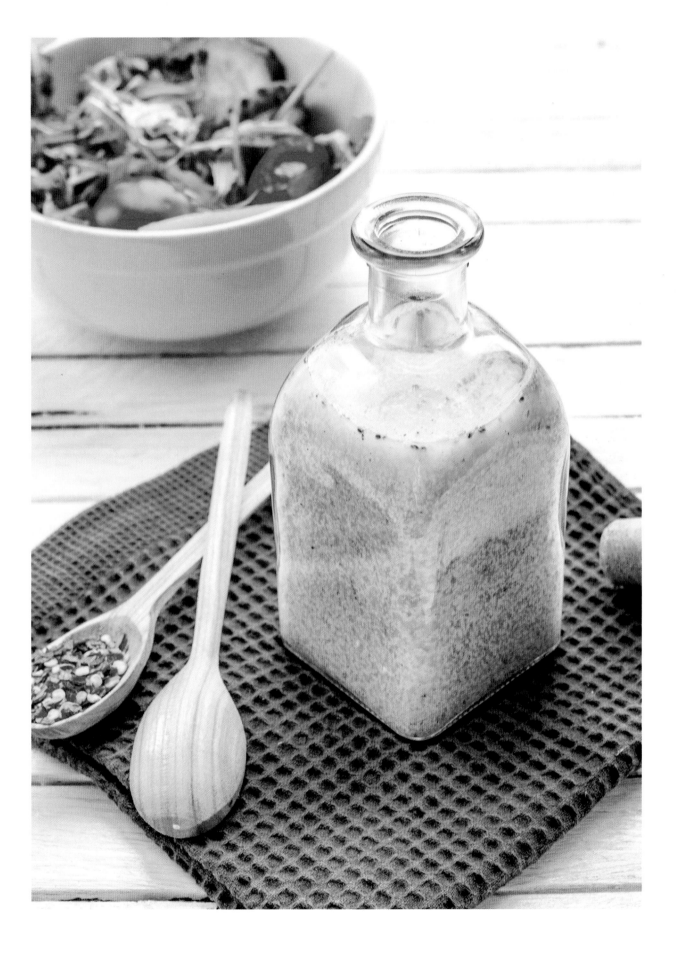

CHOCOLATE SAUCE

COCONUT-FREE • DAIRY-FREE • EGG-FREE • LOW-FODMAP • NIGHTSHADE-FREE • NUT-FREE • VEGAN • VEGETARIAN

OPTION: AIP

MAKES ¾ cup (180 ml)

PREP TIME: 1 minute

COOK TIME: –

Anywhere you want chocolate, add this sauce! My favorite way to use it is to blend it into fatty coffees, but drizzling it over chilled and whipped coconut cream, ice cream, or fresh berries is a close runner-up.

½ cup (120 ml) avocado oil

¼ cup (20 g) cocoa powder

2 tablespoons confectioners'-style erythritol, or 15 drops liquid stevia

make it AIP:
Replace the cocoa powder with carob powder and use stevia.

1. Place all the ingredients in an 8-ounce (240-ml) or larger airtight container. Cover and shake until incorporated.

2. Whisk with a fork when ready to serve.

STORE IT: *Keep in the fridge for up to 5 days or in the freezer for up to 1 month.*

THAW IT: *Set in the fridge to thaw completely before using.*

USE IN THESE RECIPES

136

Keto Breakfast Pudding

332

Chocolate Soft-Serve Ice Cream

Per tablespoon:

calories: **87** | calories from fat: **82** | total fat: **9.1g** | saturated fat: **1.4g** | cholesterol: **0mg**

sodium: **1mg** | carbs: **1.1g** | dietary fiber: **0.7g** | net carbs: **0.4g** | sugars: **0g** | protein: **0.3g**

FAT:	CARBS:	PROTEIN:
95%	5%	1%

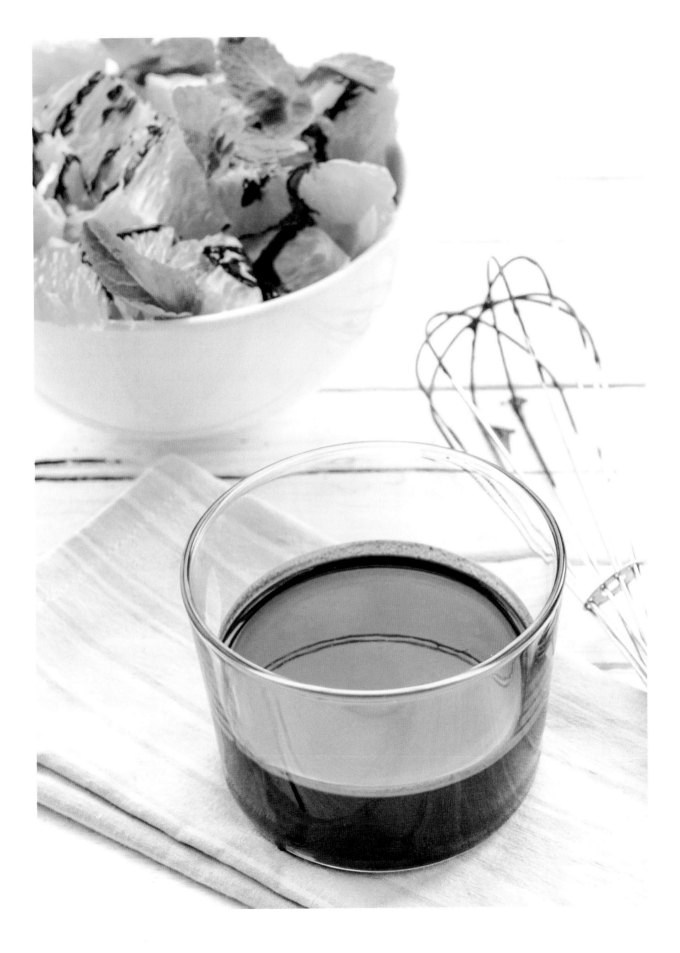

HERBY VINAIGRETTE & MARINADE

 COCONUT-FREE • DAIRY-FREE • EGG-FREE • NIGHTSHADE-FREE • NUT-FREE • VEGAN • VEGETARIAN

OPTIONS: AIP • LOW-FODMAP

MAKES 1⅓ cups (315 ml)

PREP TIME: 5 minutes

COOK TIME: –

This recipe is awesome for midsummer when fresh herbs from the garden are at their peak.

I added a healthy dose of oregano oil to this dressing because oregano oil is a potent antibiotic that has the potential to heal many ailments, and it is a great addition to any no-cook recipe that calls for oregano. In addition to its antibiotic properties, it is anti-inflammatory; aids in gut health; assists with yeast infections; balances cholesterol; helps with acne, dandruff, warts, psoriasis, muscle pain, and varicose veins; and so many other things. You can find oregano oil in many health food stores or pharmacies. It comes as a liquid or gel capsule. I like to buy the gel caps because they're more versatile. To use them in a recipe, I just cut one open and add a few drops to what I'm making.

If you don't want to use oregano oil, simply double the amount of fresh oregano.

1 cup (240 ml) light-tasting oil, such as avocado oil or light olive oil

¾ cup (180 ml) apple cider vinegar

4 cloves garlic

¼ cup (45 g) fresh rosemary leaves

2 tablespoons fresh oregano leaves

1 (½-oz/14-g) packet fresh chives

1 teaspoon finely ground sea salt

1 teaspoon ground black pepper

8 drops oregano oil, or 2 tablespoons additional fresh oregano leaves

1. Place all the ingredients in a food processor or blender. Blend until smooth.

2. Use immediately or transfer to a 14-ounce (415-ml) or larger airtight container for later use.

3. When ready to serve, give the container a little shake and enjoy.

STORE IT: *Keep in the fridge for up to 5 days.*

make it AIP:
Omit the black pepper.

make it LOW-FODMAP:
Omit the garlic and replace ¼ cup (60 ml) of the oil with garlic-infused oil.

USE IN THESE RECIPES

164
Antipasto Salad

190
BLT-Stuffed Avocados

294
Tuna Cucumber Boats

Per tablespoon, made with avocado oil:

calories: **93** | calories from fat: **84** | total fat: **9.8g** | saturated fat: **1.4g** | cholesterol: **0mg**

sodium: **91mg** | carbs: **1.1g** | dietary fiber: **0.5g** | net carbs: **0.6g** | sugars: **0.1g** | protein: **0.2g**

FAT:	CARBS:	PROTEIN:
95%	5%	1%

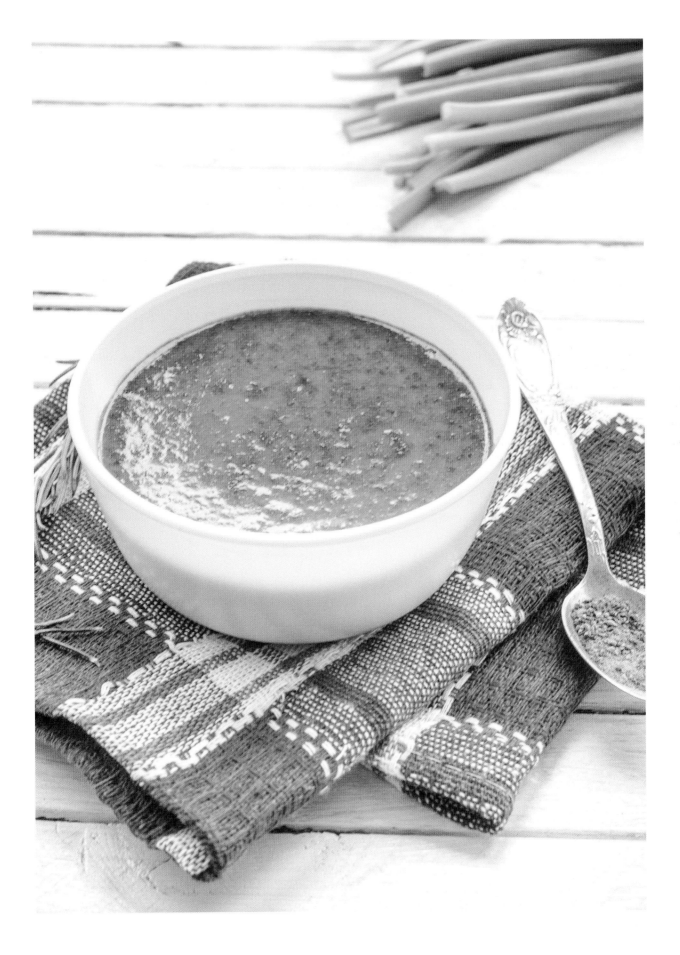

READY-IN-SECONDS HOLLANDAISE SAUCE

LOW-FODMAP • NUT-FREE • VEGETARIAN

OPTIONS: COCONUT-FREE • DAIRY-FREE • NIGHTSHADE-FREE

MAKES 1¾ cups (415 ml)
PREP TIME: 2 minutes
COOK TIME: –

This stuff is amazing on just about any type of fish, spread over the top of a Mug Biscuit (page 134), or drizzled over roasted asparagus. Unlike traditional hollandaise, where the fat is heated and the eggs are cooked, you just place all the ingredients in a blender, mix, and go to town—no cooking needed! This difference means you'll be eating raw egg yolk. If you have a concern about that, you could purchase pasteurized eggs.

Make this recipe with butter-flavored coconut oil, ghee, or unsalted butter. Being dairy-free, I opt for the former, but you can use whichever fat you'd like and it'll taste great.

1¼ cups (220 g) butter-flavored coconut oil or ghee, chilled in the fridge until hardened

6 large egg yolks

2 tablespoons lemon juice

1 teaspoon finely ground sea salt

Pinch of cayenne pepper (optional)

1. Place all the ingredients in a food processor or blender. Blend on medium speed for 15 to 25 seconds, until creamy.

2. Use immediately or transfer to an 18-ounce (530-ml) or larger airtight container for later use. When ready to serve, set the chilled sauce on the counter to come to room temperature, then transfer to the food processor or blender and blend again before using.

STORE IT: *Keep in an airtight container in the fridge for up to 5 days.*

make it COCONUT-FREE:
Use ghee.

make it DAIRY-FREE:
Use coconut oil.

make it NIGHTSHADE-FREE:
Omit the cayenne.

USE IN THIS RECIPE

Eggs Benedict

132

Per tablespoon, made with butter-flavored coconut oil:

calories: **100**	calories from fat: **96**	total fat: **10.7g**	saturated fat: **8.8g**	cholesterol: **45mg**	
sodium: **68mg**	carbs: **0.2g**	dietary fiber: **0g**	net carbs: **0.2g**	sugars: **0g**	protein: **0.6g**

FAT:	CARBS:	PROTEIN:
96%	**1%**	**2%**

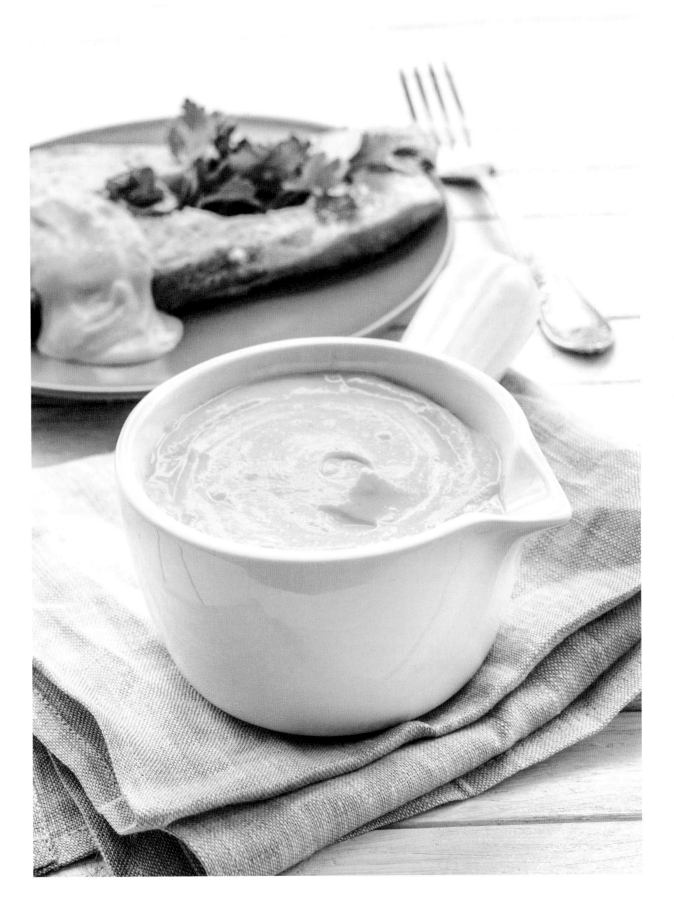

EGG-FREE MAYONNAISE

COCONUT-FREE • DAIRY-FREE • EGG-FREE • NIGHTSHADE-FREE • NUT-FREE • VEGAN • VEGETARIAN

MAKES 1¾ cups (365 g)

PREP TIME: 5 minutes

COOK TIME: –

While not completely keto diet–approved because it uses the liquid from a can of chickpeas (called aquafaba), this is a fabulous mayonnaise alternative for those who are sensitive to eggs.

- ¼ cup plus 2 tablespoons (90 ml) chickpea liquid (from a can of chickpeas)
- 2 tablespoons lemon juice
- 1 tablespoon plus 1 teaspoon Dijon mustard
- 1 tablespoon apple cider vinegar
- ½ teaspoon finely ground sea salt
- ½ teaspoon ground black pepper
- 1½ cups (350 ml) light-tasting oil, such as avocado oil or light olive oil

If using a countertop blender, put all the ingredients, except the oil, in the blender. Pulse just enough to combine. Then, with the blender running on medium speed, slowly drizzle in the oil, taking at least 2 minutes to add all the oil. After the oil has been added, continue to blend until the mixture has the consistency of mayonnaise.

If using an immersion blender, put all the ingredients, including the oil, in the blending jar or beaker. (If your immersion blender didn't come with a jar, use a wide-mouthed 1-quart/950-ml jar or similar-sized container.) Insert the blender into the jar, turn it to high speed, and keep it at the base of the jar for 25 seconds. Then move the blender up and down in the jar until the ingredients are well incorporated.

STORE IT: *Keep in an airtight container in the fridge for up to 5 days.*

USE IN THESE RECIPES

German No-Tato Salad **156**

Sammies with Basil Mayo **186**

Cucumber Salmon Coins **288**

Per 2-tablespoon serving, made with avocado oil:

calories: **199**	calories from fat: **190**	total fat: **21.9g**	saturated fat: **3.1g**	cholesterol: **0mg**
sodium: **82mg**	carbs: **0.4g**	dietary fiber: **0g**	net carbs: **0.4g**	sugars: **0g**	protein: **0.3g**

FAT:	CARBS:	PROTEIN:
99%	**1%**	**0%**

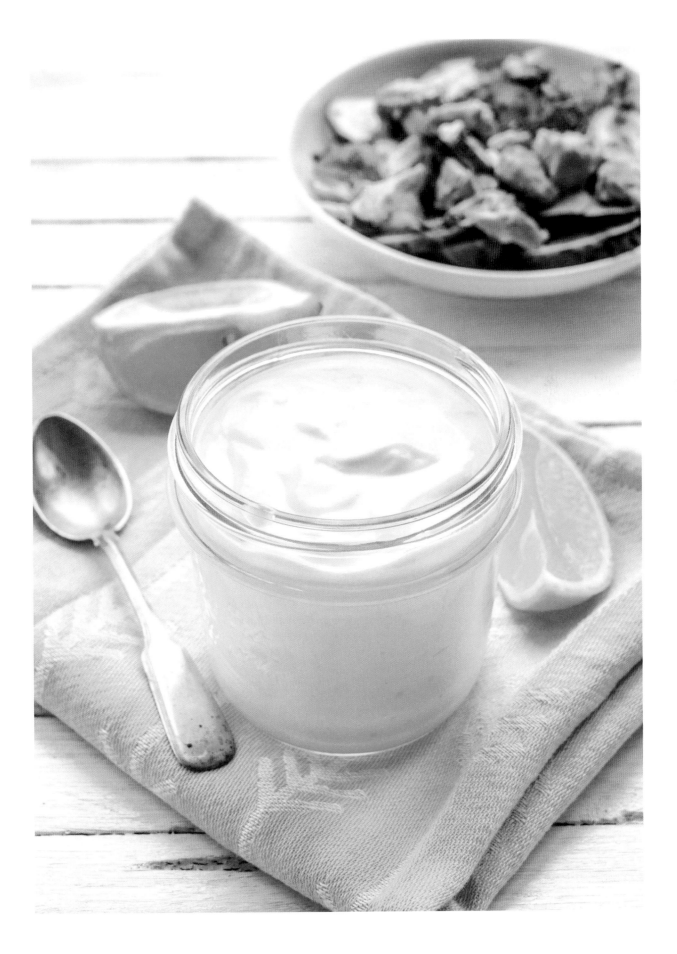

MAYONNAISE

COCONUT-FREE • DAIRY-FREE • LOW-FODMAP • NIGHTSHADE-FREE • NUT-FREE • VEGETARIAN

MAKES 1¼ cups (260 g)

PREP TIME: 5 minutes

COOK TIME: –

A keto cookbook is not complete without a mayonnaise recipe. Yes, you can buy mayonnaise; my favorite is avocado oil mayonnaise from Chosen Foods or Primal Kitchen. But if you want to save a couple dollars and make it yourself, I've got you covered!

1 large egg

2 large egg yolks

1 tablespoon plus 1 teaspoon white wine vinegar, or 1 tablespoon apple cider vinegar

1 tablespoon lemon juice

1 teaspoon Dijon mustard

¼ teaspoon finely ground sea salt

⅛ teaspoon ground black pepper

1 cup (240 ml) light-tasting oil, such as avocado oil or light olive oil

If using a countertop blender, put all the ingredients, except the oil, in the blender. Pulse just enough to combine. With the blender running on medium speed, slowly drizzle in the oil, taking at least 2 minutes to add it all. After the oil has been added, continue to blend until the mixture has the consistency of mayonnaise.

If using an immersion blender, put all the ingredients, including the oil, in the blending jar or beaker. (If your immersion blender didn't come with a jar, use a wide-mouthed quart-sized (950-ml) jar or similar-sized container.) Insert the blender into the jar, turn it to high speed, and keep it at the base of the jar for 25 seconds. Then move the blender up and down in the jar until the ingredients are well incorporated.

| **STORE IT:** *Keep in an airtight container in the fridge for up to 5 days.*

USE IN THESE RECIPES

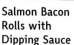

118 Salmon Bacon Rolls with Dipping Sauce

214 Creamy Spinach Zucchini Boats

292 BLT Dip

Per 2-tablespoon serving, made with avocado oil:

calories: **200**	calories from fat: **192**	total fat: **21.6g**	saturated fat: **3.4g**	cholesterol: **61mg**
sodium: **62mg**	carbs: **0.3g**	dietary fiber: **0g**	net carbs: **0.3g**	sugars: **0g**	protein: **1.2g**

FAT:	CARBS:	PROTEIN:
97%	1%	2%

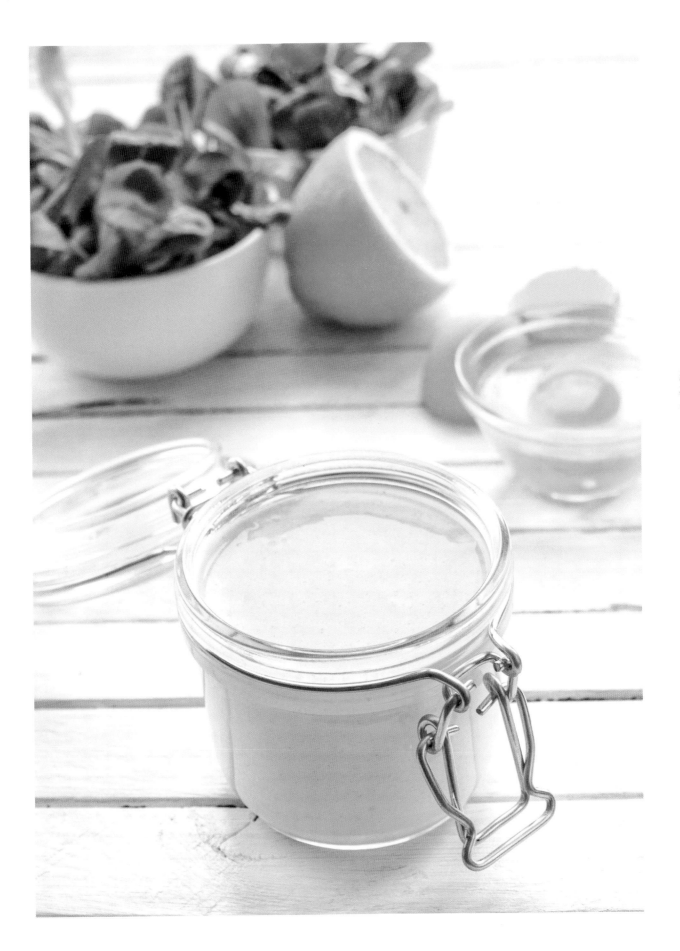

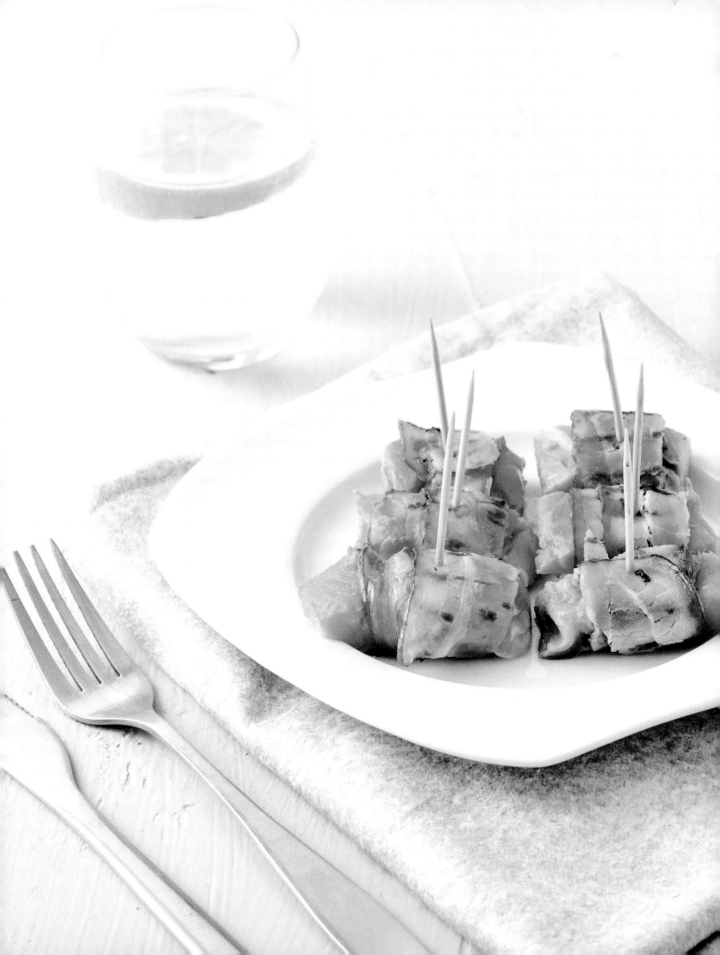

5.

BREAKFAST

CHOCOHOLIC GRANOLA / 108

AVOCADO BREAKFAST MUFFINS / 110

HERB CHICKEN SAUSAGES WITH BRAISED BOK CHOY / 112

BUFFALO CHICKEN BREAKFAST MUFFINS / 114

PROSCIUTTO BISCUITS / 116

SALMON BACON ROLLS WITH DIPPING SAUCE / 118

HEY GIRL / 120

PUMPKIN SPICE LATTE OVERNIGHT "OATS" / 122

ROCKET FUEL HOT CHOCOLATE / 124

FULL MEAL DEAL / 126

LIVER SAUSAGES & ONIONS / 128

CROSS-COUNTRY SCRAMBLER / 130

EGGS BENEDICT / 132

MUG BISCUIT / 134

KETO BREAKFAST PUDDING / 136

PEPPER SAUSAGE FRY / 138

INDIAN MASALA OMELET / 140

STICKY WRAPPED EGGS / 142

ALL DAY ANY DAY HASH / 144

SOMETHING DIFFERENT BREAKFAST SAMMY / 146

SUPER BREAKFAST COMBO / 148

COFFEE SHAKE / 150

CHOCOHOLIC GRANOLA

DAIRY-FREE • EGG-FREE • NIGHTSHADE-FREE • NUT-FREE • VEGAN • VEGETARIAN
OPTIONS: COCONUT-FREE • LOW-FODMAP

MAKES 3½ cups (290 g) (14 servings)

PREP TIME: 5 minutes, plus 20 minutes to cool

COOK TIME: 10 minutes

Laura, one of our amazing Healthful Pursuit *readers, named this recipe, and for good reason! Nothing but chocolate on this one. If you want to go over the top, you could add cacao nibs or stevia-sweetened chocolate chips. Cacao nibs are little bits of raw cacao, completely unsweetened and in its natural state.*

This recipe calls for coconut flakes. These are large flakes of coconut, much larger than standard shredded coconut. I purchase unsweetened coconut flakes from Thrive Market.

⅓ cup (65 g) erythritol

2 tablespoons water

1 teaspoon vanilla extract

⅓ cup (27 g) cocoa powder

1 teaspoon ground cinnamon

¾ teaspoon finely ground sea salt

3 cups (190 g) unsweetened coconut flakes

make it COCONUT-FREE:
Replace the coconut with 2½ cups (375 g) hulled sunflower seeds.

make it LOW-FODMAP:
Do not eat more than one serving per day.

1. Cover a cutting board or baking sheet with a piece of parchment paper and set aside.

2. Place the erythritol, water, and vanilla in a large saucepan over medium-low heat. Bring to a light simmer, stirring every 30 seconds. Continue to Step 3 if using confectioners'-style erythritol; if using granulated erythritol, continue to simmer until the granules can no longer be felt on the back of the spoon.

3. Reduce the heat to low and add the cocoa powder, cinnamon, and salt; mix until fully incorporated.

4. Add the coconut flakes and continue to stir frequently, keeping the temperature low to prevent burning. Cook for 6 to 7 minutes, until the bottom of the pan gets sticky.

5. Remove from the heat and transfer the granola to the parchment paper. Allow to cool completely, about 20 minutes, before enjoying, or transfer to a 1-quart (950-ml) or larger airtight container for storage.

STORE IT: *Keep in the fridge for up to 10 days or in the freezer for up to 1 month. You can eat it straight out of the freezer without thawing.*

Per ¼-cup/21-g serving:

calories: **106** | calories from fat: **83** | total fat: **9.2g** | saturated fat: **8.1g** | cholesterol: **0mg** | sodium: **106mg** | carbs: **5g** | dietary fiber: **2.7g** | net carbs: **2.3g** | sugars: **0.9g** | protein: **0.9g**

FAT:	CARBS:	PROTEIN:
78%	**19%**	**3%**

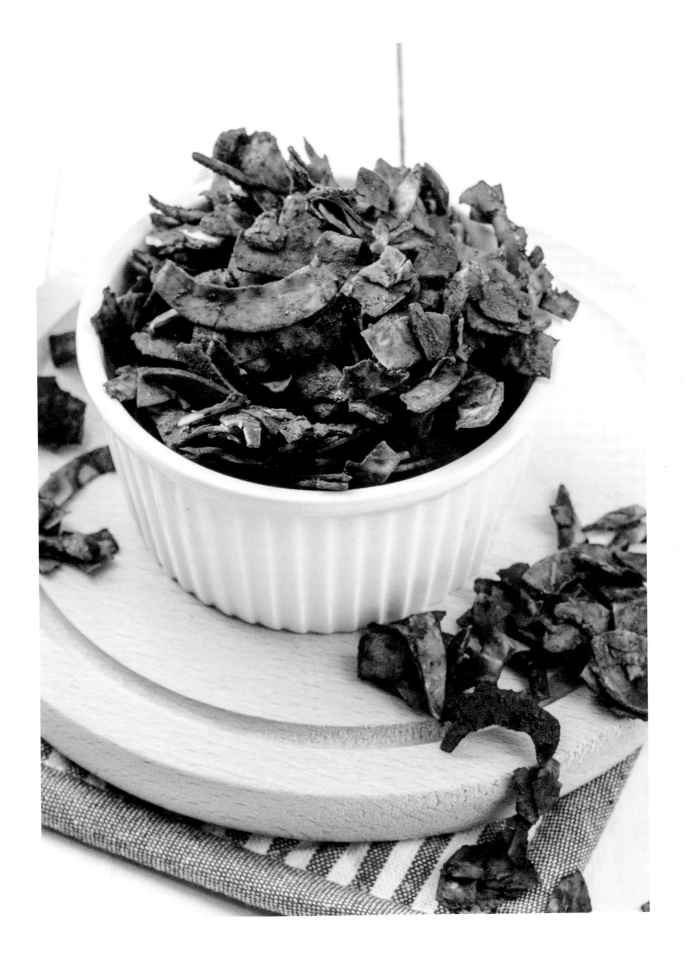

AVOCADO BREAKFAST MUFFINS

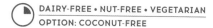 DAIRY-FREE • NUT-FREE • VEGETARIAN
OPTION: COCONUT-FREE

MAKES 12 muffins (2 per serving)

PREP TIME: 5 minutes

COOK TIME: 25 minutes

All your favorite summer flavors packed into one little muffin! Wanna get a little crazy? Serve these with salsa or sprinkle the tops with cheddar cheese (dairy-free or regular) before baking.

8 large eggs

½ cup (120 ml) full-fat coconut milk

¼ cup (20 g) finely chopped fresh cilantro leaves and stems

1 medium Hass avocado, peeled, pitted, and cubed (about 4 oz/110 g of flesh)

3 tablespoons nutritional yeast

1 jalapeño pepper, seeded and finely diced

1½ teaspoons garlic powder

1½ teaspoons onion powder

Pinch of finely ground sea salt

Pinch of ground black pepper

1. Preheat the oven to 350°F (177°C). Line a standard-size 12-well muffin pan with muffin liners, or use a silicone muffin pan, which won't require liners.

2. Place all the ingredients in a medium-sized mixing bowl and stir until combined.

3. Divide the batter evenly among the lined muffin wells, filling each about three-quarters full. Bake for 23 to 25 minutes, until a toothpick inserted into the center of a muffin comes out clean.

make it COCONUT-FREE:
Replace the coconut milk with the milk of your choice.

STORE IT: *Keep in an airtight container in the fridge for up to 5 days.*

REHEAT IT: *Place on a rimmed baking sheet and warm in a preheated 300°F (150°C) oven until heated through, about 10 minutes. Or place a single serving on a microwave-safe plate and microwave on 50% power for 1 minute. (Using 50% power ensures that the muffins won't overcook.)*

Per serving:

| calories: **160** | calories from fat: **101** | total fat: **11.2g** | saturated fat: **3.7g** | cholesterol: **248mg** |
| sodium: **135mg** | carbs: **4.4g** | dietary fiber: **1.9g** | net carbs: **2.5g** | sugars: **1.1g** | protein: **10.5g** |

FAT:	CARBS:	PROTEIN:
63%	11%	26%

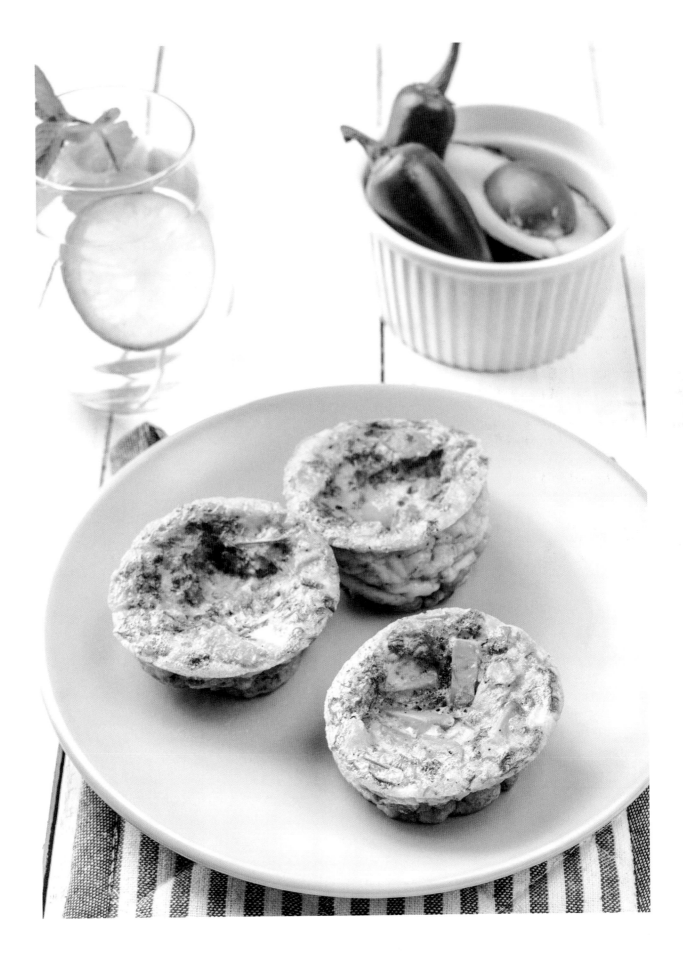

HERB CHICKEN SAUSAGES WITH BRAISED BOK CHOY

 EGG-FREE • NUT-FREE

OPTIONS: AIP • COCONUT-FREE • DAIRY-FREE • LOW-FODMAP • NIGHTSHADE-FREE

SERVES 5
PREP TIME: 5 minutes
COOK TIME: 25 minutes

There's nothing like a hot meal for breakfast, especially when it doesn't have eggs or bacon in it. Don't get me wrong, I love those things, but eggs and bacon for breakfast every day gets old. If you want to liven up this dish even more, try adding Chimichurri (page 284). The flavor combo is pretty tasty, and it'll amp up the fat content!

CHICKEN SAUSAGES:

1 pound (455 g) ground chicken

¾ teaspoon finely ground sea salt

2 tablespoons diced white onions

2 leaves fresh sage, chopped

1 tablespoon chopped fresh chives

1 tablespoon chopped fresh parsley

1 clove garlic, minced

½ teaspoon ground black pepper

½ teaspoon fresh thyme leaves

⅛ teaspoon red pepper flakes

3 tablespoons coconut oil, avocado oil, or ghee, for the pan

5 cups (350 g) chopped bok choy

1. Place all the ingredients for the sausages in a large mixing bowl and mix until fully incorporated.

2. Heat the oil in a large frying pan over medium-low heat.

3. While the oil is heating, form the chicken mixture into patties: Using a ¼-cup (60-ml) scoop, scoop up and shape the mixture with your hands to form 10 balls about 1¾ inches (4.5 cm) in diameter. Place the balls in the hot pan and press down until the patties are ¼ inch (6 mm) thick.

4. Cook the sausages for 10 minutes per side, or until golden on the outside and cooked through.

5. Transfer the cooked sausages to a serving plate. If you wish, place them in a 180°F (82°C) oven to keep warm.

6. Place the bok choy in the same pan, cover, and cook over medium heat for 5 minutes, or until fork-tender.

7. Transfer the cooked bok choy to the serving plate with the sausages and enjoy.

make it AIP:
Omit the black pepper. Do not use ghee.

make it COCONUT-FREE:
Do not use coconut oil.

make it DAIRY-FREE:
Use avocado oil.

make it LOW-FODMAP:
Omit the onions and garlic.

make it NIGHTSHADE-FREE:
Omit the red pepper flakes.

STORE IT: *Keep in an airtight container in the fridge for up to 3 days or in the freezer for up to 1 month.*

REHEAT IT: *Place in a microwave-safe dish and microwave for 2 minutes, or place in a frying pan with a drop of oil, cover, and reheat over medium heat for 5 minutes.*

THAW IT: *Set in the fridge and allow to thaw completely before using the reheating instructions above.*

Per serving, cooked in coconut oil:

| calories: **246** | calories from fat: **131** | total fat: **14.5g** | saturated fat: **6.6g** | cholesterol: **101mg** |
| sodium: **405mg** | carbs: **2.4g** | dietary fiber: **1g** | net carbs: **1.4g** | sugars: **1g** | protein: **27.6g** |

FAT:	CARBS:	PROTEIN:
52%	**4%**	**44%**

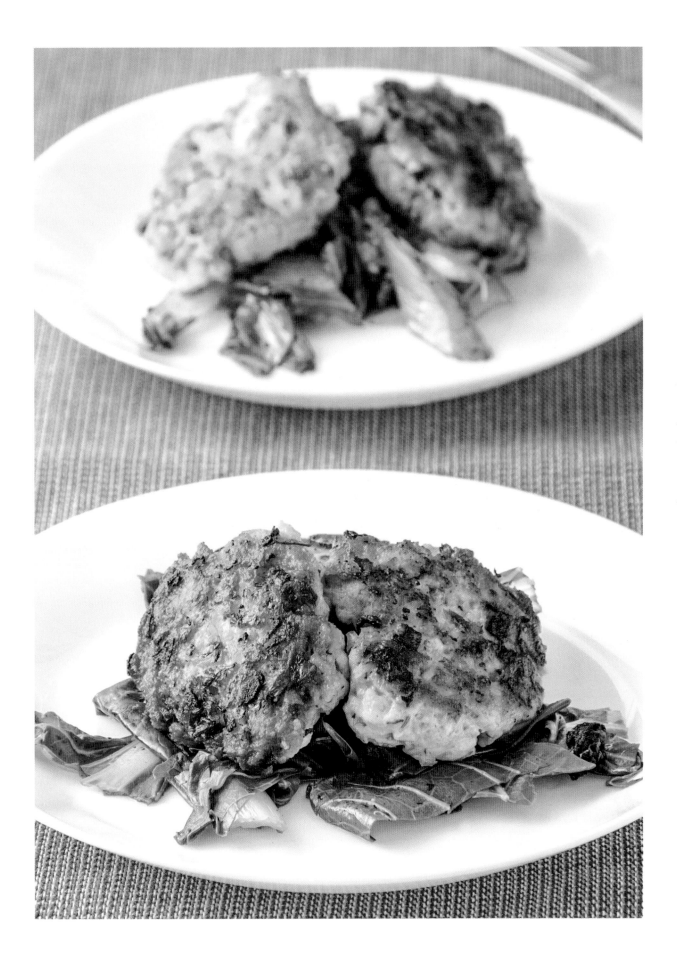

BUFFALO CHICKEN BREAKFAST MUFFINS

NUT-FREE

OPTIONS: COCONUT-FREE • DAIRY-FREE • LOW-FODMAP • NIGHTSHADE-FREE

MAKES 12 muffins (2 per serving)

PREP TIME: 5 minutes (not including time to cook chicken)

COOK TIME: 20 minutes

Muffins are the way to go when you're in a hurry, and these are some of my favorites when we have leftover chicken in the fridge that needs to be used! Rotisserie chicken is especially tasty in this recipe. If you're pressed for time and budget, canned chicken will work, too.

These muffins are awesome with Avocado Lime Dressing (page 84) or Quick 'n' Easy Barbecue Sauce (page 70) slathered on top.

1 cup (185 g) shredded cooked chicken

8 large eggs

¼ cup plus 2 tablespoons (80 g) coconut oil or ghee

4 green onions, finely chopped

1 tablespoon hot sauce

2 teaspoons garlic powder

Pinch of finely ground sea salt

Pinch of ground black pepper

1. Preheat the oven to 350°F (177°C). Line a standard-size 12-well muffin pan with muffin liners, or use a silicone muffin pan, which won't require liners.

2. Place all the ingredients in a medium-sized mixing bowl and stir until combined.

3. Divide the batter evenly among the lined muffin wells, filling each about three-quarters full. Bake for 18 to 20 minutes, until a toothpick inserted into the center of a muffin comes out clean.

STORE IT: *Keep in an airtight container in the fridge for up to 5 days.*

REHEAT IT: *Place on a rimmed baking sheet and warm in a preheated 300°F (150°C) oven until heated through, about 10 minutes. Or place a single serving on a microwave-safe plate and microwave on 50% power for 1 minute. (Using 50% power ensures that the muffins won't overcook.)*

make it COCONUT-FREE:
Use ghee.

make it DAIRY-FREE:
Use coconut oil.

make it LOW-FODMAP:
Use only the green parts of the green onions. Omit the garlic powder and replace 1 tablespoon of the coconut oil with garlic-infused oil.

make it NIGHTSHADE-FREE:
Replace the hot sauce with 2 teaspoons dried parsley leaves.

Per serving, made with coconut oil:

						FAT:	CARBS:	PROTEIN:
calories: **269**	calories from fat: **191**	total fat: **21.2g**	saturated fat: **14.1g**	cholesterol: **272mg**		**71%**	**3%**	**26%**
sodium: **155mg**	carbs: **1.9g**	dietary fiber: **0.4g**	net carbs: **1.5g**	sugars: **1g**	protein: **17.8g**			

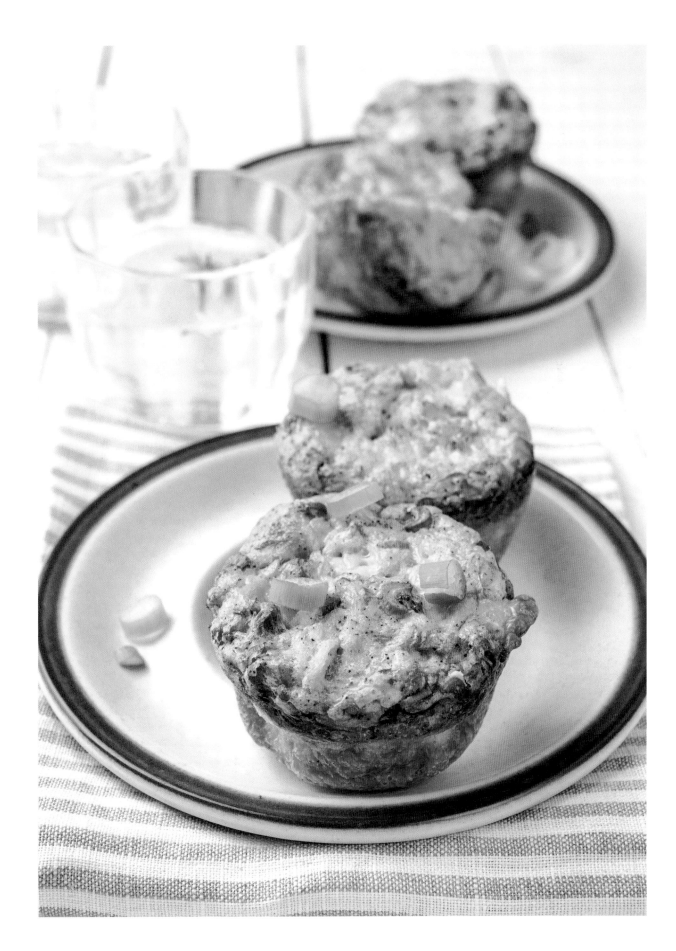

PROSCIUTTO BISCUITS

DAIRY-FREE • LOW-FODMAP • NIGHTSHADE-FREE • NUT-FREE

MAKES 12 biscuits (2 per serving)

PREP TIME: 10 minutes

COOK TIME: 20 minutes

It may seem a little weird to add mayonnaise to biscuit dough, but the end result will have you wanting to make more biscuits, with even more mayonnaise! Regardless of which mayonnaise you use, you'll be pleasantly surprised by these little breakfast treasures.

If you can eat dairy and want to incorporate it into this recipe, try folding ½ cup (57 g) of shredded cheddar cheese into the batter before dividing and baking. Don't get me wrong, though, these biscuits are 100% delicious without a spot of dairy!

¾ cup (155 g) mayonnaise

6 large eggs

1 cup (100 g) coconut flour

1½ teaspoons baking powder

12 slices prosciutto (about 3½ oz/ 100 g), finely chopped

3 green onions (green parts only), finely chopped

1. Preheat the oven to 375°F (190°C). Line a baking sheet with parchment paper or a silicone baking mat.

2. Place the mayonnaise and eggs in a small mixing bowl and whisk to combine.

3. Place the coconut flour and baking powder in a medium-sized mixing bowl and mix to combine. Add the mayonnaise mixture to the dry ingredients and stir to fully incorporate. Fold in the chopped prosciutto and green onions.

4. Divide the dough evenly into 12 pieces. Roll one piece into a ball between your palms, then place it on the lined baking sheet and press down with your palm until it's 1 inch (2.5 cm) thick. Repeat with the remaining dough pieces.

5. Bake for 15 to 20 minutes, or until the edges of the biscuits begin to turn golden and the tops crack a bit.

6. Remove from the oven and serve.

MAKE IT AT HOME

Replace store-bought mayonnaise with my homemade version.

Mayonnaise

STORE IT: *Keep in an airtight container in the fridge for up to 3 days or in the freezer for up to 1 month.*

REHEAT IT: *Place on a rimmed baking sheet and warm in a preheated 300°F (150°C) oven until heated through, about 10 minutes. Or place a single serving on a microwave-safe plate and microwave on 50% power for 30 to 45 seconds. (Using 50% power ensures that the biscuits won't overcook.)*

THAW IT: *Set the biscuits on the counter for an hour or so to defrost completely before using the reheating instructions above.*

Per serving, made with homemade mayonnaise:

calories: **299**	calories from fat: **247**	total fat: **27.4g**	saturated fat: **5.8g**	cholesterol: **208mg**	
sodium: **567mg**	carbs: **2.9g**	dietary fiber: **1.1g**	net carbs: **1.8g**	sugars: **0.7g**	protein: **10.9g**

FAT:	CARBS:	PROTEIN:
82%	**4%**	**14%**

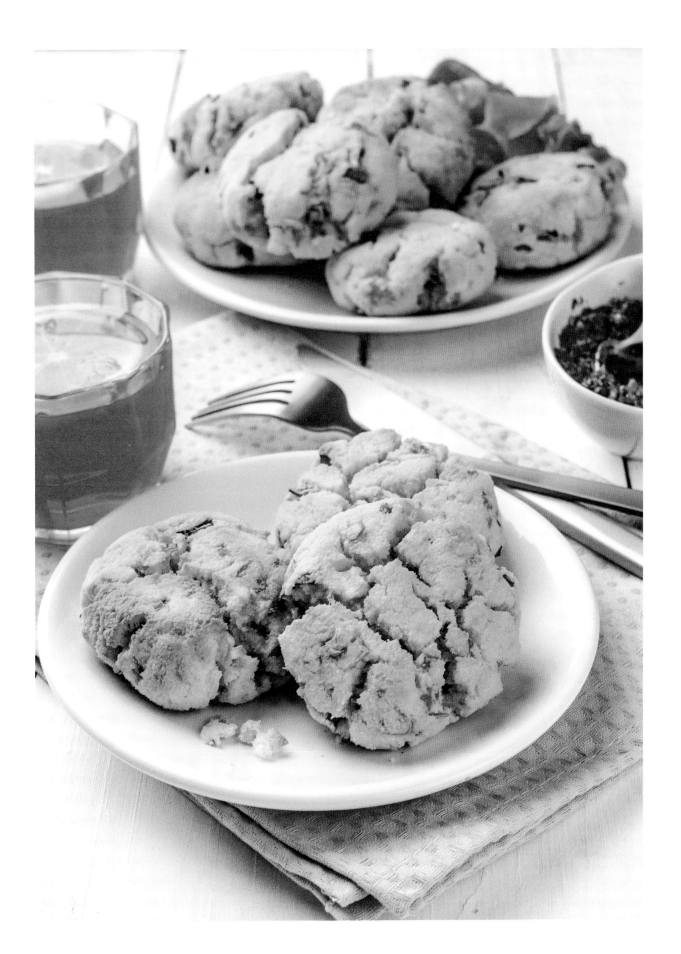

SALMON BACON ROLLS WITH DIPPING SAUCE

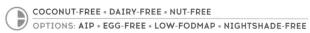

COCONUT-FREE • DAIRY-FREE • NUT-FREE

OPTIONS: AIP • EGG-FREE • LOW-FODMAP • NIGHTSHADE-FREE

MAKES 16 rolls (4 per serving)

PREP TIME: 10 minutes

COOK TIME: 10 minutes

These rolls are one of my favorite things to eat when I'm in a rush, starving, and don't want to have a second fatty coffee of the day. Because I always have a bottle of sugar-free barbecue sauce in the pantry (or, better yet, a batch of my homemade barbecue sauce in the freezer), cooked bacon in the fridge, and smoked salmon kicking about, I'm guaranteed to eat this meal at least twice a week. No flavor of smoked salmon is off-limits for this quick dish. Once I made it using salmon that'd been brined in vanilla and then smoked. What a flavor! It's my favorite so far.

If you don't want to use the dipping sauce in this recipe, try serving the rolls with Creamy Italian Dressing (page 94) or Green Speckled Dressing (page 80).

8 strips bacon (about 8 oz/225 g)

8 ounces (225 g) smoked salmon, cut into 16 squares

DIPPING SAUCE:

½ cup (105 g) mayonnaise

2 tablespoons sugar-free barbecue sauce

SPECIAL EQUIPMENT:

Toothpicks

1. Cook the bacon in a large frying pan over medium heat until much of the fat is rendered and the bacon is lightly browned but not crispy, 8 to 10 minutes. (You want the bacon to remain pliable so that you can bend it.)

2. Cut the cooked bacon in half lengthwise to create 16 narrow strips. Place a square of salmon on one end of a bacon strip. Roll the salmon in the bacon, secure with a toothpick, and place on a clean plate. Repeat with the remaining bacon and salmon, making a total of 16 rolls.

3. Make the dipping sauce: Place the mayonnaise and barbecue sauce in a small bowl and stir to combine. Serve alongside the salmon rolls.

STORE IT: *Keep the rolls and dipping sauce in separate airtight containers in the fridge for up to 3 days.*

make it AIP/LOW-FODMAP/NIGHTSHADE-FREE:
Omit the dipping sauce.

make it EGG-FREE:
Use egg-free mayonnaise (see recipe on page 102).

MAKE IT AT HOME
Replace store-bought mayonnaise and/or barbecue sauce with my homemade version(s).

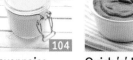

Mayonnaise   **Quick 'n' Easy Barbecue Sauce**

Per serving, made with homemade mayonnaise and Quick 'n' Easy Barbecue Sauce:

calories: **324**	calories from fat: **257**	total fat: **28.5g**	saturated fat: **6.5g**	cholesterol: **33mg**
sodium: **1492mg**	carbs: **3.2g**	dietary fiber: **0.6g**	net carbs: **2.6g**	sugars: **1.7g**	protein: **13.9g**

FAT:	CARBS:	PROTEIN:
79%	**4%**	**17%**

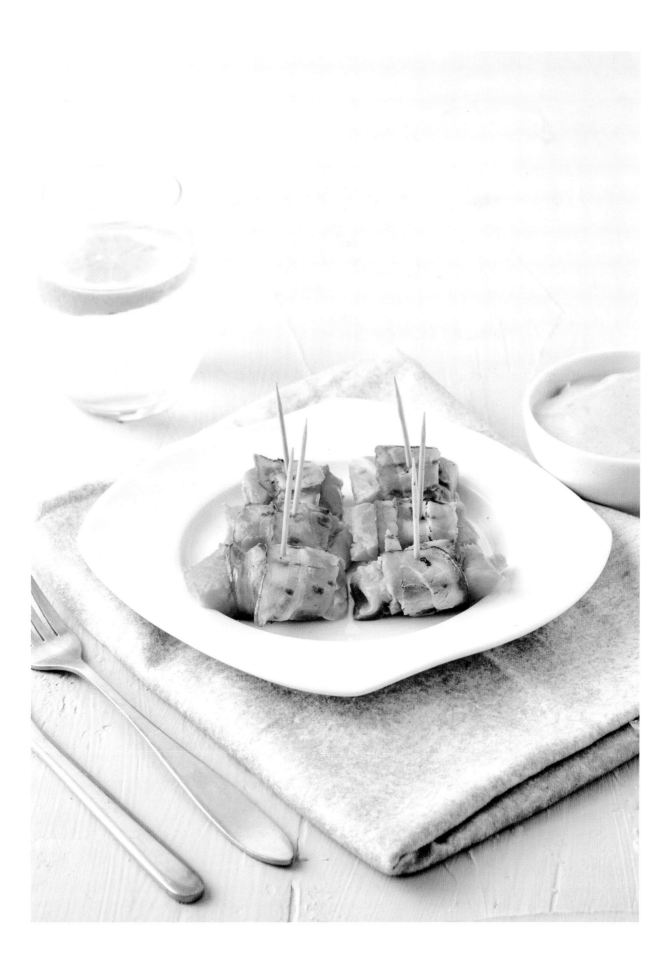

HEY GIRL

EGG-FREE • NIGHTSHADE-FREE • NUT-FREE

OPTIONS: **AIP • DAIRY-FREE • LOW-FODMAP • VEGAN • VEGETARIAN**

MAKES one 12-ounce (350-ml) serving

PREP TIME: 1 minute (not including time to brew coffee)

COOK TIME: –

I make this drink when I need a strong pep in my step come morning time. If you like the idea of exogenous ketones and are interested in learning how to incorporate them into your daily routine (aside from just adding them to a glass of water), this recipe is a perfect template. If you're looking for a good exogenous ketone brand, Perfect Keto is one that I trust. Exogenous ketones have a slightly sour taste, which is why this recipe has a touch of sweetener and vanilla extract to offset the flavor.

What is cordyceps? It's a type of fungus that can aid in the reduction of inflammation and leaky gut symptoms, improve athletic performance, and assist with detoxification. If you've always been curious about how to incorporate it into your keto diet, drinks like this and fat bombs are great ways. If you have no interest, simply omit the cordyceps. The flavor is really mild, so leaving it out it won't affect the end result.

1¼ cups (300 ml) brewed coffee (decaf or regular), hot

2 tablespoons full-fat coconut milk

2 tablespoons coconut oil, unflavored MCT oil powder, or ghee

2 tablespoons collagen peptides or protein powder

1 teaspoon erythritol, or 2 drops liquid stevia

½ teaspoon exogenous ketones

¼ teaspoon vanilla extract

0.1 ounce (3 g) cordyceps (optional)

1. Place all the ingredients in a blender or food processor and blend for 20 to 30 seconds, until incorporated. Alternatively, place all the ingredients in a stainless-steel bottle or Thermos, seal, and shake for 10 seconds.

2. Transfer to a 12-ounce (350-ml) or larger coffee mug. Best enjoyed immediately.

---

make it **AIP/LOW-FODMAP:**
Do not use ghee. Opt for stevia.

make it **DAIRY-FREE:**
Do not use ghee.

make it **VEGAN:**
Do not use ghee or collagen. Opt for a plant-based protein powder.

make it **VEGETARIAN:**
Do not use collagen. Opt for a plant- or egg-based protein powder.

STORE IT: If there are leftovers or you need to make the drink ahead of time, store it in an airtight container in the fridge for up to 3 days. When ready to enjoy, give it a little shake and drink it cold or follow the reheating instructions below.

REHEAT IT: Transfer to a 12-ounce (350-ml) or larger microwave-safe mug and microwave for 1½ minutes, or place in a saucepan, cover, and reheat over low heat for 5 minutes.

Per serving, made with coconut oil and collagen, without cordyceps:

| calories: **334** | calories from fat: **259** | total fat: **28.8g** | saturated fat: **24.9g** | cholesterol: **0mg** | | FAT: | CARBS: | PROTEIN: |
| sodium: **224mg** | carbs: **0.4g** | dietary fiber: **0g** | net carbs: **0.4g** | sugars: **0.3g** | protein: **18.5g** | **78%** | **0%** | **22%** |

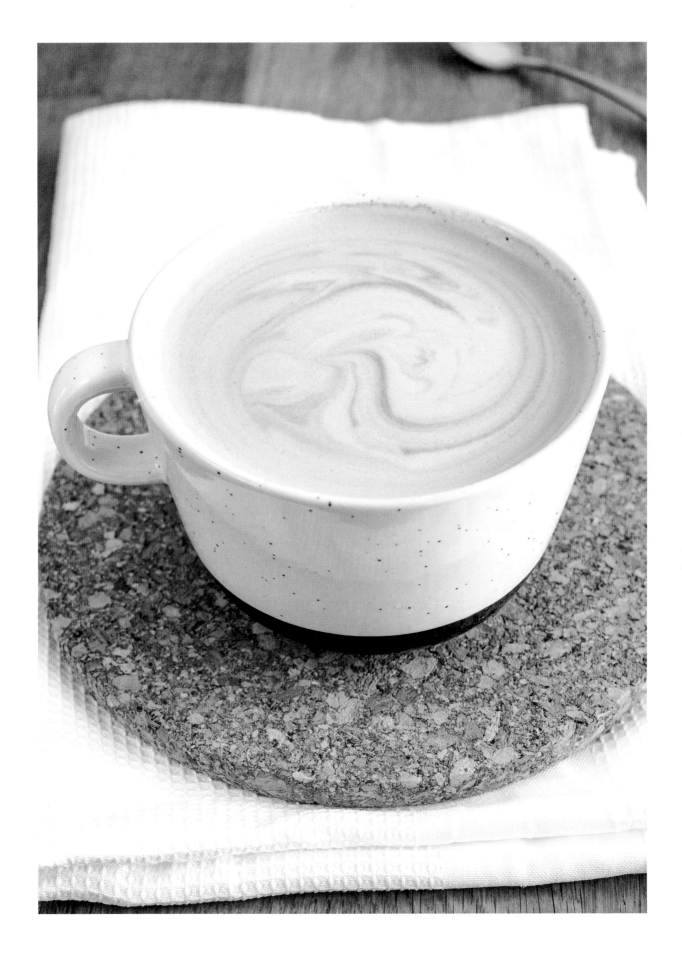

PUMPKIN SPICE LATTE OVERNIGHT "OATS"

EGG-FREE • LOW-FODMAP • NIGHTSHADE-FREE • VEGETARIAN
OPTIONS: COCONUT-FREE • DAIRY-FREE • NUT-FREE • VEGAN

SERVES 2

PREP TIME: 5 minutes, plus 8 hours to soak (not including time to brew coffee)

COOK TIME: –

Missing your oat-filled bowls of overnight oats? If so, you're going to love this keto-friendly, low-carb, Paleo version! Made perfect with hulled hemp seeds (aka hemp hearts), these grain-free breakfast bowls are a total win in my book. Just soak the ingredients overnight, as you would with oats, and enjoy in the morning, adding an extra splash of milk before consuming. If you have pumpkin pie spice kicking around, feel free to replace the individual spices with ¾ teaspoon pumpkin pie spice.

½ cup (75 g) hulled hemp seeds

⅓ cup (80 ml) milk (nondairy or regular), plus more for serving

⅓ cup (80 ml) brewed coffee (decaf or regular)

2 tablespoons canned pumpkin puree

1 tablespoon chia seeds

2 teaspoons erythritol, or 3 drops liquid stevia

½ teaspoon vanilla extract

½ teaspoon ground cinnamon

¼ teaspoon ground nutmeg

⅛ teaspoon ground cloves

Pinch of finely ground sea salt

TOPPINGS (optional):

Chopped raw or roasted pecans

Ground cinnamon

Additional hulled hemp seeds

Toasted unsweetened shredded coconut

make it COCONUT-FREE:
Do not use coconut milk or top with shredded coconut.

make it DAIRY-FREE/VEGAN:
Use a nondairy milk.

make it NUT-FREE:
Use coconut milk or a seed-based nondairy milk. Do not top with pecans.

1. Place all the ingredients in a 12-ounce (350-ml) or larger container with a lid and stir until combined. Cover and set in the fridge to soak overnight, or for at least 8 hours.

2. The following day, add more milk until the desired consistency is reached. Divide between 2 small bowls, top as desired, and enjoy.

STORE IT: *Keep in an airtight container in the fridge for up to 3 days.*

Per serving, made with full-fat coconut milk, without toppings:

calories: **337** | calories from fat: **240** | total fat: **26.7g** | saturated fat: **9.6g** | cholesterol: **0mg**
sodium: **89mg** | carbs: **9.4g** | dietary fiber: **6.8g** | net carbs: **2.6g** | sugars: **1.4g** | protein: **15g**

FAT:	CARBS:	PROTEIN:
71%	**11%**	**18%**

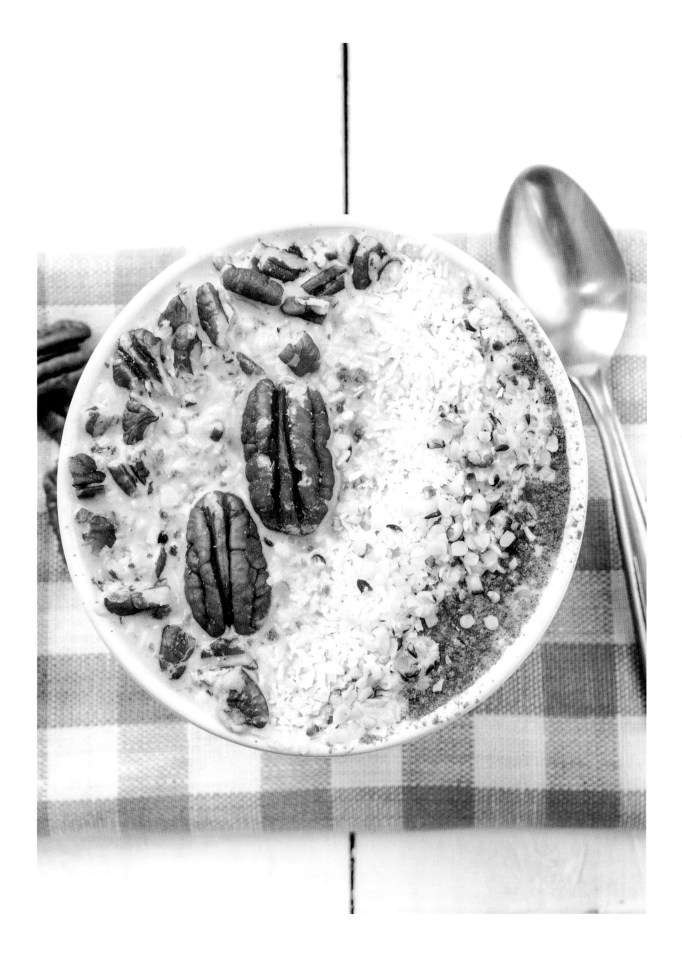

ROCKET FUEL HOT CHOCOLATE

EGG-FREE · LOW-FODMAP · NIGHTSHADE-FREE · NUT-FREE

OPTIONS: AIP · DAIRY-FREE · VEGAN · VEGETARIAN

MAKES two 10-ounce (300-ml) servings

PREP TIME: 5 minutes

COOK TIME: –

This drink is so rich and perfect that a full batch is best shared with a friend. Or save half for the next day!

2 cups (475 ml) milk (nondairy or regular), hot

2 tablespoons cocoa powder

2 tablespoons collagen peptides or protein powder

2 tablespoons coconut oil, MCT oil, unflavored MCT oil powder, or ghee

1 tablespoon coconut butter

1 tablespoon erythritol, or 4 drops liquid stevia

Pinch of ground cinnamon (optional)

1. Place all the ingredients in a blender and blend for 10 seconds, or until the ingredients are fully incorporated.

2. Divide between 2 mugs, sprinkle with cinnamon if you'd like, and enjoy!

STORE IT: *Keep in an airtight container in the fridge for up to 3 days.*

REHEAT IT: *Transfer to a 12-ounce (350-ml) or larger microwave-safe mug and microwave for 1½ minutes, or place in a saucepan, cover, and reheat over low heat for 5 minutes.*

make it AIP:
Replace the cocoa powder with carob powder. Do not use ghee. Opt for stevia.

make it DAIRY-FREE:
Use a nondairy milk. Do not use ghee.

make it VEGAN:
Use a nondairy milk. Do not use collagen or ghee. Opt for a plant-based protein powder.

make it VEGETARIAN:
Do not use collagen. Opt for a plant- or egg-based protein powder.

Per serving, made with lite coconut milk, collagen, and coconut oil:

				FAT:	CARBS:	PROTEIN:
calories: **357**	calories from fat: **222**	total fat: **29.3g**	saturated fat: **25.8g**	cholesterol: **0mg**	**74%**	**12%**	**14%**
sodium: **144mg**	carbs: **11g**	dietary fiber: **4.1g**	net carbs: **6.9g**	sugars: **1.1g**	protein: **12.5g**		

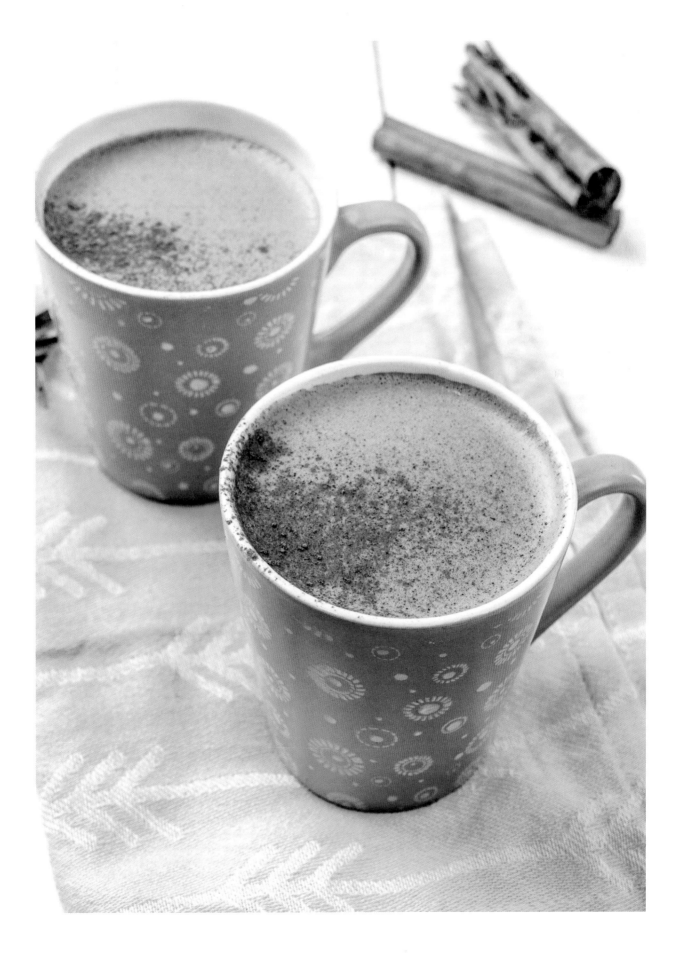

FULL MEAL DEAL

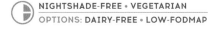 NIGHTSHADE-FREE • VEGETARIAN
OPTIONS: DAIRY-FREE • LOW-FODMAP

SERVES 4

PREP TIME: 10 minutes
(not including time
to make biscuits or
chimichurri)

COOK TIME: 3 minutes

It's not a bad idea to make a bunch of mug biscuits, cut them in half, and store them in the freezer for this recipe precisely!

If you're making this meal for your lunch kit, keep the mashed avocado from browning by sprinkling it with lemon juice and tightly covering it with plastic wrap. Storing the avocado with the pit helps, too.

2 Mug Biscuits (page 134)

1 large Hass avocado, peeled, pitted, and mashed (about 6 oz/170 g of flesh)

1 tablespoon avocado oil

2 cups (140 g) fresh spinach

½ cup (105 g) Chimichurri (page 284)

1. Cut the biscuits in half and set each half on a separate plate. Top each half with an equal portion of the mashed avocado.

2. Place the oil in a medium-sized frying pan over medium heat. Add the spinach and sauté until lightly wilted, about 3 minutes.

3. Place the wilted spinach on top of the avocado, then drizzle each serving with 2 tablespoons of chimichurri. Enjoy immediately.

make it DAIRY-FREE:
Use the dairy-free modifications for the Mug Biscuits on page 134.

make it LOW-FODMAP:
Use the low-FODMAP modifications for the Chimichurri on page 284.

Per serving:

calories: **358** | calories from fat: **299** | total fat: **33.8g** | saturated fat: **9.7g** | cholesterol: **82mg**
sodium: **348mg** | carbs: **6.5g** | dietary fiber: **3.3g** | net carbs: **3.2g** | sugars: **1.1g** | protein: **7.1g**

FAT:	CARBS:	PROTEIN:
85%	7%	8%

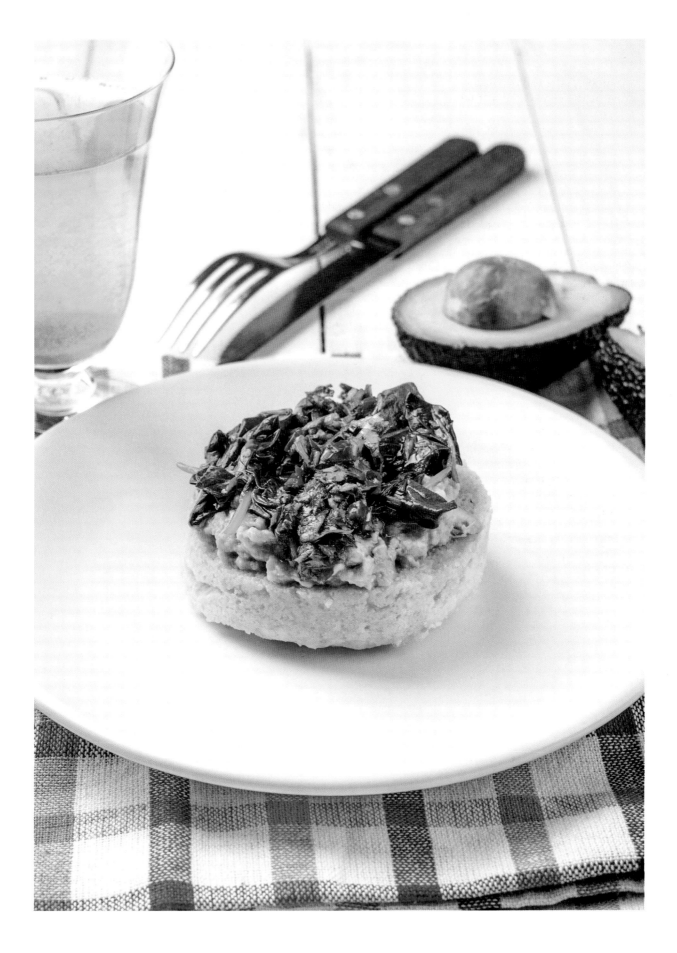

LIVER SAUSAGES & ONIONS

COCONUT-FREE • EGG-FREE • NIGHTSHADE-FREE • NUT-FREE

OPTIONS: AIP • DAIRY-FREE

SERVES 6

PREP TIME: 10 minutes, plus 24 hours to soak livers

COOK TIME: 26 minutes

Cooking these sausages creates an amazing caramelized coating on the pan that's perfect for cooking some onions. Don't love onions? Replace them with chard, kale, asparagus, bell peppers, or whatever you have.

This recipe will taste heaps and bounds better if you soak the livers in water for 24 to 48 hours before cooking them. When livers are soaked, their taste becomes far less punchy. The result: You will find yourself enjoying, and eating more, liver since that metallic taste that turns people off from eating liver in the first place disappears.

Hate pan-frying things? You can make this recipe in a preheated 350°F (177°C) oven. Make the patties as described below and place them on a rimmed baking sheet. Toss the onions in the oil and distribute them around the sausage patties. Bake for 25 to 30 minutes, until the patties are golden brown.

SAUSAGES:

8 ounces (225 g) chicken livers

1 tablespoon apple cider vinegar

1 pound (455 g) ground beef

1 pound (455 g) ground pork

2½ teaspoons dried rubbed sage

1¼ teaspoons dried rosemary leaves

1 teaspoon dried thyme leaves

1 teaspoon finely ground sea salt

¾ teaspoon ground black pepper

4 cloves garlic, minced

¼ cup (60 ml) avocado oil, or ¼ cup (55 g) coconut oil or ghee, for the pan

2 medium-sized white onions, thinly sliced

make it AIP:
Omit the black pepper. Do not use ghee.

make it DAIRY-FREE:
Do not use ghee.

1. Place the chicken livers in a medium-sized bowl and cover with water. Add the vinegar. Cover and place in the fridge to soak for 24 to 48 hours.

2. Rinse and drain the livers, then place them in a blender or food processor. Blend until smooth.

3. Transfer the pureed livers to a large mixing bowl and add the remaining ingredients for the sausages. Mix thoroughly with your hands to combine.

4. Heat the oil in a large frying pan over medium-low heat.

5. While the oil is heating, form the liver mixture into patties: Using a ¼-cup (60-ml) scoop, scoop up portions of the mixture and roll between your hands to form into 12 balls about 1¾ inches (4.5 cm) in diameter. Place the balls in the hot pan and press down until they're ½ inch (1.25 cm) thick. Do not overcrowd the pan; you may have to cook the sausages in two batches if they don't all fit comfortably.

6. Cook the sausages for 8 minutes per side, or until no longer pink in the center.

7. Place the cooked sausages on a serving plate. Set in a 180°F (82°C) oven to keep warm, if you wish.

8. Once the sausages are done, place the sliced onions in the same pan and cook for 10 minutes, or until translucent, stirring every minute or so.

9. Transfer the cooked onions to the serving plate with the sausages and enjoy.

Per serving, cooked in avocado oil:

| calories: **392** | calories from fat: **197** | total fat: **21.9g** | saturated fat: **8g** | cholesterol: **320mg** | | FAT: | CARBS: | PROTEIN: |
| sodium: **437mg** | carbs: **5.6g** | dietary fiber: **1.6g** | net carbs: **4g** | sugars: **1.6g** | protein: **43.2g** | **50%** | **6%** | **43.2%** |

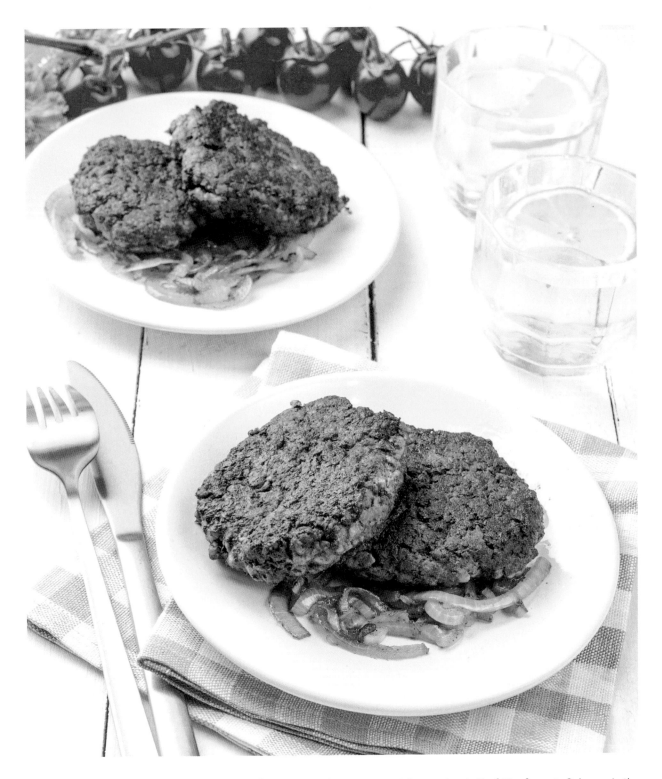

STORE IT: *Keep in an airtight container in the fridge for up to 3 days or in the freezer for up to 1 month.*

REHEAT IT: *Transfer a single serving to a microwave-safe dish, cover, and microwave for 2 minutes, or place in a frying pan with a drop of oil, cover, and reheat over medium heat for 5 minutes.*

THAW IT: *Set in the fridge and allow to thaw completely before using the reheating instructions above.*

CROSS-COUNTRY SCRAMBLER

 COCONUT-FREE • DAIRY-FREE • LOW-FODMAP • NUT-FREE

SERVES 2

PREP TIME: 5 minutes

COOK TIME: 28 minutes

We ate this scrambled egg dish a lot when we lived in the RV exploring the country. It's easy, delicious, and, if you can eat cheese, great with cheese. Or so I'm told. If you have a batch of Avocado Lime Dressing (page 84) or Basil Vinaigrette & Marinade (page 88) on hand, drizzle some over the top!

8 strips bacon (about 8 oz/225 g)

1 packed cup spiral-sliced butternut squash (about 5¼ oz/150 g)

½ green bell pepper, diced

6 large eggs, beaten

½ cup (40 g) sliced green onions (green parts only)

¼ teaspoon ground black pepper

1. Cook the bacon in a large frying pan over medium heat until crispy, about 15 minutes. Remove the bacon from the pan, leaving the grease in the pan. When the bacon has cooled, crumble it.

2. Add the squash and bell pepper to the pan with the bacon grease. Cover and cook over medium-low heat for 8 minutes, or until the vegetables are fork-tender.

3. Add the beaten eggs, green onions, and black pepper. Mix with a large spoon until fully incorporated.

4. Cook, uncovered, for 5 minutes, stirring every minute, or until the eggs are cooked to your liking. Once complete, fold in half of the crumbled bacon.

5. Divide evenly between 2 plates, top with remaining crumbled bacon, and dig in!

> **STORE IT:** *Keep in an airtight container in the fridge for up to 3 days.*
>
> **REHEAT IT:** *Transfer a single serving to a microwave-safe dish, cover, and microwave for 2 minutes, or place in a frying pan with a drop of oil, cover, and reheat over medium heat for 5 minutes.*

Per serving:

calories: **395** | calories from fat: **243** | total fat: **27g** | saturated fat: **8.6g** | cholesterol: **578mg** | sodium: **474mg** | carbs: **11.7g** | dietary fiber: **2.5g** | net carbs: **9.2g** | sugars: **1.8g** | protein: **26.3g**

FAT:	CARBS:	PROTEIN:
62%	12%	26%

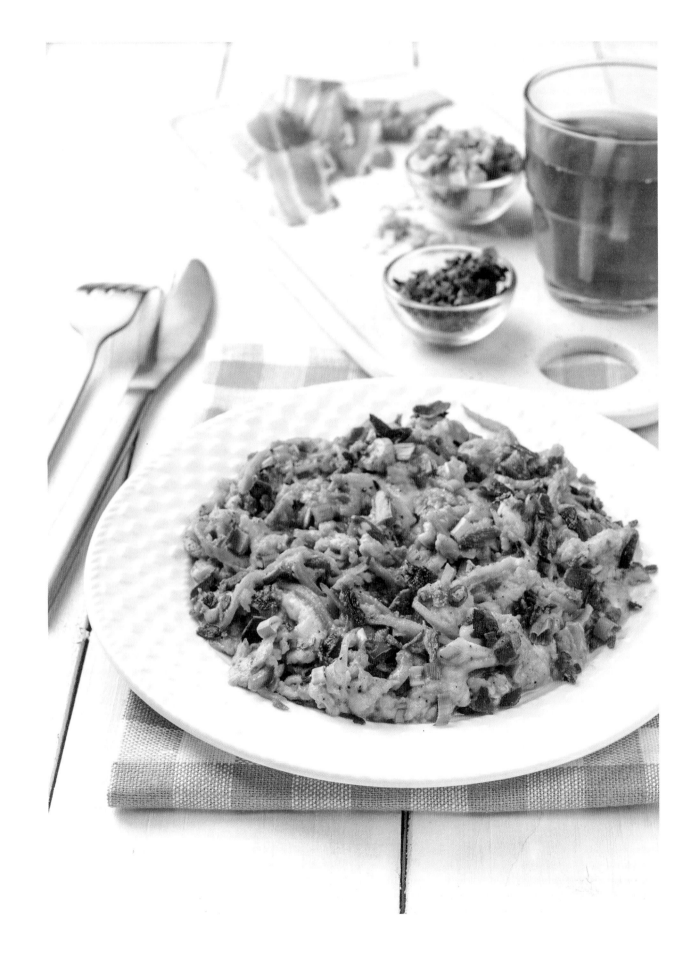

EGGS BENEDICT

LOW-FODMAP • NIGHTSHADE-FREE

OPTIONS: **COCONUT-FREE • DAIRY-FREE • NUT-FREE**

SERVES 4

PREP TIME: 10 minutes
(not including time
to make biscuits or
hollandaise)

COOK TIME: 16 minutes

If you have friends and family around and want to impress them with how awesome keto is, this is your recipe! Or you could make a batch for yourself and revel in how good all the layers are. Don't have time to make biscuits or poach eggs? Cut corners by following the nut-free recommendations and fry the eggs over-easy instead of poaching them.

The timing for this recipe is based on having the hollandaise sauce already made. Thankfully, and just like the name implies, my hollandaise recipe is ready in seconds. So, if you don't want to make it ahead and store it in the fridge for safekeeping, we're not talking about a bunch of added time here; just add 2 minutes to the total prep time for this recipe. When we have guests, I make the sauce fresh because it saves me from having to remember to take it out of the fridge ahead of time to bring it to room temperature and then rewhip it when they arrive.

2 Mug Biscuits (page 134)

2 teaspoons apple cider vinegar

4 large eggs

4 slices Canadian bacon

½ cup (120 ml) Ready-in-Seconds Hollandaise Sauce (page 100)

2 tablespoons finely chopped fresh parsley, for garnish

make it COCONUT-FREE/ NUT-FREE:
Replace the biscuits with 2 large avocados (peeled, pitted, and cut in half crosswise) and put the toppings on the cut sides of the avocados.

make it DAIRY-FREE:
Follow the dairy-free instructions for the Mug Biscuits on page 134.

1. Cut the biscuits in half and set each half on a separate plate.

2. Fill a large saucepan two-thirds full with water and bring to a light simmer over medium-low heat. Once simmering, add the vinegar.

3. Crack each egg into a separate small bowl, then gently slide an egg into the lightly simmering water. Once the egg begins to turn white, add another egg, and so on until all the eggs are in the saucepan. Cook for 2 minutes, then turn off the heat and allow the eggs to sit in the hot water bath for 8 minutes before removing with a slotted spoon.

4. Meanwhile, place the Canadian bacon in a large frying pan and fry over medium heat for 3 minutes per side, or until lightly golden.

5. Top each biscuit half with a slice of the pan-fried Canadian bacon and a poached egg, finishing each with 2 tablespoons of hollandaise sauce.

6. Sprinkle with the parsley and enjoy immediately.

Per serving:

calories: **399** | calories from fat: **343** | total fat: **38.2g** | saturated fat: **24.9g** | cholesterol: **172mg**
sodium: **404mg** | carbs: **5.7g** | dietary fiber: **2.8g** | net carbs: **2.9g** | sugars: **1g** | protein: **8.1g**

FAT:	CARBS:	PROTEIN:
86%	6%	8%

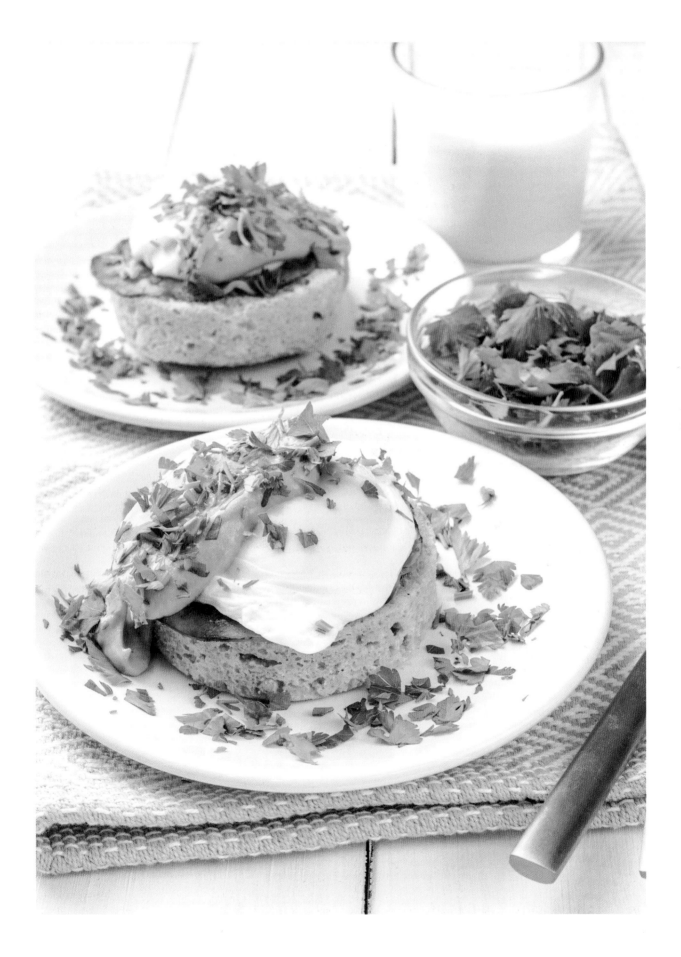

MUG BISCUIT

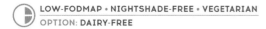

LOW-FODMAP • NIGHTSHADE-FREE • VEGETARIAN
OPTION: DAIRY-FREE

SERVES 1

PREP TIME: 1 minute

COOK TIME: 2 minutes

In five minutes, you can have a freshly made biscuit in your belly using this incredibly easy and versatile recipe! I've become obsessed with making myself one of these biscuits, slathering it with mayonnaise, and then stuffing it with sandwich goodies like avocado, bacon, ham, and tomato. You can use any size mug you want for this recipe; I like a wide-based mug so I get a wider biscuit. Also, since every microwave is a little different, it's best to err on the side of caution and cook the biscuit for the minimum amount of time, check it for doneness, and then cook it longer if needed. After you've made this recipe once or twice, you'll know exactly how long it takes to cook a biscuit to perfection in your microwave.

¼ cup (28 g) blanched almond flour

1 tablespoon coconut flour

½ teaspoon baking powder

¼ teaspoon finely ground sea salt

1 large egg

1 tablespoon softened coconut oil or ghee, plus more for serving if desired

1 teaspoon apple cider vinegar

1. Place all the ingredients in a microwave-safe mug with a base at least 2 inches (5 cm) in diameter. Mix until fully incorporated, then flatten with the back of a spoon.

2. Place the mug in the microwave and cook on high for 1 minute 30 seconds.

3. Remove the mug from the microwave and insert a toothpick. It should come out clean. If batter is clinging to the toothpick, microwave the biscuit for an additional 15 to 30 seconds.

4. Flip the mug over a clean plate and shake it a bit until the biscuit releases from the mug. If desired, slather the biscuit with the fat of your choice while still warm.

make it **DAIRY-FREE:**
Do not use ghee.

STORE IT: *Keep in an airtight container in the fridge for up to 3 days or in the freezer for up to 2 months.*

REHEAT IT: *Best toasted in a toaster oven, but also can be microwaved for 15 seconds.*

THAW IT: *Set in the fridge and allow to thaw completely before using the reheating instructions above.*

PREP AHEAD: *Mix batches of the dry ingredients and store in tightly sealed baggies in the pantry until ready to use.*

Per biscuit, made with coconut oil:

calories: **399**	calories from fat: **302**	total fat: **33.5g**	saturated fat: **14.6g**	cholesterol: **164mg**
sodium: **535mg**	carbs: **10.6g**	dietary fiber: **5.5g**	net carbs: **5.1g**	sugars: **1.9g**	protein: **13.8g**

FAT:	CARBS:	PROTEIN:
76%	**10%**	**14%**

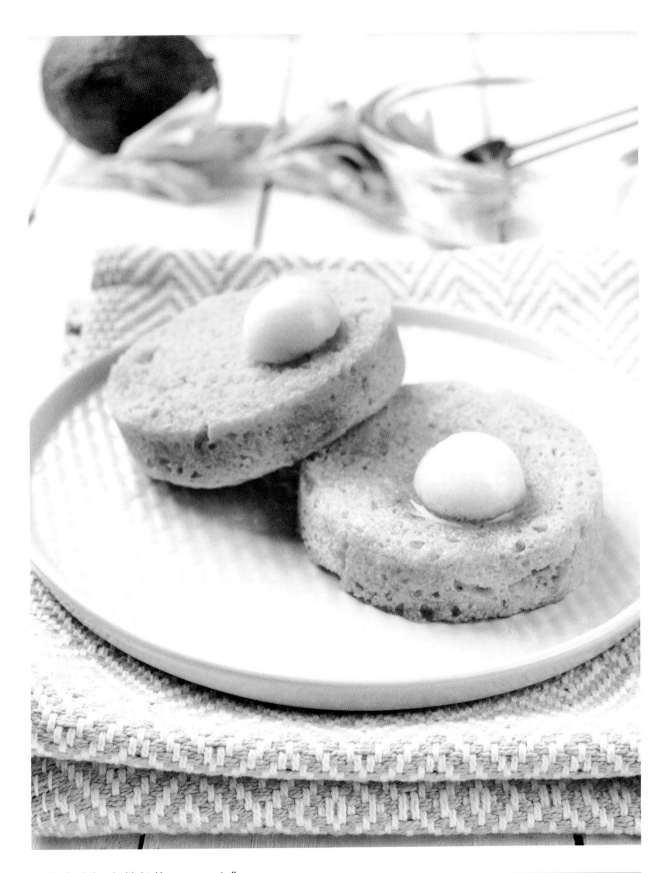

Per biscuit, slathered with 1 tablespoon coconut oil:

calories: **496** | calories from fat: **428** | total fat: **47.5g** | saturated fat: **26.6g** | cholesterol: **164mg**
sodium: **535mg** | carbs: **10.6g** | dietary fiber: **5.5g** | net carbs: **5.1g** | sugars: **1.9g** | protein: **13.8g**

FAT:	CARBS:	PROTEIN:
81%	8%	11%

KETO BREAKFAST PUDDING

DAIRY-FREE • EGG-FREE • NIGHTSHADE-FREE • NUT-FREE
OPTIONS: LOW-FODMAP • VEGAN • VEGETARIAN

SERVES 3

PREP TIME: 5 minutes

COOK TIME: –

Before you go thinking that this pudding couldn't possibly be keto with "all that sugar" from the raspberries, take a gander at the nutrition information below and think again. Just because a food "isn't keto" on its own doesn't mean that it can't hold a place in your ketogenic diet. Here, I've used a spot of raspberries for flavor and sweetness and doubled up on fats to compensate. This is the best trick for enjoying some of your favorite whole foods without worrying too much about the carbs.

If you want to make this pudding a bit more decadent, try it with a drizzle of Chocolate Sauce (page 96).

1½ cups (350 ml) full-fat coconut milk

1 cup (110 g) frozen raspberries

¼ cup (60 ml) MCT oil or melted coconut oil, or ¼ cup (40 g) unflavored MCT oil powder

¼ cup (40 g) collagen peptides or protein powder

2 tablespoons chia seeds

1 tablespoon apple cider vinegar

1 teaspoon vanilla extract

1 tablespoon erythritol, or 4 drops liquid stevia

TOPPINGS (optional):

Unsweetened shredded coconut

Hulled hemp seeds

Fresh berries of choice

Place all the pudding ingredients in a blender or food processor and blend until smooth. Serve in bowls with your favorite toppings, if desired.

STORE IT: *Keep in an airtight container in the fridge for up to 3 days.*

make it LOW-FODMAP:
Replace the coconut milk with almond, macadamia nut, or hemp milk.

make it VEGAN:
Do not use collagen. Opt for a plant-based protein powder.

make it VEGETARIAN:
Do not use collagen. Opt for a plant- or egg-based protein powder.

Per serving, made with MCT oil and collagen, without toppings:

| calories: **403** | calories from fat: **308** | total fat: **34.2g** | saturated fat: **30.8g** | cholesterol: **0mg** |
| sodium: **99mg** | carbs: **8.8g** | dietary fiber: **3.1g** | net carbs: **5.7g** | sugars: **3.4g** | protein: **15.2g** |

FAT:	CARBS:	PROTEIN:
76%	**9%**	**15%**

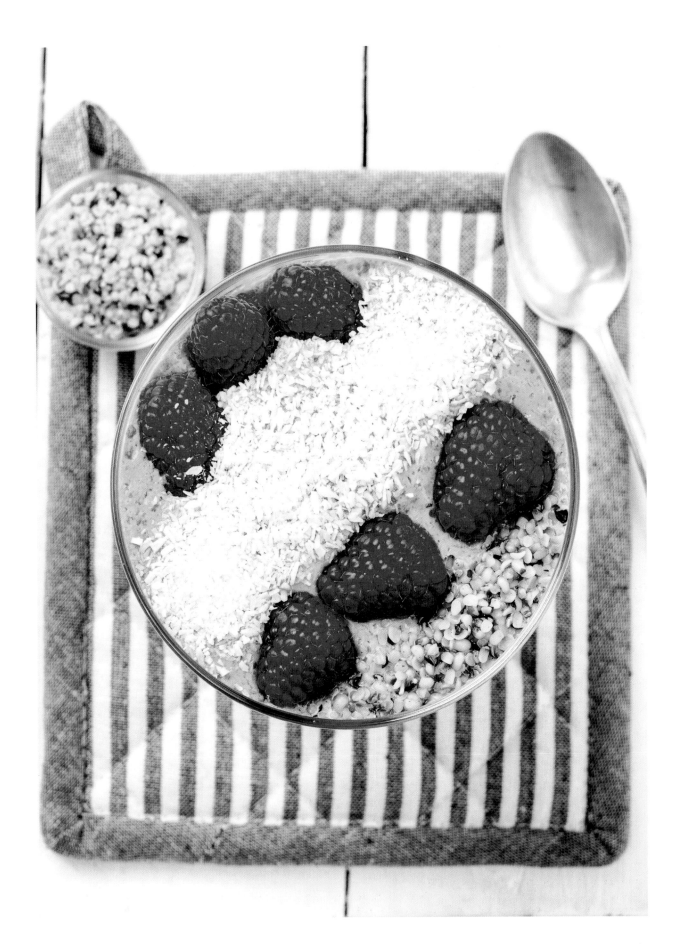

PEPPER SAUSAGE FRY

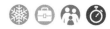

DAIRY-FREE • EGG-FREE • NUT-FREE

OPTIONS: AIP • COCONUT-FREE • LOW-FODMAP • NIGHTSHADE-FREE

SERVES 4

PREP TIME: 5 minutes

COOK TIME: 20 minutes

Any smoked or cured sausages will work for this recipe. Even hot dogs are okay!

¼ cup (60 ml) avocado oil, or ¼ cup (55 g) coconut oil

12 ounces (340 g) smoked sausages, thinly sliced

1 small green bell pepper, thinly sliced

1 small red bell pepper, thinly sliced

1½ teaspoons garlic powder

1 teaspoon dried oregano leaves

1 teaspoon paprika

¼ teaspoon finely ground sea salt

¼ teaspoon ground black pepper

¼ cup (17 g) chopped fresh parsley

1. Heat the oil in a large frying pan over medium-low heat until it shimmers.

2. When the oil is shimmering, add the rest of the ingredients, except the parsley. Cover and cook for 15 minutes, until the bell peppers are fork-tender.

3. Remove the lid and continue to cook for 5 to 6 minutes, until the liquid evaporates.

4. Remove from the heat, stir in the parsley, and serve.

make it AIP/NIGHTSHADE-FREE:
Ensure that the sausage is compliant, replace the bell peppers with 2 sliced zucchinis, and use turmeric in place of the paprika. For AIP, also omit the black pepper.

make it COCONUT-FREE:
Use avocado oil.

make it LOW-FODMAP:
Omit the garlic powder and replace 2 tablespoons of the avocado oil with garlic-infused oil.

PRESSURE COOK IT: *Use the sauté mode to heat the oil in Step 1. In Step 2, seal the lid and cook on high pressure for 10 minutes. Allow the pressure to release naturally before removing the lid, then set the cooker to the sauté mode for 3 minutes. Continue with Step 4.*

STORE IT: *Keep in an airtight container in the fridge for up to 3 days or in the freezer for up to 1 month.*

REHEAT IT: *Transfer a single serving to a microwave-safe dish, cover, and microwave for 2 minutes, or place in a frying pan with a drop of oil, cover, and reheat over medium heat for 5 minutes.*

THAW IT: *Set in the fridge and allow to thaw completely before using the reheating instructions above.*

Per serving, made with avocado oil and pork sausage:

calories: **411**	calories from fat: **345**	total fat: **38.3g**	saturated fat: **9.9g**	cholesterol: **49mg**
sodium: **903mg**	carbs: **6.3g**	dietary fiber: **1.5g**	net carbs: **4.8g**	sugars: **1.9g**	protein: **11.1g**

FAT:	CARBS:	PROTEIN:
84%	6%	10%

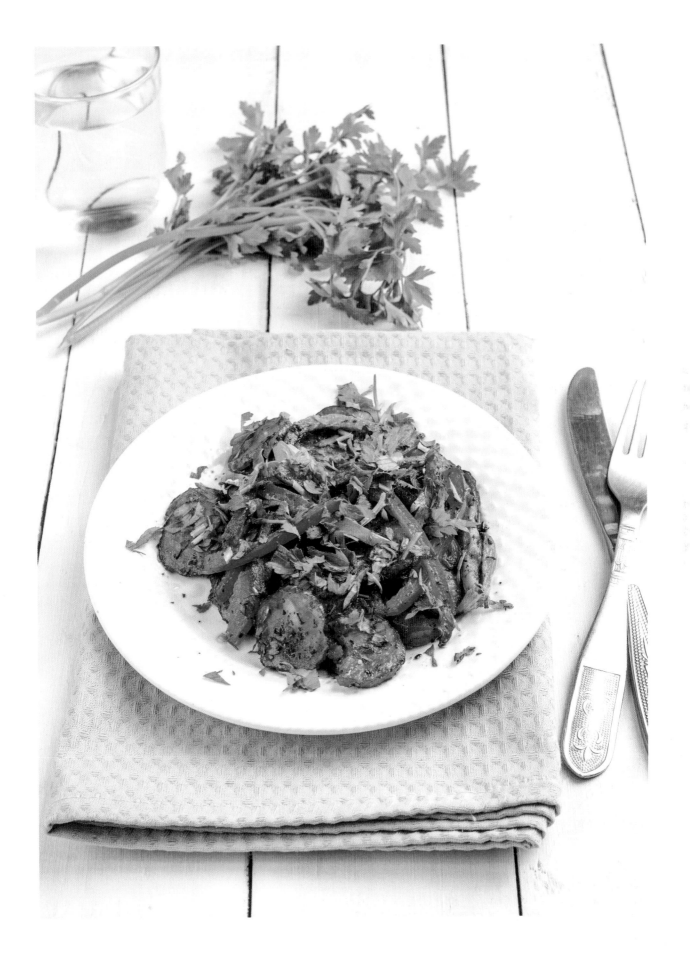

INDIAN MASALA OMELET

COCONUT-FREE · NUT-FREE · VEGETARIAN
OPTION: DAIRY-FREE

MAKES 1 large omelet
(2 servings)

PREP TIME: 8 minutes

COOK TIME: 25 minutes

This omelet is amazing served with Chilled Chai (page 360).

3 tablespoons avocado oil, coconut oil, or ghee

¼ cup (20 g) sliced green onions

1 clove garlic, minced

1 small tomato, diced

1 green chili pepper, seeded and finely diced

1½ teaspoons curry powder

½ teaspoon garam masala

6 large eggs, beaten

¼ cup (15 g) chopped fresh cilantro leaves and stems

1. Heat the oil in a large frying pan over medium heat until it shimmers. When the oil is shimmering, add the green onions, garlic, tomato, and chili pepper. Cook for 10 minutes, or until the liquid from the tomatoes has evaporated.

2. Reduce the heat to low and sprinkle the tomato mixture with the curry powder and garam masala. Stir to incorporate, then drizzle the beaten eggs over the top.

3. Cover and cook for 5 minutes, or until the edges are cooked through.

4. Sprinkle with the cilantro, fold one side over the other, cover, and cook for another 10 minutes.

5. Remove from the heat, cut in half, and serve.

make it **DAIRY-FREE:**
Do not use ghee.

STORE IT: *Keep in an airtight container in the fridge for up to 3 days.*

REHEAT IT: *Place a single serving on a microwave-safe plate, cover, and microwave for 2 minutes, or place in a frying pan with a drop of oil, cover, and reheat over medium heat for 5 minutes.*

Per serving, made with avocado oil:

| calories: **438** | calories from fat: **327** | total fat: **36.3g** | saturated fat: **7.1g** | cholesterol: **558mg** | FAT: | CARBS: | PROTEIN: |
| sodium: **279mg** | carbs: **7.7g** | dietary fiber: **1.9g** | net carbs: **5.8g** | sugars: **4.2g** | protein: **20.2g** | **75%** | **7%** | **18%** |

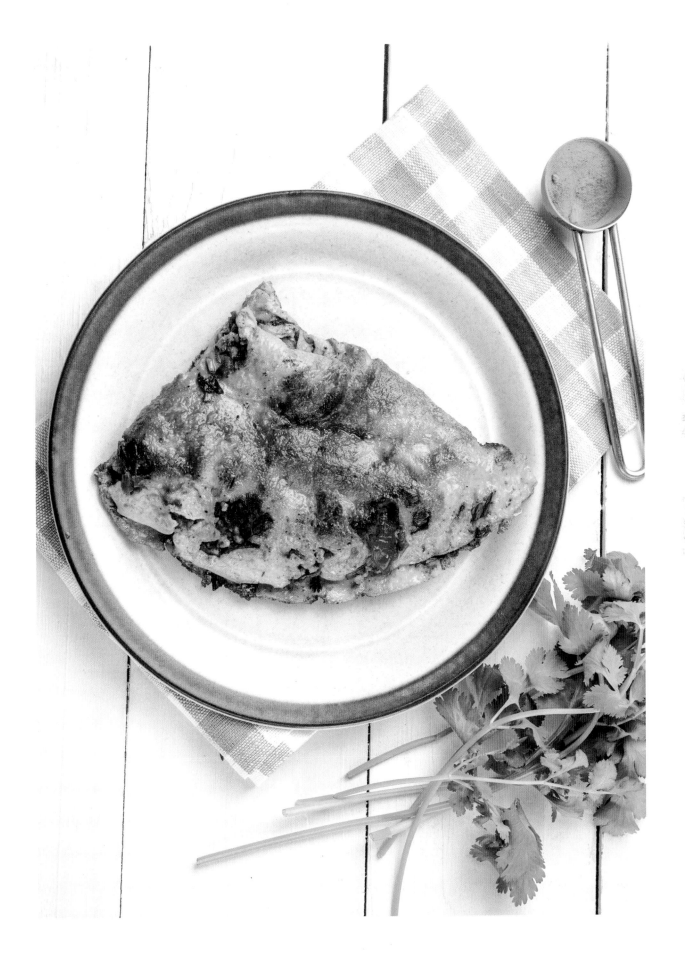

STICKY WRAPPED EGGS

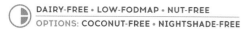

DAIRY-FREE • LOW-FODMAP • NUT-FREE

OPTIONS: COCONUT-FREE • NIGHTSHADE-FREE

MAKES 12 wrapped eggs (2 per serving)

PREP TIME: 10 minutes (not including time to hard-boil eggs)

COOK TIME: 30 minutes

I was wasting time on social media one day and found a low-carb recipe in which avocados are cut in half and pitted. Then a hard-boiled egg goes into the hole where the pit was, and the entire thing is wrapped in bacon. That's what this recipe was supposed to be, but...have you ever tried to wrap an entire avocado in bacon and then fry it? It's next to impossible. The bacon was all over the place, not adhering well to the avocado, and about halfway through frying, the egg popped out somehow!

I figured if I couldn't master the recipe on the first go, it wasn't a good fit for this book, so I changed it up a little. This method is easier and doesn't lead to bacon grease being splattered all over your (or my) clean kitchen.

Pro tip: If you have a pressure cooker, use it to hard-boil the eggs! Set a steamer rack inside your pressure cooker. Place the eggs on top, pour in enough water to cover the eggs, and add 1 tablespoon of vinegar (which will make the eggs easier to peel). Seal the lid and set the cooker to the egg mode for 5 minutes. Allow the pressure to release naturally before removing the lid. The eggs will be perfect!

¼ cup (60 ml) coconut aminos

2 tablespoons hot sauce

12 hard-boiled eggs

12 strips bacon (about 12 oz/340 g)

6 cups (100 g) arugula

1. Preheat the oven to 400°F (205°C). Line a standard-size 12-well muffin pan with muffin liners, or use a silicone muffin pan, which won't require liners.

2. Place the coconut aminos and hot sauce in a small bowl and whisk to combine. Set the bowl close to the muffin pan.

3. Peel the hard-boiled eggs. One at a time, wrap each egg in a strip of bacon, then dunk it in the hot sauce mixture and place it in a well of the muffin pan.

4. Bake for 30 minutes, flipping the eggs over halfway through.

5. Divide the arugula evenly among 6 small serving plates. Top each with 2 sticky eggs and the sauce from their muffin liners.

make it COCONUT-FREE:
Replace the coconut aminos with 2 tablespoons soy sauce and 2 tablespoons water.

make it NIGHTSHADE-FREE:
Omit the hot sauce.

STORE IT: *Keep the eggs and arugula in separate airtight containers in the fridge for up to 5 days.*

REHEAT IT: *Enjoy cold, or place the wrapped eggs in a frying pan with a drop of oil, cover, and reheat over medium-low heat for 5 minutes.*

PREP AHEAD: *Prepare the hot sauce mixture up to 5 days ahead and the hard-boiled eggs up to 2 days before using in this recipe.*

Per serving:

calories: **438** | calories from fat: **293** | total fat: **32.5g** | saturated fat: **1.5g** | cholesterol: **390mg**
sodium: **1498mg** | carbs: **4.1g** | dietary fiber: **0.3g** | net carbs: **3.8g** | sugars: **1g** | protein: **32.5g**

FAT:	CARBS:	PROTEIN:
67%	**3%**	**30%**

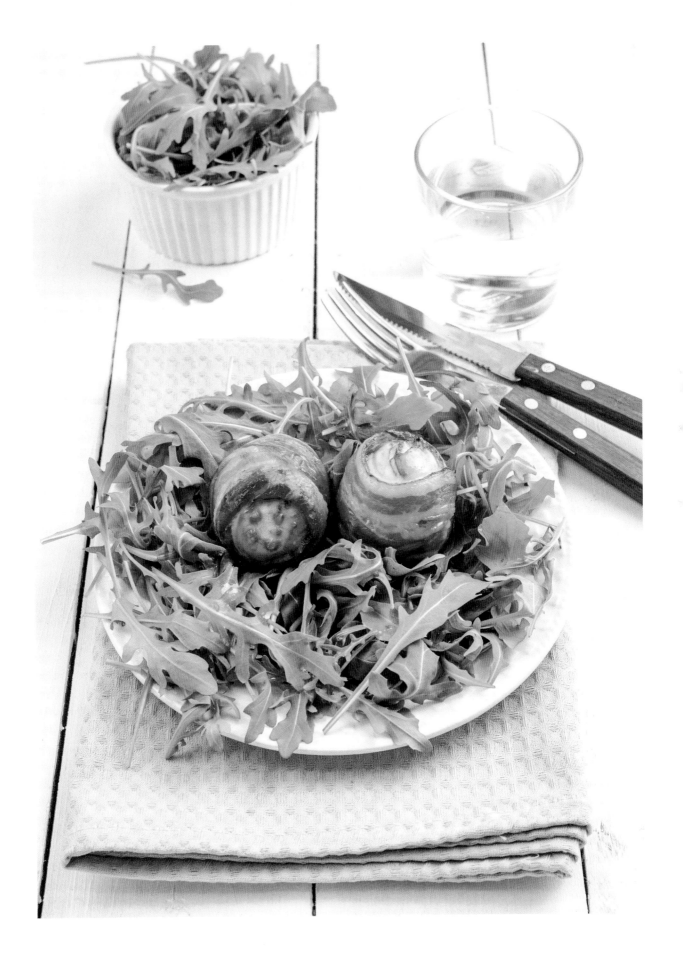

ALL DAY ANY DAY HASH

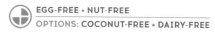 EGG-FREE • NUT-FREE

OPTIONS: COCONUT-FREE • DAIRY-FREE

SERVES 4

PREP TIME: 10 minutes

COOK TIME: 25 minutes

Living on a sailboat full-time, we are a little obsessed about easy one-pan meals, especially when they yield leftovers so that I have to cook only twice as opposed to three times a day. This hash is a household favorite! I think it'll become one of yours, too. We love it with creamy Italian dressing, but mayonnaise (store-bought or homemade, page 94) or my Lemon Turmeric Dressing & Marinade (page 86) would also be amazing.

I like to use bottom round steak in this recipe, but you can have your pick!

¼ cup (55 g) coconut oil or ghee

⅔ cup (100 g) sliced white onions

3 cloves garlic, minced

3 medium turnips (about 1 lb/455 g), peeled and cubed

2 medium carrots (about 5 oz/140 g), diced

1 red bell pepper, diced

8 ounces (225 g) boneless steak, thinly sliced

⅓ cup (25 g) crushed pork rinds

2 tablespoons chopped fresh parsley leaves

1 teaspoon fresh thyme leaves

¼ teaspoon finely ground sea salt

⅛ teaspoon ground black pepper

½ cup (120 ml) creamy Italian dressing

1. Heat the oil in a large frying pan over medium heat. Add the onions and garlic and cook until the onions are translucent, 5 to 7 minutes.

2. Add the turnips, carrots, bell pepper, and steak. Toss to coat, cover, and cook for 15 to 18 minutes, stirring every 3 minutes, until the turnips are fork-tender and the steak is cooked to your liking. Remove the pan from the heat.

3. Add the crushed pork rinds, parsley, thyme, salt, and pepper and toss to coat.

4. Divide the hash evenly among 4 bowls and drizzle each bowl with 2 tablespoons of dressing just before serving.

make it COCONUT-FREE: Do not use coconut oil.

make it DAIRY-FREE: Do not use ghee.

MAKE IT AT HOME

Replace store-bought creamy Italian dressing with my homemade version.

Creamy Italian Dressing

PRESSURE COOK IT: *Use the sauté mode for Step 1. In Step 2, add ¼ cup (60 ml) of beef bone broth, seal the lid, and cook on high pressure for 10 minutes. Allow the pressure to release naturally before removing the lid, then continue with Steps 3 and 4.*

STORE IT: *Keep in an airtight container in the fridge for up to 3 days or in the freezer for up to 1 month.*

REHEAT IT: *Transfer a single serving to a microwave-safe dish, cover, and microwave for 2 minutes, or place in a frying pan with a drop of oil, cover, and reheat over medium heat for 5 minutes.*

THAW IT: *Set in the fridge and allow to thaw completely before using the reheating instructions above.*

Per serving, made with coconut oil and bottom round steak, with homemade creamy Italian dressing:

| calories: **512** | calories from fat: **335** | total fat: **37.4g** | saturated fat: **16.1g** | cholesterol: **62mg** |
| sodium: **454mg** | carbs: **17.4g** | dietary fiber: **4.1g** | net carbs: **13.3g** | sugars: **9.1g** | protein: **26.6g** |

FAT:	CARBS:	PROTEIN:
66%	13%	21%

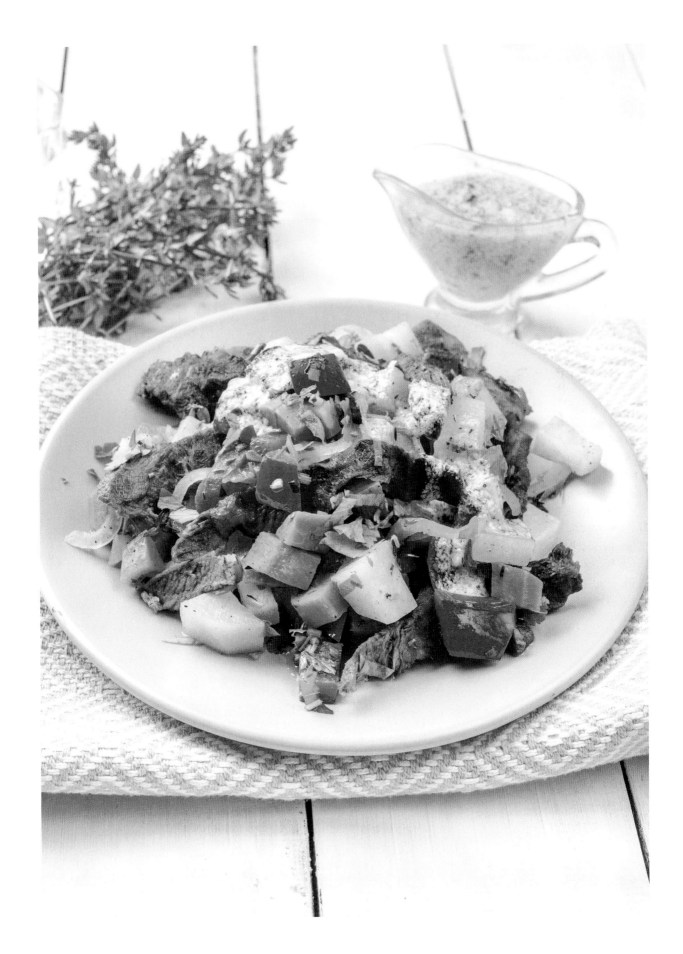

SOMETHING DIFFERENT BREAKFAST SAMMY

COCONUT-FREE · DAIRY-FREE · NUT-FREE

OPTIONS: EGG-FREE · NIGHTSHADE-FREE · VEGAN · VEGETARIAN

SERVES 1

PREP TIME: 5 minutes

COOK TIME: 10 minutes

On a recent cross-country trip, driving from our hometown of Calgary, Alberta, in Canada to Fort Lauderdale, Florida, in the U.S., I discovered a new thing: avocado sandwiches. Our food budget was tight, so eating breakfast at grungy diners was the way to go. Grungy diners don't always have the best keto options on the menu, but you can just about bet that they have bacon, lettuce, tomatoes, onions, and, if you're lucky, a little avocado. In our case, we lucked out every time. Instead of packing all the ingredients inside a lettuce wrap, I tried something different, and it stuck. Welcome, avocado sandwich! What will you put in yours? This is my favorite, and the simplest, combination.

Pressed for time in the morning? I like to precook bacon on Sundays so I have lots to use in recipes like this during the week.

Sick and tired of mayonnaise? It happens. This sandwich is also really good with Green Speckled Dressing (page 80) or Quick 'n' Easy Barbecue Sauce (page 70).

1 medium Hass avocado, peeled and pitted (about 4 oz/110 g of flesh)

1 lettuce leaf, torn in half

1 tablespoon mayonnaise

2 strips bacon (about 2 oz/55 g), cooked until crispy

1 red onion ring

1 tomato slice

Pinch of finely ground sea salt

Pinch of ground black pepper

Pinch of sesame seeds or poppy seeds (optional)

1. Cook the bacon in a medium-sized frying pan over medium heat until crispy, about 10 minutes.

2. Place the avocado halves cut side up on a plate.

3. Lay the lettuce pieces on top of one of the avocado halves, then slather the mayonnaise on the lettuce. Top the lettuce with the bacon, onion, and tomato, then sprinkle with the salt and pepper.

4. Cover the stack with the other avocado half and sprinkle with the seeds, if using. Enjoy immediately!

make it EGG-FREE:
Use egg-free mayonnaise (see recipe on page 102).

make it NIGHTSHADE-FREE:
Omit the tomato.

make it VEGAN/VEGETARIAN:
Omit the bacon. For vegan, also use egg-free mayonnaise (see recipe on page 102).

MAKE IT AT HOME

Replace store-bought mayonnaise with my homemade version.

104

Mayonnaise

Per serving, made with homemade mayonnaise, with sesame seeds:

| calories: **545** | calories from fat: **391** | total fat: **43.4g** | saturated fat: **11.2g** | cholesterol: **60mg** | | FAT: | CARBS: | PROTEIN: |
| sodium: **1407mg** | carbs: **19.8g** | dietary fiber: **8.8g** | net carbs: **11g** | sugars: **7.8g** | protein: **18.9g** | **72%** | **14%** | **14%** |

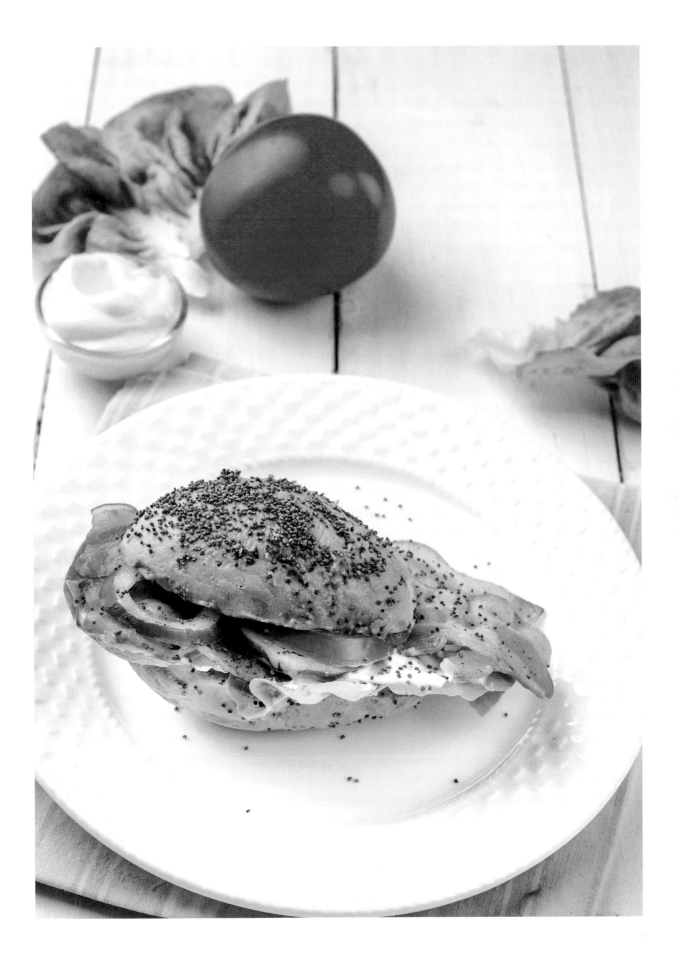

SUPER BREAKFAST COMBO

DAIRY-FREE • EGG-FREE • NIGHTSHADE-FREE

OPTIONS: AIP • COCONUT-FREE • LOW-FODMAP • NUT-FREE • VEGAN • VEGETARIAN

SERVES 1

PREP TIME: 10 minutes

COOK TIME: –

Some days I wake up really hungry, and other days I don't. On days when fasting until noon or later sounds like a horrible idea, this is one of my go-to breakfasts. It's mega fatty and keeps you full for hours on end, making it awesome for days that are so busy that lunch may not be an option. You can have the latte only or pair it with the fat bombs. I like to keep little fat bombs like these in the freezer for fast access so my mornings unfold with ease!

You'll notice that I call for maca and chaga or ashwagandha powders, all superfoods with a purpose, but they are not required for the latte to turn out well. Maca is an herb that helps with hormone balance; chaga is a type of mushroom that helps balance stress and supports immune function; and ashwagandha is an herb that helps support adrenal function. When added to recipes like this, or to homemade keto ice pops, shakes, smoothies, and fatty coffees, they boost the overall nutrition without affecting the taste. And hey, if I can support my adrenals by drinking a matcha latte, I'm all for it!

CHOCOLATE FAT BOMBS:

1 tablespoon coconut butter

2 teaspoons coconut oil

1 teaspoon cocoa powder

½ teaspoon confectioners'-style erythritol, or 1 drop liquid stevia

MATCHA LATTE:

1 cup (240 ml) boiling water

2 tablespoons collagen peptides or protein powder

1 tablespoon coconut butter, coconut oil, or nut butter

1 teaspoon erythritol, or 2 drops liquid stevia

1 teaspoon matcha powder

½ teaspoon maca powder (optional)

¼ teaspoon chaga powder or ashwagandha powder (optional)

1¼ cups (300 ml) full-fat coconut milk, hot

1. To prepare the fat bomb, place all the ingredients in a bowl and either set out in the sun to melt or microwave for 20 to 30 seconds. Once the coconut butter has melted, whisk thoroughly and transfer to a paper muffin liner, a silicone mold, a plastic container—anything will do. Place in the freezer for 5 minutes, or until hardened.

2. Meanwhile, place the boiling water, collagen, coconut butter, sweetener, matcha, and maca and chaga, if using, in a 20-ounce (600-ml) or larger mug. Whisk until the ingredients are incorporated and the lumps are gone, about 1 minute. Stir in the hot coconut milk.

3. Serve the latte with the chilled fat bomb.

STORE IT: *Store the latte in the fridge for up to 3 days and the fat bomb in the freezer for up to 1 month. The fat bomb can be eaten directly from the freezer.*

REHEAT IT: *Transfer the latte to a 10-ounce (295-ml) or larger microwave-safe mug and microwave for 1½ minutes, or place the latte in a saucepan, cover, and reheat over low heat for 5 minutes.*

Latte made with collagen, coconut butter, and superfood powders, with fat bomb:

| calories: **740** | calories from fat: **589** | total fat: **65.4g** | saturated fat: **24g** | cholesterol: **0mg** | FAT: | CARBS: | PROTEIN: |
| sodium: **233mg** | carbs: **11.6g** | dietary fiber: **9.3g** | net carbs: **2.3g** | sugars: **2.1g** | protein: **26.3g** | **80%** | **6%** | **14%** |

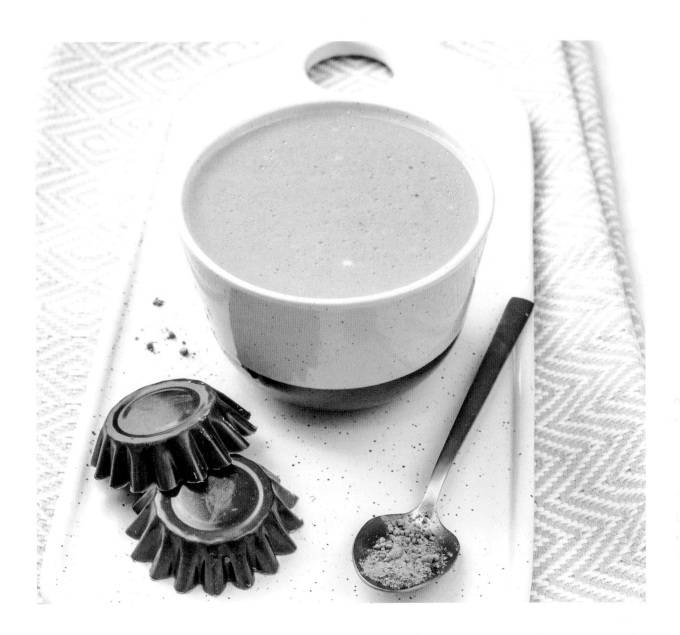

make it AIP:
Use carob powder in place of the cocoa powder in the fat bomb and use stevia in both the fat bomb and the latte.

make it COCONUT-FREE:
For the fat bomb, replace the coconut butter with a nut butter and replace the coconut oil with ghee or cocoa butter. For the latte, use a nut butter and replace the coconut milk with another milk of your choice. Cashew Milk (page 342) is a great alternative.

make it LOW-FODMAP:
Replace the coconut milk with almond, macadamia nut, or hemp milk.

make it NUT-FREE:
Use coconut butter or coconut oil in the latte.

make it VEGAN:
Do not use collagen. Opt for a plant-based protein powder.

make it VEGETARIAN:
Do not use collagen. Opt for a plant- or egg-based protein powder.

Latte only:

calories: **546** | calories from fat: **424** | total fat: **47.1g** | saturated fat: **8g** | cholesterol: **0mg**
sodium: **228mg** | carbs: **6.3g** | dietary fiber: **5.7g** | net carbs: **0.6g** | sugars: **1.2g** | protein: **24.4g**

FAT:	CARBS:	PROTEIN:
78%	4%	18%

COFFEE SHAKE

EGG-FREE • NIGHTSHADE-FREE • NUT-FREE • VEGETARIAN

OPTIONS: COCONUT-FREE • DAIRY-FREE • LOW-FODMAP • VEGAN

MAKES one 14-ounce (415-ml) serving

PREP TIME: 5 minutes

COOK TIME: –

I love using mushroom coffee in this recipe because it tastes great, has healing properties, and doesn't contain caffeine. But any type of coffee will do the trick, even freshly ground coffee beans instead of the instant stuff. You could even play around with using your favorite tea leaves in place of the coffee. Black tea or rooibos leaves are amazing.

1 cup (240 ml) full-fat coconut milk

½ cup (120 ml) water

4 ice cubes

2 tablespoons coconut oil, unflavored MCT oil powder, or ghee

1½ tablespoons cocoa powder

1½ teaspoons erythritol, or 2 drops liquid stevia

½ teaspoon instant coffee granules

1. Place all the ingredients in a blender or food processor. Blend on high until the ice is broken up completely and the texture of the shake is smooth.

2. Transfer to a 14-ounce (415-ml) or larger glass. Best enjoyed immediately.

make it COCONUT-FREE:
Use heavy cream instead of coconut milk.

make it DAIRY-FREE/VEGAN:
Do not use ghee.

make it LOW-FODMAP:
Replace the coconut milk with almond, macadamia nut, or hemp milk.

STORE IT: *If there are leftovers or you need to make the shake ahead of time, store it in an airtight container in the fridge for up to 3 days. When ready to enjoy, give it a little shake. Alternatively, pour the leftovers into ice pop molds and freeze.*

Per serving, made with coconut oil:

calories: **757**	calories from fat: **684**	total fat: **76g**	saturated fat: **67.9g**	cholesterol: **0mg**	FAT:	CARBS:	PROTEIN:
sodium: **60mg**	carbs: **12.3g**	dietary fiber: **2.7g**	net carbs: **9.6g**	sugars: **4g**	protein: **6.1g**	**91%**	**6%**	**3%**

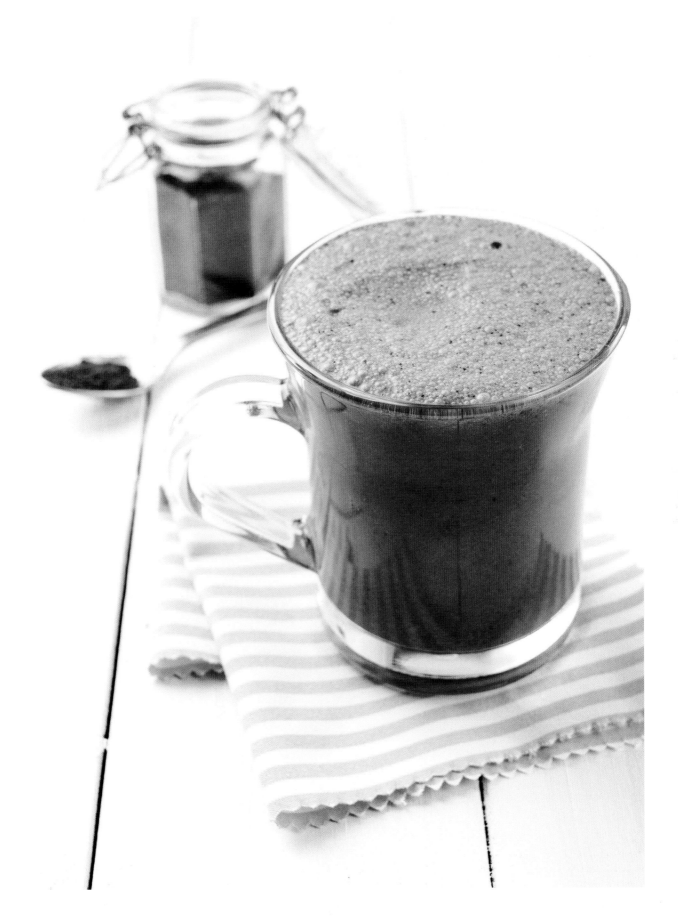

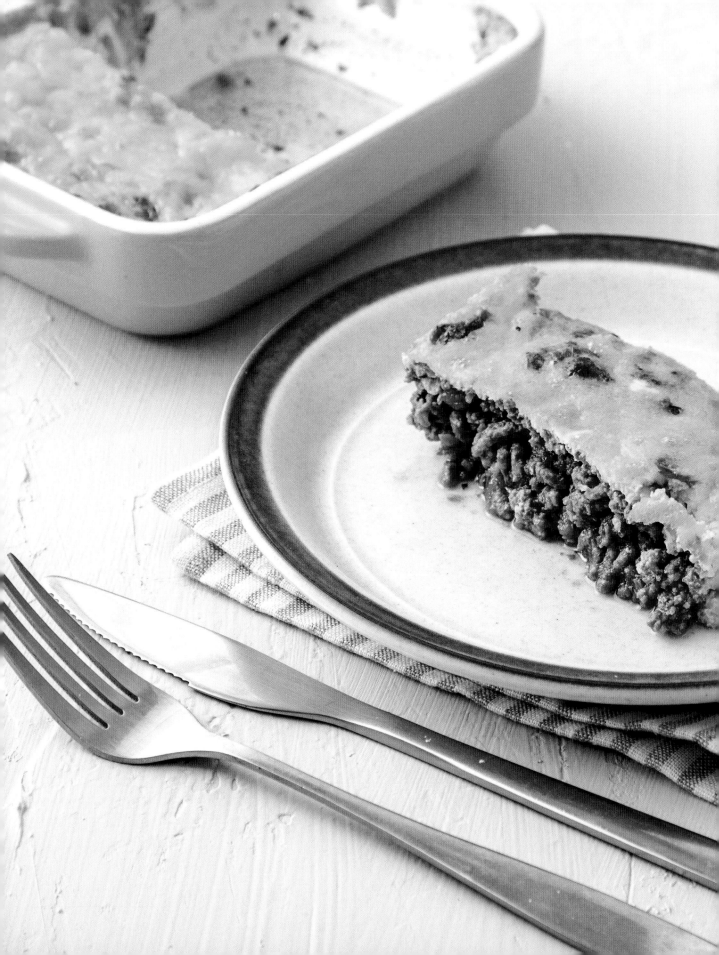

6.

LUNCH

CHILI LIME CHICKEN BOWLS

 COCONUT-FREE • DAIRY-FREE • EGG-FREE • NUT-FREE

SERVES 4
PREP TIME: 15 minutes
COOK TIME: 30 minutes

While moving into our new place, we got a little too obsessed with going to Whole Foods for their epic lunch buffet and eating until we couldn't eat any more. One of my favorites quickly became their Cilantro Cauliflower Rice. Unlike most cauliflower rice dishes I'd tried, it was served cold. I had that rice every darn day and never got sick of it. Paired with spicy chicken thighs as it is in this recipe, it can't be beat!

If you want to bump up the fat content, Avocado Lime Dressing (page 84) is awesome drizzled over the top of these bowls.

CILANTRO CAULIFLOWER RICE SALAD:

1 medium head cauliflower (about 1½ lbs/680 g), or 3 cups (375 g) pre-riced cauliflower

⅓ packed cup (27 g) chopped fresh cilantro leaves and stems

¼ cup (60 ml) avocado oil

2 tablespoons lime juice

2 green onions, sliced

½ teaspoon finely ground sea salt

¼ teaspoon ground black pepper

CHILI LIME CHICKEN:

2 tablespoons avocado oil

1 tablespoon lime juice

1½ teaspoons chili powder

1 teaspoon garlic powder

2 teaspoons erythritol

2 teaspoons hot sauce

¾ teaspoon ground cumin

½ teaspoon paprika

¾ teaspoon finely ground sea salt

¼ teaspoon ground black pepper

1 pound (455 g) boneless, skinless chicken thighs

1. If you're using pre-riced cauliflower, skip ahead to Step 2. Otherwise, cut the base off the head of cauliflower and remove the florets. Transfer the florets to a food processor or blender and pulse 3 or 4 times to break them up into small (¼-inch/6-mm) pieces.

2. Put the riced cauliflower in a large saucepan and cover completely with water. Cover with the lid and bring to a boil over high heat, then reduce the heat to medium and simmer for 5 minutes, until fork-tender. (You don't want to let it get mushy!) Once done, drain, pressing the cauliflower with the back of a spoon to get out as much water as possible. Transfer the drained cauliflower to a large mixing bowl and place in the fridge to cool.

3. Make the chili lime chicken: Combine all the ingredients but the chicken thighs in a large frying pan. Whisk to combine, then add the chicken and turn to coat. Cover and set over low heat for 25 minutes, until the chicken reaches an internal temperature of 165°F (74°C).

4. After 20 minutes, pull the cooked cauliflower out of the fridge and add the remaining ingredients for the cauliflower rice salad. Toss to coat, then divide evenly among 4 bowls. Top each bowl with one-quarter of the chili lime chicken and drizzle with a bit of the pan sauce. Serve!

Per serving:

calories: **268**	calories from fat: **124**	total fat: **13.8g**	saturated fat: **2.5g**	cholesterol: **96mg**
sodium: **454mg**	carbs: **10.4g**	dietary fiber: **5g**	net carbs: **5.4g**	sugars: **4g**	protein: **25.7g**

FAT:	CARBS:	PROTEIN:
46%	16%	38%

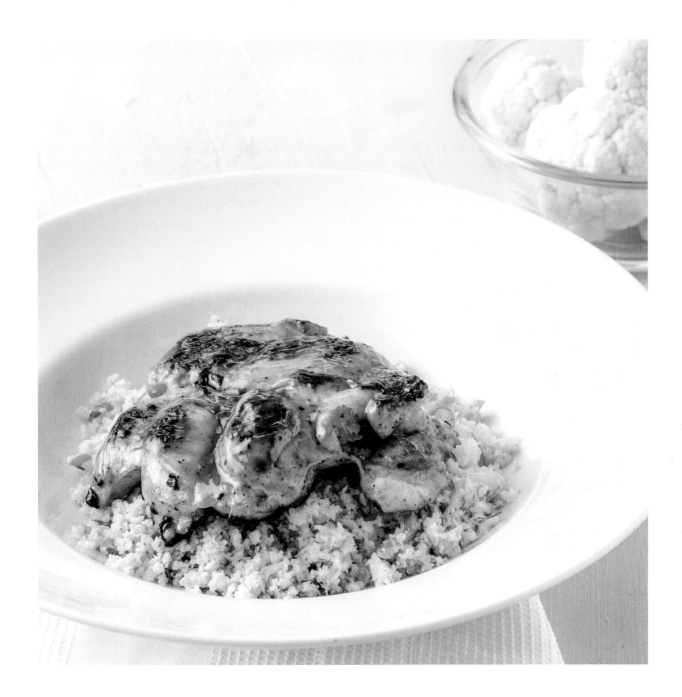

STORE IT: *Keep the chicken and cauliflower rice salad in separate airtight containers in the fridge for up to 3 days or in the freezer for up to 1 month.*

REHEAT IT: *Wonderful enjoyed cold, or transfer a single serving of the chicken to a microwave-safe dish, cover, and microwave for 1 minute. Serve the chicken alongside the chilled cauliflower rice salad.*

THAW IT: *Place in the fridge and allow to thaw completely, then follow the reheating instructions above.*

PREP AHEAD: *To prepare the cauliflower for the salad ahead, complete Steps 1 and 2 and store in the fridge for up to 1 day before serving.*

To prepare the chile lime chicken ahead, place all the ingredients for the chicken in a large zip-top freezer bag and freeze for up to 1 month. When ready to make the rest of the recipe, thaw the chicken completely in the fridge before picking up at Step 3.

GERMAN NO-TATO SALAD

COCONUT-FREE • DAIRY-FREE • NIGHTSHADE-FREE • NUT-FREE
OPTIONS: EGG-FREE • LOW-FODMAP

SERVES 5
PREP TIME: 10 minutes
COOK TIME: 10 minutes

Served hot or cold, this salad is one of our favorites here at home. We like to enjoy it warm when I first make a batch, then cold for all the leftovers. To make a full meal out of this salad, I generally serve it with sliced deli meat and a simple mustard sauce.

2 medium rutabaga (2 lbs/910 g), peeled

1 teaspoon finely ground sea salt

1 small red onion, finely diced

¼ cup (60 ml) apple cider vinegar

¼ cup (60 ml) avocado oil or olive oil

4 green onions, sliced

1 tablespoon Dijon mustard

1 teaspoon erythritol

¾ teaspoon ground black pepper

FOR SERVING:

1 tablespoon plus 2 teaspoons Dijon mustard

1 tablespoon plus 2 teaspoons mayonnaise

10 ounces (285 g) thinly sliced deli ham or other meat of choice

1. Cut the rutabaga into ½-inch (1.25-cm) cubes, place in a large saucepan, cover completely with water, and add the salt. Cover with the lid, bring to a boil over high heat, then reduce the heat to a simmer and cook for 10 minutes, or until fork-tender.

2. Meanwhile, place the remaining ingredients in a large salad bowl. Once the rutabaga is cooked, drain completely and transfer to the salad bowl. Toss to combine, then divide among 5 plates.

3. In a small bowl, mix together the mustard and mayonnaise.

4. Serve the ham slices alongside the salad with 2 teaspoons of the mustard sauce.

STORE IT: *Keep in an airtight container in the fridge for up to 3 days.*

make it **EGG-FREE:**
Use egg-free mayonnaise (see recipe on page 102).

make it **LOW-FODMAP:**
Omit the red onion. Use only the green parts of the green onions. Check the ingredients of the ham to ensure it's safe.

MAKE IT AT HOME

Replace store-bought mayonnaise with my homemade version.

Mayonnaise

Per serving, made with avocado oil and homemade mayonnaise, with ham:

calories: **296** | calories from fat: **167** | total fat: **18.8g** | saturated fat: **3.2g** | cholesterol: **33mg**
sodium: **1377mg** | carbs: **19g** | dietary fiber: **5g** | net carbs: **14g** | sugars: **10g** | protein: **14g**

FAT: **57%** | CARBS: **25%** | PROTEIN: **19%**

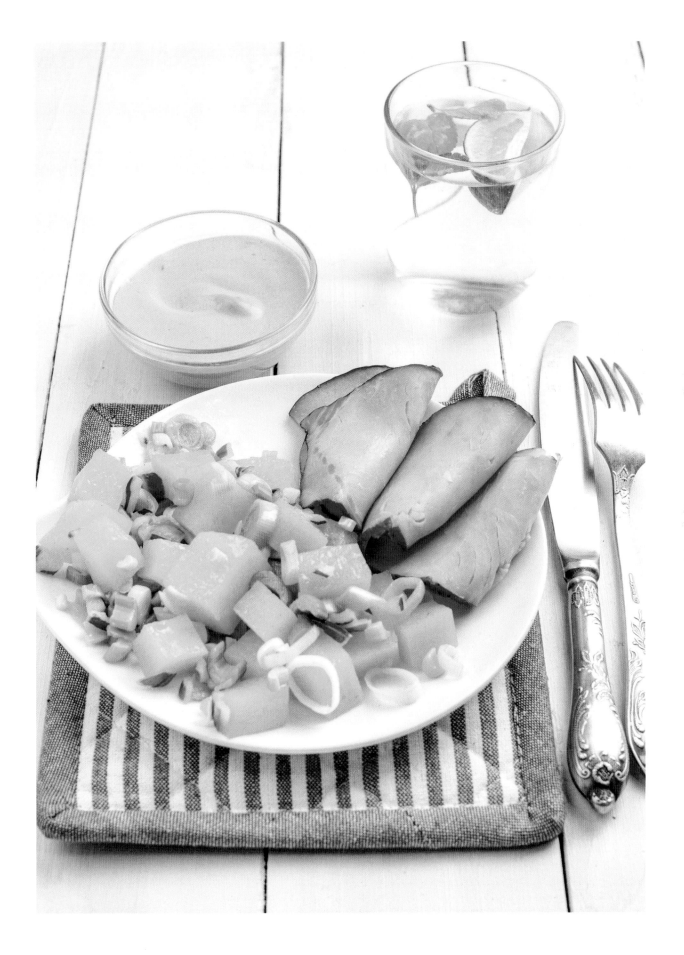

SALMON SALAD CUPS

COCONUT-FREE • DAIRY-FREE • LOW-FODMAP • NIGHTSHADE-FREE • NUT-FREE
OPTIONS: AIP • EGG-FREE

SERVES 4

PREP TIME: 10 minutes

COOK TIME: –

A perfectly light lunch for any day of the year! I stock up on canned salmon when it's on sale and save it for recipes like this one—easy to make and loaded with calcium. If you don't want to use mayonnaise, try using Herby Vinaigrette & Marinade (page 98) or Lemon Turmeric Dressing & Marinade (page 86) in its place.

12 ounces (340 g) canned salmon (no salt added)

3 tablespoons prepared horseradish

1 tablespoon chopped fresh dill

2 teaspoons lemon juice

½ teaspoon finely ground sea salt

½ teaspoon ground black pepper

12 butter lettuce leaves (from 1 head)

½ cup (105 g) mayonnaise

1. Place the salmon, horseradish, dill, lemon juice, salt, and pepper in a medium-sized bowl. Stir until the ingredients are fully incorporated.

2. Set the lettuce leaves on a serving plate. Fill each leaf with 2 tablespoons of the salmon salad mixture and top with 2 teaspoons of mayonnaise.

STORE IT: *Keep in an airtight container in the fridge for up to 3 days.*

make it AIP:
Omit the black pepper. Replace the mayonnaise with Lemon Turmeric Dressing & Marinade (page 86).

make it EGG-FREE:
Use egg-free mayonnaise (see recipe on page 102).

MAKE IT AT HOME

Replace store-bought mayonnaise with my homemade version.

104

Mayonnaise

Per serving of 3 filled lettuce cups, made with homemade mayonnaise:

| calories: **314** | calories from fat: **239** | total fat: **26.5g** | saturated fat: **4.6g** | cholesterol: **33mg** | | FAT: | CARBS: | PROTEIN: |
| sodium: **526mg** | carbs: **4.4g** | dietary fiber: **1.1g** | net carbs: **3.3g** | sugars: **1.8g** | protein: **14.6g** | **76%** | **6%** | **19%** |

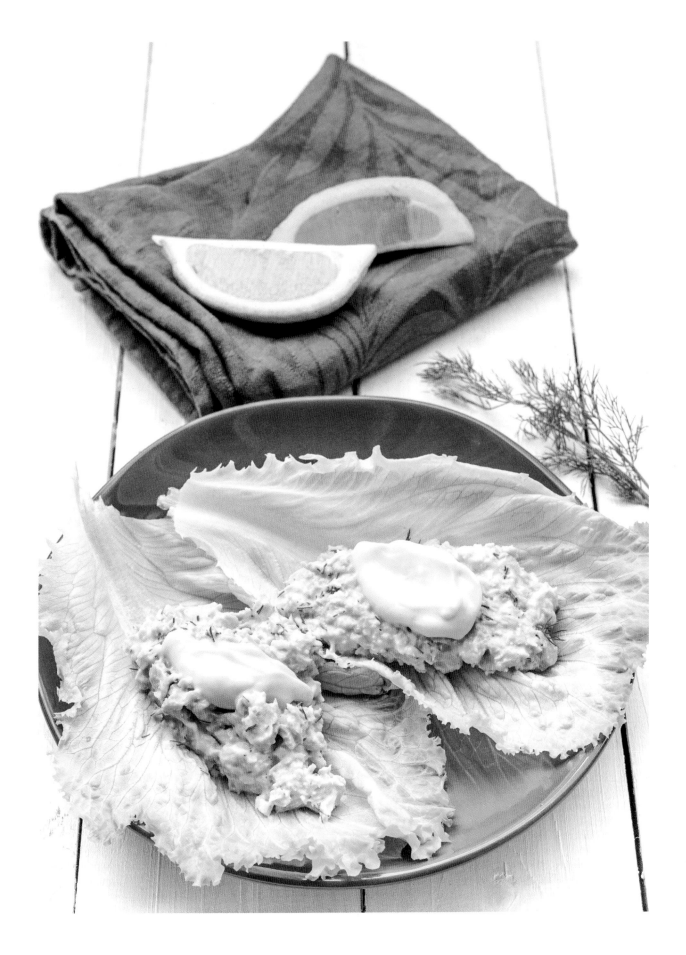

STEAK FRY CUPS

DAIRY-FREE • EGG-FREE • NUT-FREE
OPTION: COCONUT-FREE

SERVES 6

PREP TIME: 10 minutes,
plus 2 hours to marinate

COOK TIME: 8 minutes

The marinade in this recipe is legit! I've used it for pork, chicken, and beef, and each time I make a batch, I wish I'd doubled it for later. You can use coconut aminos or soy sauce here; I chose coconut aminos just because it turns a bit syrup-like when heated, which adds to the deliciousness of the final result. Also, you could go a step further by adding a drizzle of ranch dressing to each cup.

¼ cup plus 2 tablespoons (90 ml) avocado oil

¼ cup (60 ml) coconut aminos

2 tablespoons hot sauce

2 tablespoons lime juice

6 cloves garlic, minced

½ teaspoon ground black pepper

1 pound (455 g) top sirloin steak, cubed

1 red onion, diced

1 yellow bell pepper, sliced

36 endive leaves (from about 6 heads endive)

¼ cup (17 g) chopped fresh parsley leaves

1. Place the oil, coconut aminos, hot sauce, lime juice, garlic, and black pepper in a medium-sized bowl. Whisk to combine, then add the steak, onion, and bell pepper and toss to coat. Cover and place in the refrigerator to marinate for at least 2 hours or overnight.

2. When ready to cook the steak, transfer the entire contents of the bowl to a large frying pan. Cook over medium heat, stirring frequently, until the steak is cooked through, about 8 minutes.

3. Meanwhile, divide the endive leaves evenly among 6 plates. To serve, fill each leaf with about 2 tablespoons of the steak mixture. Sprinkle with the parsley and enjoy.

make it COCONUT-FREE:
Replace the coconut aminos with 2 tablespoons of soy sauce and 2 tablespoons of water.

PRESSURE COOK IT: *Complete Step 1. For Step 2, place the contents of the bowl in a pressure cooker. Seal the lid and cook on high pressure for 10 minutes. Allow the pressure to release naturally before removing the lid, then move on to Step 3.*

STORE IT: *Keep the steak and endive leaves in separate airtight containers in the fridge for up to 3 days. The steak mixture can be frozen for up to 1 month.*

REHEAT IT: *Wonderful enjoyed cold, or place a single serving of the steak mixture in a microwave-safe dish, cover, and microwave for 2 minutes before placing in the endive leaves.*

THAW IT: *Place the steak mixture in the fridge and allow to defrost completely. Once defrosted, enjoy cold or follow the reheating instructions above.*

PREP AHEAD: *Prepare the marinade and place the steak and vegetables in the marinade. Freeze the mixture for up to 1 month before completing the recipe. When ready to prepare, allow to thaw completely in the fridge before picking up at Step 2.*

Per serving of 6 filled endive cups:

calories: **325** | calories from fat: **173** | total fat: **19.2g** | saturated fat: **3.9g** | cholesterol: **68mg**
sodium: **229mg** | carbs: **12.3g** | dietary fiber: **6.2g** | net carbs: **6.1g** | sugars: **2.3g** | protein: **25.8g**

FAT:	CARBS:	PROTEIN:
53%	15%	32%

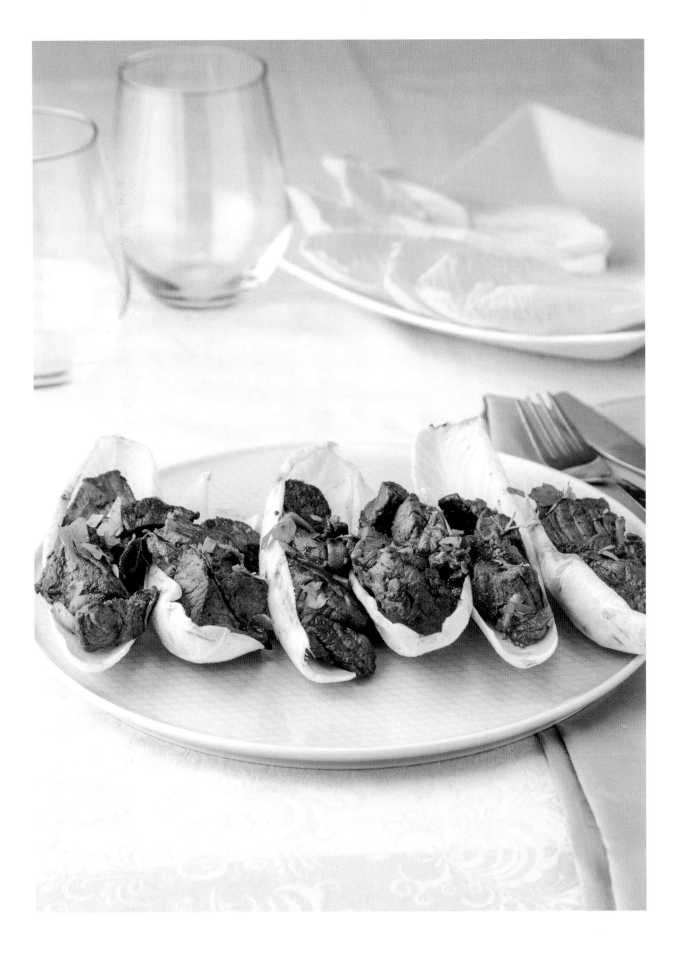

BROCCOLI GINGER SOUP

DAIRY-FREE • EGG-FREE • NUT-FREE
OPTION: **AIP**

SERVES 4
PREP TIME: 5 minutes
COOK TIME: 25 minutes

The color of this soup doesn't look like much, I know, but the taste is great! You can swap out the broccoli for an equal amount of cauliflower if the color has you or your little family members totally weirded out. The flavor won't change too much, and it'll be more yellow than anything.

3 tablespoons coconut oil or avocado oil

1 small white onion, sliced

2 cloves garlic, minced

5 cups (420 g) broccoli florets

1 (13½-oz/400-ml) can full-fat coconut milk

1½ cups (355 ml) chicken bone broth

1 (2-in/5-cm) piece fresh ginger root, peeled and minced

1½ teaspoons turmeric powder

¾ teaspoon finely ground sea salt

⅓ cup (55 g) collagen peptides (optional)

¼ cup (40 g) sesame seeds

1. Melt the oil in a large frying pan over medium heat. Add the onion and garlic and cook until translucent, about 10 minutes.

2. Add the broccoli, coconut milk, broth, ginger, turmeric, and salt. Cover and cook for 15 minutes, or until the broccoli is tender.

3. Transfer the broccoli mixture to a blender or food processor. Add the collagen, if using, and blend until smooth.

4. Divide among 4 bowls, top each bowl with 1 tablespoon of sesame seeds, and enjoy!

make it AIP:
Omit the sesame seeds.

PRESSURE COOK IT: *Use the sauté mode for Step 1. For Step 2, place everything in a pressure cooker, seal the lid, and either set the cooker to the soup mode or cook on high pressure for 10 minutes. Allow the pressure to release naturally before removing the lid, then pick up with Step 3.*

STORE IT: *Keep in an airtight container in the fridge for up to 3 days or in the freezer for up to 1 month.*

REHEAT IT: *Transfer a single serving to a microwave-safe bowl, cover, and microwave for 2 minutes; or place in a saucepan and reheat over low heat for 5 minutes.*

THAW IT: *Place in the fridge and allow to defrost completely, then follow the reheating instructions above.*

Per 1-cup/240-ml serving, made with coconut oil and collagen:

calories: **344**	calories from fat: **241**	total fat: **26.8g**	saturated fat: **4.6g**	cholesterol: **4mg**
sodium: **548mg**	carbs: **12.4g**	dietary fiber: **4.5g**	net carbs: **7.9g**	sugars: **2.9g**	protein: **13.3g**

FAT:	CARBS:	PROTEIN:
70%	14%	15%

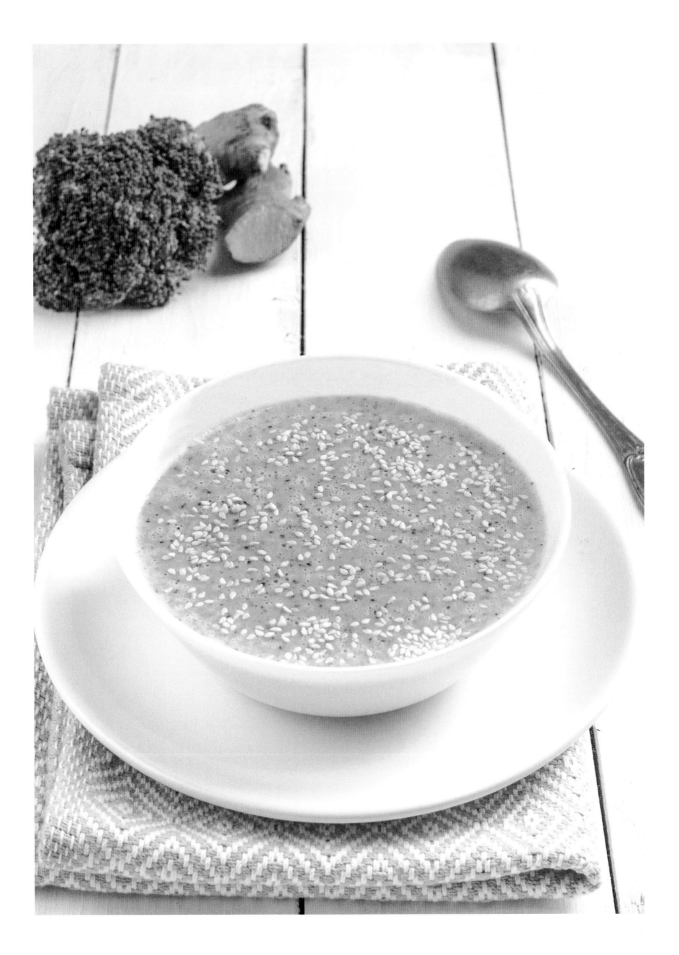

ANTIPASTO SALAD

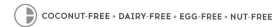 COCONUT-FREE · DAIRY-FREE · EGG-FREE · NUT-FREE

SERVES 4

PREP TIME: 10 minutes

COOK TIME: –

This salad is great on its own, served on a bed of greens, or as a side to something a bit more substantial, like grilled steak.

1 (12-oz/340-g) jar roasted red peppers, drained and roughly chopped

1 (6½-oz/185-g) jar marinated artichoke quarters, drained and roughly chopped

1 (4-oz/113-g) can sliced cremini mushrooms, drained

4 ounces (115 g) salami, sliced

3 tablespoons capers, drained

¾ cup (210 ml) vinaigrette of choice

Place all the ingredients in a large mixing bowl. Toss to coat, then serve.

STORE IT: *Keep in an airtight container in the fridge for up to 3 days.*

MAKE IT AT HOME

Replace store-bought vinaigrette with one of my homemade versions. My favorite for this recipe is the Herby Vinaigrette.

98

Herby Vinaigrette & Marinade

Per serving, made with Herby Vinaigrette & Marinade:

calories: **433**	calories from fat: **338**	total fat: **38.9g**	saturated fat: **7g**	cholesterol: **20mg**
sodium: **1335mg**	carbs: **13.5g**	dietary fiber: **4.4g**	net carbs: **9.1g**	sugars: **5g**	protein: **7.3g**

FAT:	CARBS:	PROTEIN:
81%	**12%**	**7%**

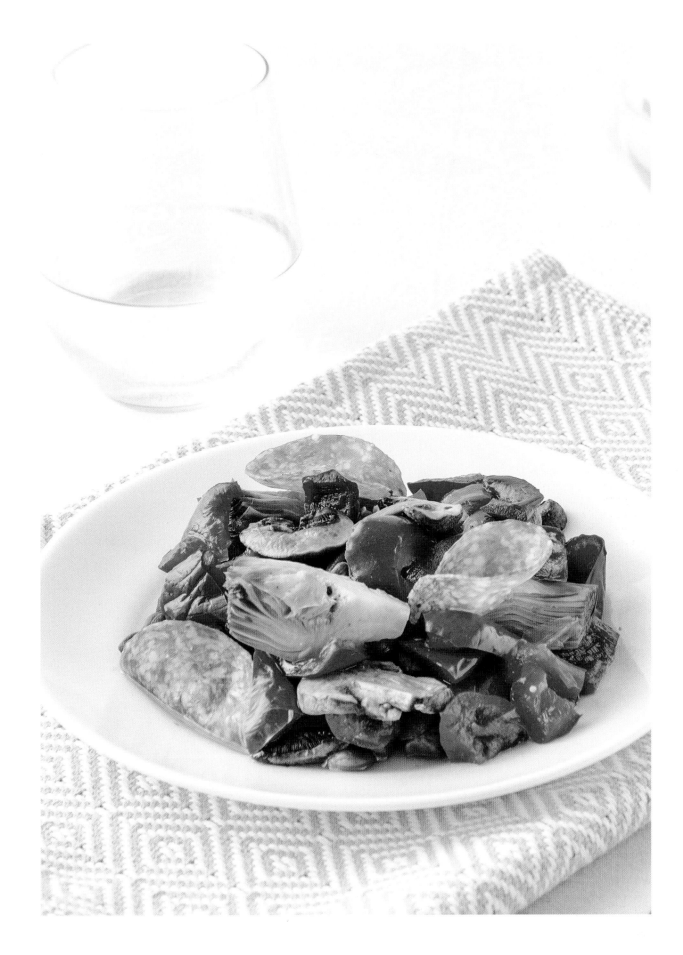

SAUERKRAUT SOUP

COCONUT-FREE • DAIRY-FREE • EGG-FREE • NIGHTSHADE-FREE • NUT-FREE
OPTION: AIP

SERVES 4

PREP TIME: 2 minutes

COOK TIME: 25 minutes

We all have the best intentions to eat as much sauerkraut as we can, but sometimes it just doesn't happen. Adding it to soups and stews is a great way to get your kraut in without having to overdo it on salads and sandwiches.

1 pound (455 g) ground beef

1 small white onion, thinly sliced

1 clove garlic, minced

1¼ teaspoons ground cumin

3 cups (710 ml) beef bone broth

1 cup (235 g) sauerkraut

½ teaspoon finely ground sea salt

1. Place the ground beef, onion, garlic, and cumin in a saucepan. Sauté over medium heat until the onion is translucent, about 10 minutes.

2. Add the broth, sauerkraut, and salt. Cover and cook, still over medium heat, for 15 minutes, until the onion is soft and the soup is fragrant.

3. Divide the soup evenly among 4 bowls and serve.

make it AIP:
Replace the cumin with dried oregano leaves.

PRESSURE COOK IT: *Use the sauté mode for Step 1. For Step 2, place everything in the pressure cooker, seal the lid, and either set to the soup mode or cook on high pressure for 10 minutes. Allow the pressure to release naturally before removing the lid, then serve.*

STORE IT: *Keep in an airtight container in the fridge for up to 3 days or in the freezer for up to 1 month.*

REHEAT IT: *Wonderful enjoyed cold. To reheat, transfer a single serving to a microwave-safe bowl, cover, and microwave for 2½ minutes; or place in a saucepan and reheat over medium heat for 5 minutes.*

THAW IT: *Place in the fridge to thaw completely, then follow the reheating instructions above.*

Per 1-cup/240-ml serving:

calories: **469**	calories from fat: **243**	total fat: **27g**	saturated fat: **8g**	cholesterol: **131mg**
sodium: **4150mg**	carbs: **7.7g**	dietary fiber: **2.2g**	net carbs: **5.5g**	sugars: **3.9g**	protein: **48.8g**

FAT:	CARBS:	PROTEIN:
52%	7%	42%

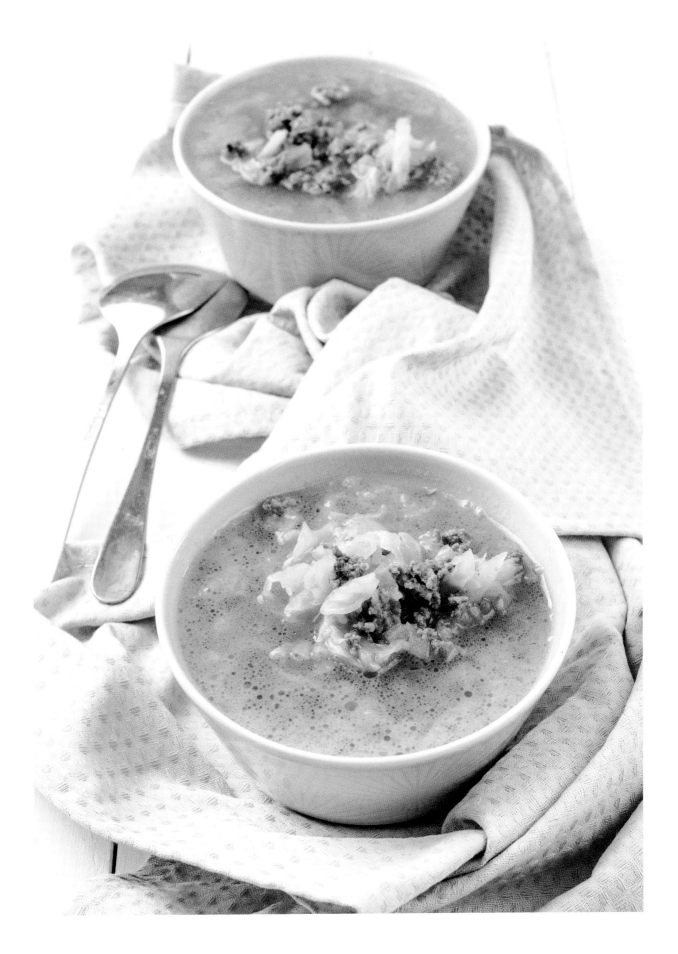

EASY CHOPPED SALAD

COCONUT-FREE • DAIRY-FREE • EGG-FREE • NUT-FREE • VEGAN • VEGETARIAN
OPTIONS: AIP • NIGHTSHADE-FREE

SERVES 1

PREP TIME: 10 minutes

COOK TIME: –

Fresh! Fresh! Sometimes you need a bunch of crunch-tastic veggies, and this salad gives you just that. This recipe is meant to show you just how easy it is to whip up a satisfying keto salad for one, with whatever you have on hand. Get creative here! Use this recipe as a guide, or go wild with your own keto ingredients.

1 small head romaine lettuce, chopped

8 cherry or grape tomatoes, halved

½ cucumber, seeded and chopped

1 celery stick, chopped

¼ cup (45 g) pitted black olives, chopped

2 tablespoons diced red onions

2 tablespoons chopped fresh mint

¼ cup (60 ml) vinaigrette of choice

Place the lettuce in a large serving bowl. Top with the remaining salad ingredients, then drizzle with the vinaigrette and enjoy.

STORE IT: *Store the salad and vinaigrette in separate airtight containers for up to 3 days.*

make it AIP/NIGHTSHADE-FREE:
Omit the tomatoes.

MAKE IT AT HOME

Replace store-bought vinaigrette with one of my homemade versions. My favorite for this recipe is the Basil Vinaigrette.

88

Basil Vinaigrette & Marinade

Per salad, made with Basil Vinaigrette & Marinade:

calories: **476** | calories from fat: **378** | total fat: **42g** | saturated fat: **5.1g** | cholesterol: **0mg**
sodium: **608mg** | carbs: **18g** | dietary fiber: **6.5g** | net carbs: **11.5g** | sugars: **7.1g** | protein: **6.5g**

FAT:	CARBS:	PROTEIN:
79%	**15%**	**5%**

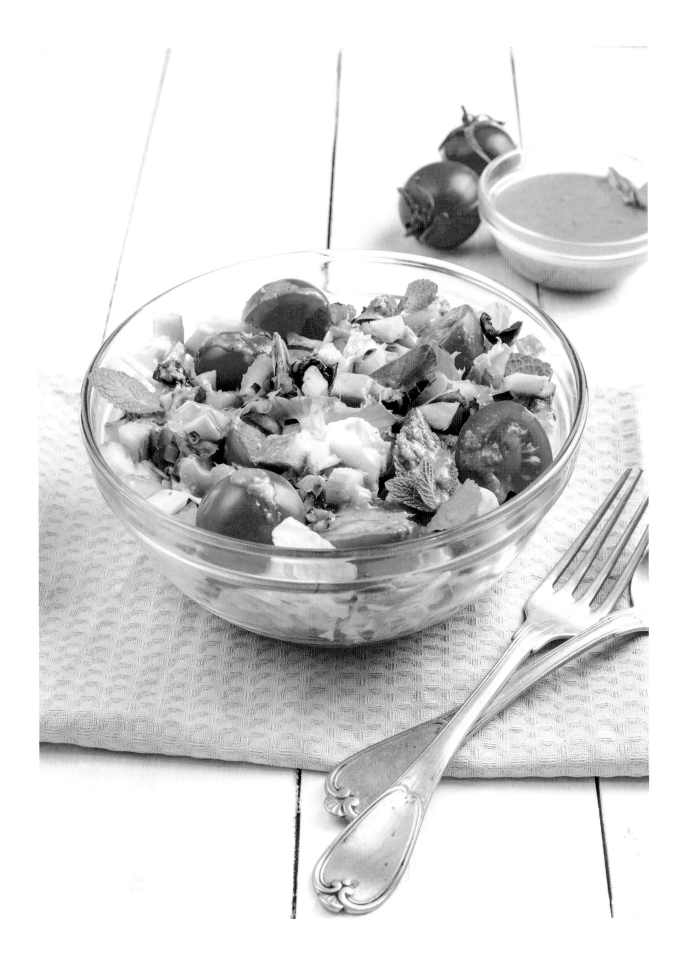

CAJUN SHRIMP SALAD

COCONUT-FREE · DAIRY-FREE · EGG-FREE · NUT-FREE

SERVES 4

PREP TIME: 5 minutes

COOK TIME: 15 minutes

Shrimp is such an underrated protein option, especially when you are on a budget and need a break from bacon and beef. This salad is great warm or cold and is awesome to take with you on a busy day.

1 pound (455 g) large shrimp, peeled and deveined

2 tablespoons avocado oil

2 cloves garlic, minced

2 teaspoons dried basil

1 teaspoon dried thyme leaves

1¾ teaspoons paprika

¾ teaspoon ground black pepper

½ teaspoon finely ground sea salt

⅛ teaspoon cayenne pepper

1 bunch asparagus, woody ends snapped off, cut in half crosswise

SALAD:

1 large head butter lettuce, chopped

1 medium Hass avocado, peeled, pitted, and sliced (about 4 oz/110 g of flesh)

1 small red onion, thinly sliced

½ cup (120 ml) creamy Italian dressing or other creamy salad dressing of choice

1. Place the shrimp, oil, garlic, basil, thyme, paprika, black pepper, salt, and cayenne in a large frying pan. Toss to coat the shrimp, then turn the heat to medium and cook until the shrimp is pink, about 5 minutes.

2. Add the asparagus, cover, and cook for 10 minutes, or until the asparagus is fork-tender.

3. Meanwhile, divide the lettuce, avocado, and onion evenly among 4 salad plates. When the shrimp and asparagus are done, divide the mixture evenly among the plates, drizzle each salad with 2 tablespoons of dressing, and enjoy!

STORE IT: *Keep the shrimp and asparagus mixture, cold salad ingredients, and dressing in separate airtight containers in the fridge for up to 3 days. Do not add the avocado to the recipe until you're ready to serve it.*

PREP AHEAD: *It is always a good idea to have a bottle of creamy Italian dressing on hand—store-bought or homemade!*

MAKE IT AT HOME

Replace store-bought creamy Italian dressing with my homemade version.

94

Creamy Italian Dressing

Per serving, made with homemade creamy Italian dressing:

| calories: **485** | calories from fat: **279** | total fat: **31g** | saturated fat: **4.5g** | cholesterol: **242mg** | FAT: | CARBS: | PROTEIN: |
| sodium: **636mg** | carbs: **19.4g** | dietary fiber: **7.2g** | net carbs: **12.2g** | sugars: **5.4g** | protein: **32.2g** | **58%** | **16%** | **27%** |

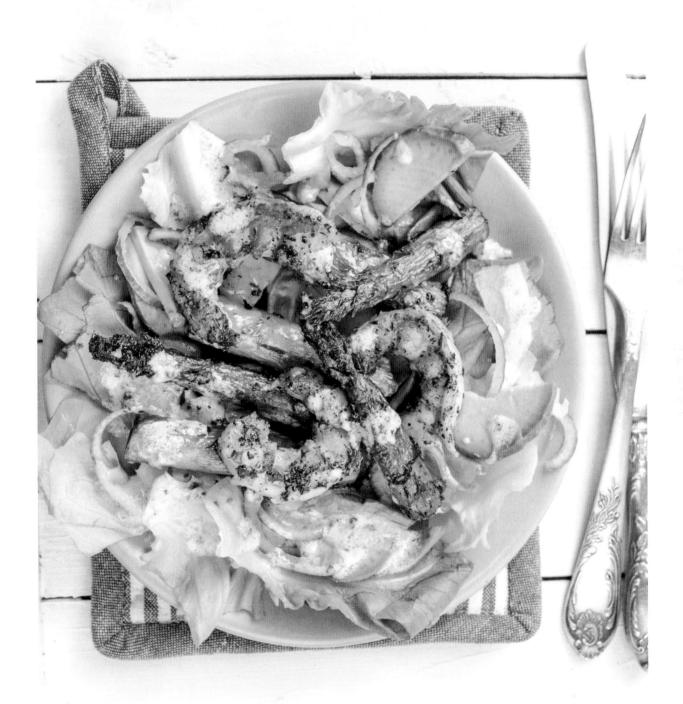

SPECKLED SALAD

COCONUT-FREE • DAIRY-FREE • EGG-FREE • NIGHTSHADE-FREE • NUT-FREE • VEGAN • VEGETARIAN
OPTIONS: AIP • LOW-FODMAP

SERVES 1
PREP TIME: 10 minutes
COOK TIME: –

Have you ever ordered a restaurant salad with high hopes of chowing down on a huge bowl of greens and instead got a measly amount of veggies swimming in a pool of dressing? How restaurants think this is appealing is beyond me.

Well, this salad is the complete opposite. It's loaded with greens, it's packed with nutrients, and you don't need a rubber dinghy to make your way across your plate. It's the queen of all salads, the Mack Daddy of them all.

But maybe you're thinking, "Leanne, it's just a salad...what makes this one so special?"

I wondered the same thing when I had it for the first time in New York in 2012. It was like magic on my taste buds—the lemon, healthy oils, fresh herbs...the...mint? Mint in a salad? Weird. Who else is totally boggled by this concept? You won't be after making this salad. I've been making this very same salad ever since, so I figured it deserved a spot in this book. It's a winner!

If you don't want to make the dressing as outlined below, this salad is also amazing with Lemon Turmeric Dressing & Marinade (page 86) or Honey Mustard Dressing & Marinade (page 78).

DRESSING:

¼ cup (60 ml) lemon juice

2 tablespoons plus 2 teaspoons olive oil

1 teaspoon peeled and minced fresh ginger root

2 cloves garlic, minced

Pinch of finely ground sea salt

Pinch of ground black pepper

SALAD:

1 cup (60 g) destemmed kale leaves, roughly chopped

3 cups (85 g) mixed salad greens

¼ cup (38 g) hulled hemp seeds

Handful of fresh cilantro leaves, chopped

Handful of fresh flat-leaf parsley leaves, chopped

Handful of fresh mint leaves, chopped

1. Place the dressing ingredients in a large salad bowl and stir until blended.

2. For the salad, rinse the chopped kale under hot water for 30 seconds or so to soften it up and make it easier to digest, then dry well. Add the dried kale leaves along with the rest of the salad ingredients to the bowl with the dressing. Toss to coat, then serve.

STORE IT: *Keep the salad, stored separately from the dressing, in airtight containers in the fridge for up to 3 days.*

make it AIP:
Omit the black pepper. Replace the hemp seeds with chopped cooked chicken thighs.

make it LOW-FODMAP:
Replace the olive oil with garlic-infused oil and omit the garlic.

Per salad:

calories: **496**	calories from fat: **367**	total fat: **40.8g**	saturated fat: **6g**	cholesterol: **0mg**	
sodium: **187mg**	carbs: **23g**	dietary fiber: **5.6g**	net carbs: **17.4g**	sugars: **4.4g**	protein: **9.3g**

FAT:	CARBS:	PROTEIN:
74%	18%	8%

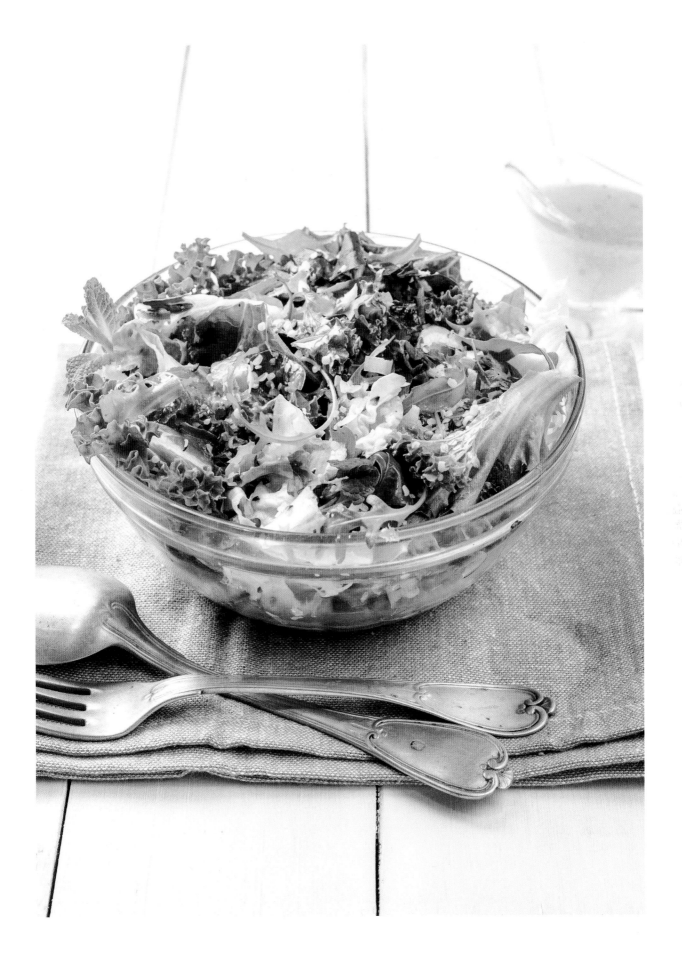

KETO LASAGNA CASSEROLE

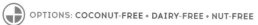 OPTIONS: COCONUT-FREE • DAIRY-FREE • NUT-FREE

SERVES 6

PREP TIME: 10 minutes

COOK TIME: 30 minutes

My husband, Kevin, loves, loves lasagna, even more than pizza. Making pans of lasagna isn't my cup of tea (too much work!), so I started making this super-easy keto lasagna casserole, which we just spoon into bowls and eat. There's more lasagna in his life, and I'm not going crazy in the kitchen slicing and layering ingredients and cooking for days on end.

If dairy is part of your keto diet, or you're just not ready to see what life would be like without dairy, feel free to omit the dairy-free "cheese" topping and top this bad boy with 1 cup (113 g) of shredded mozzarella cheese (simply cook, covered, until the cheese has melted). Alternatively, if you're not a cheese person or you want to shave time off this recipe, simply omit the topping altogether. This lasagna tastes great with or without the topping. How you approach the recipe depends entirely on what you're feeling like when you're making it!

I've shared two cheese sauce–like recipes in this book: the "cheese" topping used here and the Melty "Cheese" in the Noodle Bake recipe on page 243. They are slightly different: This one doesn't require make-ahead preparation, calls for egg yolks only, and has no starch, whereas the Melty "Cheese" requires that you heat it up on the stove, calls for whole eggs, and contains starch. Both of them are tasty—they are just different ways of preparing a similar thing.

MEAT SAUCE:

3 tablespoons avocado oil, coconut oil, or ghee

1 pound (455 g) ground beef

1 (14½-oz/410-g) can fire-roasted crushed tomatoes

1 (6-oz/170-g) can tomato paste

2 teaspoons apple cider vinegar

2 teaspoons dried basil

1 teaspoon garlic powder

1 teaspoon dried oregano leaves

1 bay leaf

¾ teaspoon finely ground sea salt

½ teaspoon onion powder

¼ teaspoon red pepper flakes

¼ teaspoon dried rosemary leaves

¼ teaspoon dried thyme leaves

"CHEESE" TOPPING:

¼ cup (60 ml) avocado oil or melted coconut oil or ghee

¼ cup (60 ml) nondairy milk

¼ cup (17 g) nutritional yeast

4 large egg yolks

1 teaspoon Dijon mustard

1 teaspoon lemon juice

½ teaspoon garlic powder

½ teaspoon onion powder

¼ cup (10 g) fresh parsley leaves, finely chopped, for garnish

1. Heat the oil in a large frying pan over medium heat. Add the ground beef and cook until no longer pink, 5 to 7 minutes, stirring to crumble the meat as it cooks.

2. Add the crushed tomatoes, tomato paste, vinegar, basil, garlic powder, oregano, bay leaf, salt, onion powder, red pepper flakes, rosemary, and thyme. Cover and cook over low heat for 15 minutes.

3. Meanwhile, prepare the "cheese" topping: Place all the ingredients in a small bowl and whisk until smooth.

4. When the meat sauce is done, remove the bay leaf, smooth out the meat, and pour the "cheese" topping over the top.

5. Cover and cook on low for 10 minutes, or until the topping is cooked through and no longer gooey.

6. Divide among 6 plates or bowls and sprinkle with the parsley.

Per serving, made with avocado oil and almond milk:

						FAT:	CARBS:	PROTEIN:
calories: **507**	calories from fat: **293**	total fat: **32.6g**	saturated fat: **6.8g**	cholesterol: **249mg**		**58%**	**14%**	**28%**
sodium: **545mg**	carbs: **18.1g**	dietary fiber: **5.2g**	net carbs: **12.9g**	sugars: **8.3g**	protein: **35.3g**			

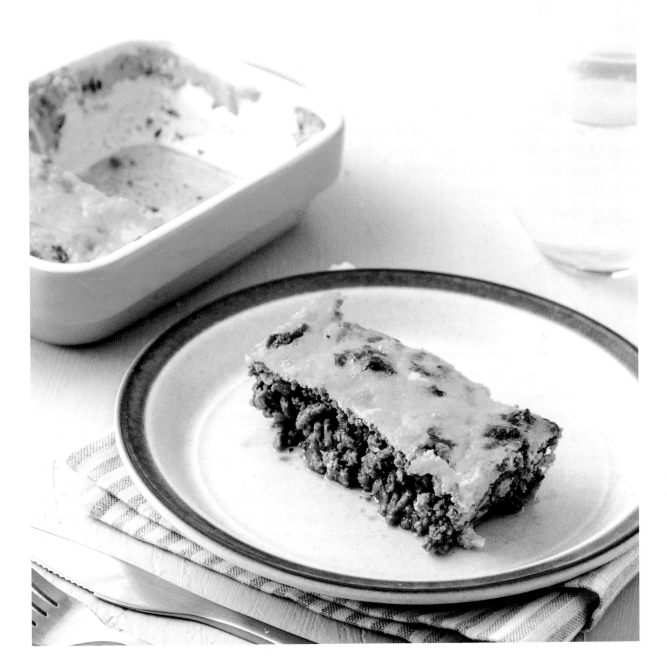

make it COCONUT-FREE:
Do not use coconut oil. Opt for a nondairy milk not made from coconut, like almond or hazelnut milk.

make it DAIRY-FREE:
Do not use ghee.

make it NUT-FREE:
Opt for a nondairy milk not made from nuts, like coconut milk.

PRESSURE COOK IT: *Use the sauté mode for Step 1. Add the ingredients listed in Step 2, then seal the lid and cook on high pressure for 10 minutes. Meanwhile, complete Step 3. Allow the pressure to release naturally before removing the lid from the pressure cooker, then complete Step 4. Set the lid back on but leave the cooker off. Allow to sit for 10 minutes, until the topping is cooked through, then serve.*

STORE IT: *Keep in an airtight container in the fridge for up to 3 days or in the freezer for up to 1 month.*

REHEAT IT: *Transfer a single serving to a microwave-safe dish, cover, and microwave for 2 minutes, or place in a saucepan, cover, and reheat over medium heat for 5 minutes.*

THAW IT: *Place in the fridge and allow to defrost completely, then follow the reheating instructions above.*

KALE SALAD WITH SPICY LIME-TAHINI DRESSING

 COCONUT-FREE • DAIRY-FREE • EGG-FREE • NUT-FREE • VEGAN • VEGETARIAN

SERVES 4

PREP TIME: 15 minutes

COOK TIME: –

If you're not into kale, look beyond this salad recipe and appreciate the dressing that pairs with it. It's off the hook! It's awesome with veggies, pork rinds—anything, really. If tahini doesn't excite you like it does me, you can swap out the dressing with 1 cup (240 ml) of Thai Dressing (page 72).

DRESSING:

½ cup (120 ml) avocado oil

¼ cup (60 ml) lime juice

¼ cup (60 ml) tahini

2 cloves garlic, minced

1 jalapeño pepper, seeded and finely diced

Handful of fresh cilantro leaves, chopped

½ teaspoon ground cumin

½ teaspoon finely ground sea salt

¼ teaspoon red pepper flakes

SALAD:

6 cups (360 g) destemmed kale leaves, roughly chopped

12 radishes, thinly sliced

1 green bell pepper, sliced

1 medium Hass avocado, peeled, pitted, and cubed (about 4 oz/110 g of flesh)

¼ cup (30 g) hulled pumpkin seeds

1. Make the dressing: Place the dressing ingredients in a medium-sized bowl and whisk to combine. Set aside.

2. Make the salad: Rinse the kale under hot water for about 30 seconds to soften it and make it easier to digest. Dry the kale well, then place it in a large salad bowl. Add the remaining salad ingredients and toss to combine.

3. Divide the salad evenly among 4 bowls. Drizzle each bowl with ¼ cup (60 ml) of the dressing and serve.

STORE IT: *Keep the salad and dressing in separate airtight containers in the fridge for up to 5 days. Do not add the avocado to the recipe until you're ready to serve it.*

Per serving:

calories: **517** | calories from fat: **423** | total fat: **47g** | saturated fat: **6g** | cholesterol: **0mg**
sodium: **373mg** | carbs: **20.9g** | dietary fiber: **9.4g** | net carbs: **11.5g** | sugars: **3.9g** | protein: **10.7g**

FAT:	CARBS:	PROTEIN:
79%	**15%**	**6%**

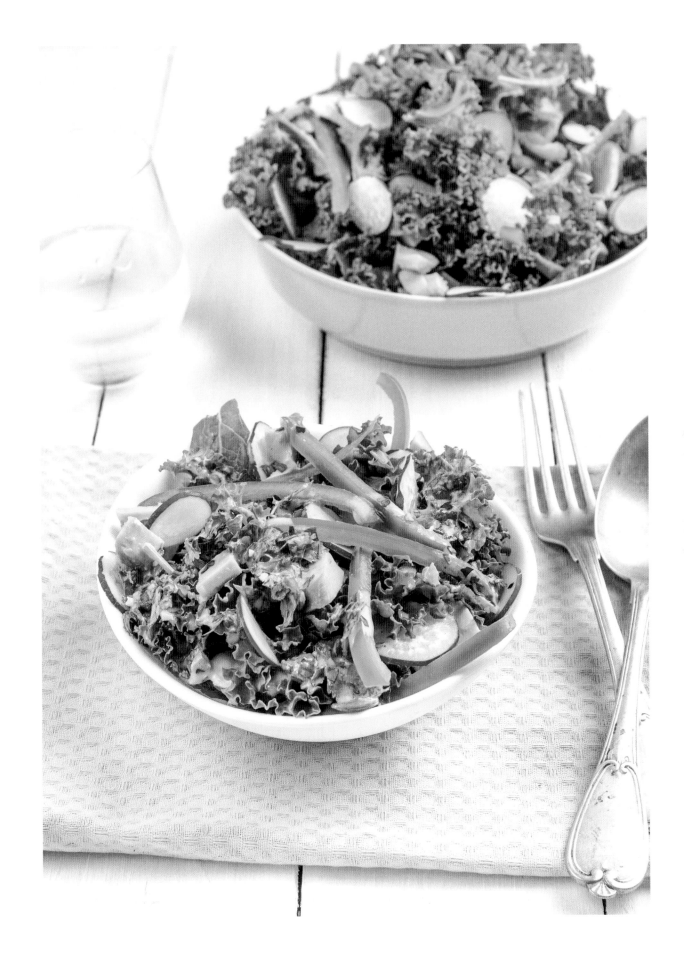

ZUCCHINI PASTA SALAD

COCONUT-FREE • DAIRY-FREE • LOW-FODMAP • VEGETARIAN
OPTIONS: EGG-FREE • NUT-FREE • VEGAN

SERVES 4

PREP TIME: 5 minutes

COOK TIME: –

When you're in an all-plant mood, this recipe is a saving grace!

4 medium zucchinis, spiral sliced

12 ounces (340 g) pitted black olives, cut in half lengthwise

1 pint (290 g) cherry tomatoes, cut in half lengthwise

½ cup (75 g) pine nuts

¼ cup plus 2 tablespoons (55 g) sesame seeds

⅔ cup (160 ml) creamy Italian dressing or other creamy salad dressing of choice

Place all the ingredients in a large mixing bowl. Toss to coat, then divide evenly between 4 serving plates or bowls.

STORE IT: *Keep in an airtight container in the fridge for up to 3 days.*

make it **EGG-FREE/VEGAN:**
Make sure the creamy Italian dressing you're using is egg-free, or use another dressing of your choice.

make it **NUT-FREE:**
Omit the pine nuts.

MAKE IT AT HOME

Replace store-bought creamy Italian dressing with my homemade version.

Creamy Italian Dressing

Per serving, made with homemade creamy Italian dressing:

calories: **562** | calories from fat: **471** | total fat: **53g** | saturated fat: **6.3g** | cholesterol: **2.7mg**
sodium: **886mg** | carbs: **22g** | dietary fiber: **8.5g** | net carbs: **13.5g** | sugars: **6.7g** | protein: **8.9g**

FAT:	CARBS:	PROTEIN:
79%	**15%**	**6%**

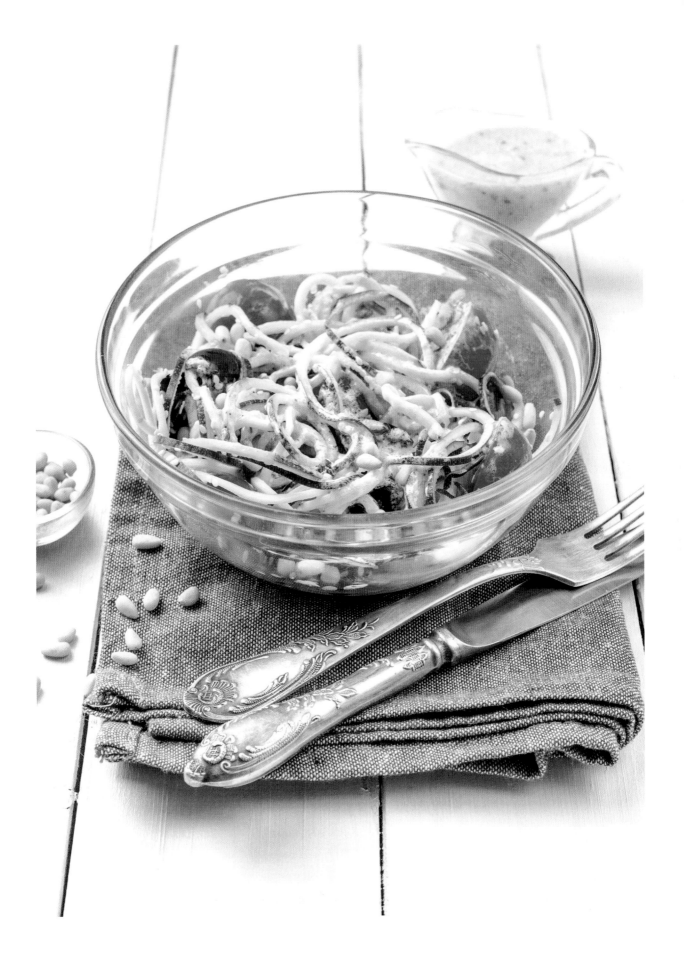

COCONUT RED CURRY SOUP

 DAIRY-FREE • EGG-FREE • NUT-FREE
OPTION: AIP

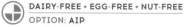

SERVES 4
PREP TIME: 10 minutes
COOK TIME: 20 minutes

This soup is everything on a cold day when all you want is a warm, comforting lunch. I make multiple batches in one day and freeze individual servings for quick and easy lunches throughout the week. Don't worry, the zucchini noodles and toppings will make it through the freezer and back!

¼ cup (55 g) coconut oil, or ¼ cup (60 ml) avocado oil

2 cloves garlic, minced

1 (2-in/5-cm) piece fresh ginger root, peeled and minced

1 pound (455 g) boneless, skinless chicken thighs, cut into small cubes

2 cups (475 ml) chicken bone broth

1 cup (240 ml) full-fat coconut milk

⅓ cup (80 g) red curry paste

1 teaspoon finely ground sea salt

FOR SERVING:

2 medium zucchinis, spiral sliced

3 green onions, sliced

¼ cup (15 g) fresh cilantro leaves, chopped

make it AIP:
Omit the red curry paste.

1. Heat the oil in a large saucepan over medium-low heat. Add the garlic and ginger and cook until fragrant, about 2 minutes.

2. Add the chicken thighs, broth, coconut milk, curry paste, and salt. Stir to combine, cover, and bring to a light simmer over medium-high heat. Once simmering, reduce the heat and continue to simmer for 15 minutes, until the flavors meld.

3. Divide the spiral-sliced zucchinis among 4 bowls and top with the curry soup. Sprinkle with the green onions and cilantro before serving.

PRESSURE COOK IT: *For Step 1, use the sauté mode to cook the garlic and ginger until fragrant. Then add the rest of the soup ingredients, seal the lid, and either set to the soup mode or cook on high pressure for 10 minutes. Allow the pressure to release naturally before removing the lid, then pick up with Step 3.*

STORE IT: *Keep in an airtight container in the fridge for up to 3 days or in the freezer for up to 1 month.*

REHEAT IT: *Transfer a single serving to a microwave-safe bowl, cover, and microwave for 2 minutes; or place in a saucepan and reheat over low heat for 5 minutes.*

THAW IT: *Place in the fridge and allow to defrost completely, then follow the reheating instructions above.*

Per 1¼-cup/300-ml serving, made with coconut oil:

calories: **567**	calories from fat: **363**	total fat: **40.3g**	saturated fat: **27.2g**	cholesterol: **101mg**
sodium: **168mg**	carbs: **11.3g**	dietary fiber: **1.5g**	net carbs: **9.8g**	sugars: **3g**	protein: **40g**

FAT:	CARBS:	PROTEIN:
64%	8%	28%

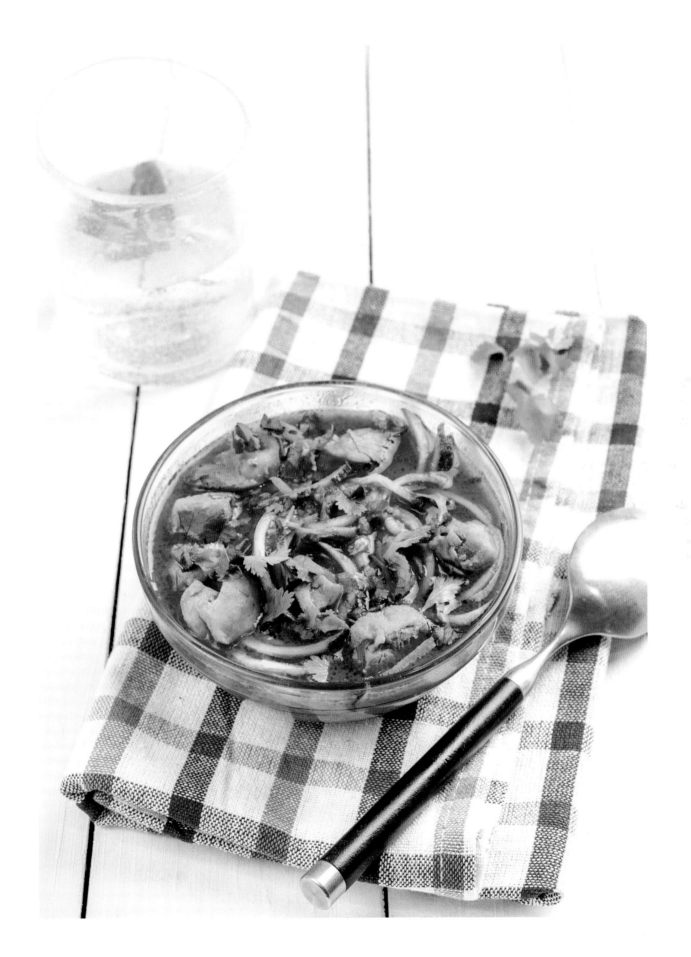

CHIMICHURRI STEAK BUNWICHES

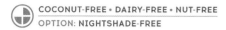 COCONUT-FREE • DAIRY-FREE • NUT-FREE
OPTION: NIGHTSHADE-FREE

**MAKES 4 bunwiches
(1 per serving)**

PREP TIME: 10 minutes
(not including time to
make chimichurri or cook
steak)

COOK TIME: 5 minutes

Calling all sandwich lovers! This book shows you how to make keto sandwiches with lettuce leaves, avocado halves, and even pounded chicken thighs, but have you made them with eggs? If you're like me and you don't like spending a lot of time baking, all these solutions for sandwich making are answers to your frustrations. No more making keto-friendly buns with a bunch of random flours and extra ingredients. Have eggs? You can make this!

Also, if you're like our keto household and you always have a bit of leftover steak from last night's meal, you'll love this lunch recipe. It does a great job of sprucing up leftover steak in a pinch. However, if you don't have leftover steak lying around begging to be made into a sandwich, simply grill some up. The steak can be served hot or cold in this sandwich.

If the chimichurri isn't calling your name, replace it with 1 cup (240 ml) of Bacon Dressing (page 82) or Ranch Dressing (page 76).

8 large eggs

½ teaspoon garlic powder

½ teaspoon onion powder

¼ teaspoon finely ground sea salt

¼ teaspoon ground black pepper

2 tablespoons avocado oil

1 cup (212 g) Chimichurri (page 284), divided

1 pound (455 g) skirt steak or flank steak, grilled and thinly sliced

4 cups (113 g) mixed greens

SPECIAL EQUIPMENT:

8 mason jar lid rings without the tops

make it NIGHTSHADE-FREE:
Follow the nightshade-free instructions in the chimichurri recipe.

1. Crack the eggs into a medium-sized bowl. Add the garlic powder, onion powder, salt, and pepper and whisk until just combined.

2. Drizzle the oil into a large frying pan. Before heating, use your fingers to oil the insides of the lid rings. Place the oiled rings flat side down in the pan and turn the heat to medium-low. Allow the pan to heat up for 1 minute before dividing the egg mixture among the rings, pouring about ¼ cup (60 ml) into each ring, or until the egg mixture just reaches the rim.

3. Cover and cook for 5 minutes, or until the eggs are cooked through. Remove from the heat and let sit for 2 minutes, then use a spatula to remove the lid rings and cooked eggs from the pan. Carefully remove the egg buns from the rings.

4. To assemble the bunwiches, spoon 2 tablespoons of the chimichurri onto an egg bun, then place one-quarter of the steak on the chimichurri. Take a second egg bun and place it on top of the steak. Repeat to make a total of 4 sandwiches.

5. Serve each bunwich with 1 cup of the greens, and top each portion of greens with 2 tablespoons of chimichurri. Enjoy!

Per sandwich, made with skirt steak:

calories: **593** | calories from fat: **386** | total fat: **43g** | saturated fat: **10.3g** | cholesterol: **435mg**
sodium: **411mg** | carbs: **6.2g** | dietary fiber: **1.9g** | net carbs: **4.3g** | sugars: **2.1g** | protein: **45.3g**

FAT:	CARBS:	PROTEIN:
65%	4%	31%

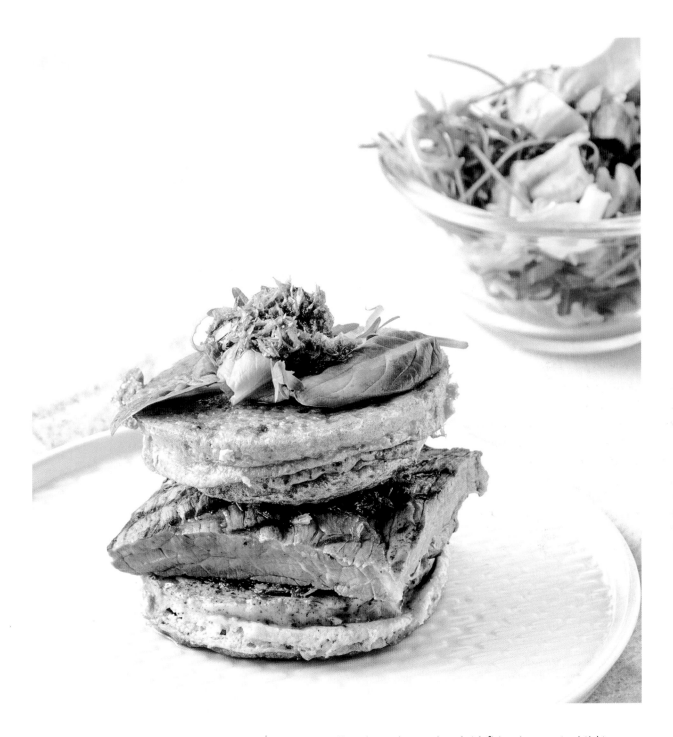

STORE IT: *Keep the egg buns and sandwich fixings in separate airtight containers in the fridge for up to 3 days. The steak and egg buns can be frozen for up to 1 month.*

THAW IT: *Place the steak in the fridge and the buns on the counter and allow to defrost completely. Once defrosted, reheat in a frying pan over medium heat for 2 to 3 minutes.*

PREP AHEAD: *Make a whole batch of egg buns, freeze them individually or layered between sheets of parchment paper, and take out two at a time anytime you want a sandwich. Purchase steak already cooked, or grill up a bunch and store it in the freezer until ready to use.*

MEXICAN CHICKEN SOUP

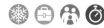

EGG-FREE • NUT-FREE

OPTIONS: COCONUT-FREE • DAIRY-FREE

SERVES 4

PREP TIME: 5 minutes

COOK TIME: 20 minutes

The first time I made this soup, I was watching Riverdale *(guilty pleasure) and got so wrapped up in "who is the Black Hood?!" that I added both ground beef and chicken breast to the pressure cooker and set it to the soup mode. I didn't realize my mistake until I opened the lid. I can tell you that this soup is good with both proteins, but for simplicity's sake, I made it again with just chicken.*

The cheese is not essential whatsoever. The soup is fabulous with or without it. If you like dairy and it's part of your keto diet, load up the soup with cheese! If you like cheese but it doesn't like you, opt for a dairy-free shredded cheese. Or, if you would just rather not, omit it and you'll still love the end result.

¼ cup (60 ml) avocado oil

1 small white onion, diced

2 cloves garlic, minced

1 red bell pepper, diced

1 pound (455 g) boneless, skinless chicken breasts, thinly sliced

1 (14½-oz/410-g) can fire-roasted whole tomatoes

1½ cups (355 ml) chicken bone broth

1 cup (240 ml) full-fat coconut milk

1 tablespoon apple cider vinegar

1 teaspoon ground cumin

1 teaspoon dried oregano leaves

1 teaspoon paprika

¾ teaspoon finely ground sea salt

1 cup (140 g) shredded cheddar cheese (dairy-free or regular) (optional)

2 medium Hass avocados, peeled, pitted, and sliced (about 8 oz/220 g of flesh)

Handful of fresh cilantro leaves

1. Heat the oil in a large saucepan over medium heat. Add the onion, garlic, and bell pepper and sauté until fragrant, about 5 minutes.

2. Add the chicken, tomatoes, broth, coconut milk, vinegar, cumin, oregano, paprika, and salt. Stir to combine, cover, and bring to a light simmer over medium-high heat. Once simmering, reduce the heat and continue to simmer for 15 minutes, until the chicken is cooked through and the bell peppers are soft.

3. When the soup is done, divide evenly among 4 bowls. Top each bowl with ¼ cup (35 g) of the cheese (if using), one-quarter of the avocado slices, and a sprinkle of cilantro.

PRESSURE COOK IT: *Use the sauté mode for Step 1, then place everything listed in Step 2 in the pressure cooker, seal the lid, and either set to the soup mode or cook on high pressure for 10 minutes. Allow the pressure to release naturally before removing the lid, then pick up with Step 3.*

STORE IT: *Keep in an airtight container in the fridge for up to 3 days or in the freezer for up to 1 month. Do not add the avocado to the soup until you're ready to serve it.*

REHEAT IT: *Transfer a single serving to a microwave-safe bowl, cover, and microwave for 2 minutes; or place in a saucepan and reheat over low heat for 5 minutes. It's best to add the fresh ingredients after reheating, but it's okay if they're already mixed in and reheated together.*

THAW IT: *Place in the fridge and allow to defrost completely, then follow the reheating instructions above.*

make it COCONUT-FREE:
Replace the coconut milk with the milk of your choice. If using dairy-free cheese, make sure it's also coconut-free.

make it DAIRY-FREE:
Use dairy-free cheese.

Per 1½-cup/350-ml serving, made with dairy-free cheese:

| calories: 602 | calories from fat: 389 | total fat: 44.6g | saturated fat: 18.3g | cholesterol: 83mg |
| sodium: 805mg | carbs: 21g | dietary fiber: 13g | net carbs: 8g | sugars: 5g | protein: 31.4g |

| FAT: | CARBS: | PROTEIN: |
| 66% | 14% | 21% |

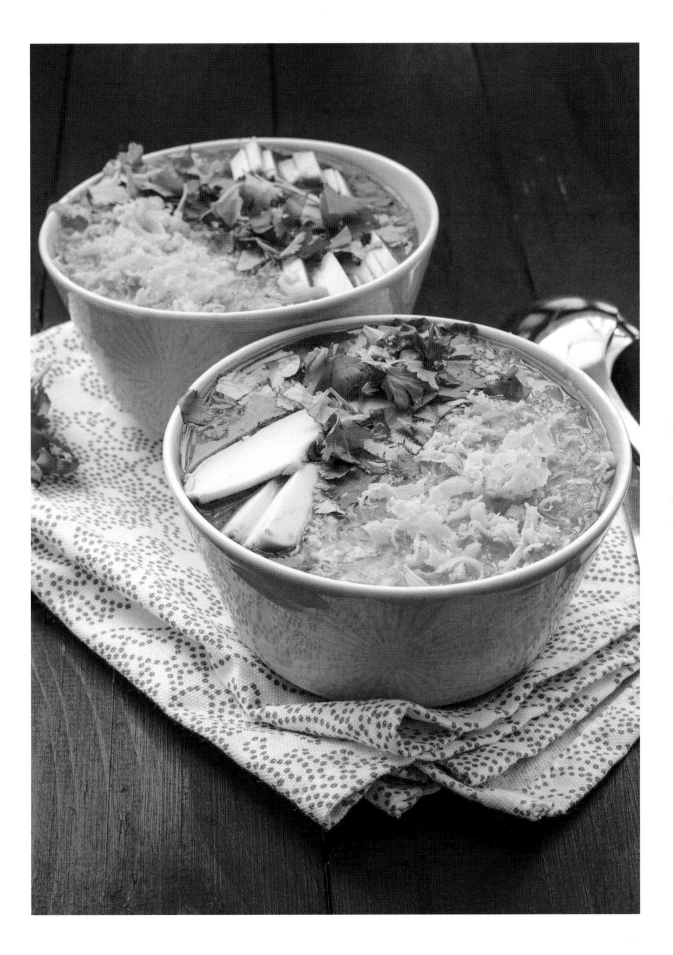

SAMMIES WITH BASIL MAYO

COCONUT-FREE • DAIRY-FREE • NIGHTSHADE-FREE • NUT-FREE
OPTION: EGG-FREE

**MAKES 2 sandwiches
(1 per serving)**

PREP TIME: 10 minutes

COOK TIME: –

Who doesn't love a good sandwich? When there's a crazy-good sauce all up in there, it's the best lunch a girl could ask for. For the deli turkey and ham, opt for nitrate-free versions if you can. If you're not feeling the Basil Mayo, you can replace it with ½ cup (120 ml) of Basil Vinaigrette & Marinade (page 88).

BASIL MAYO:

½ cup (105 g) mayonnaise

8 large fresh basil leaves, finely chopped

1 tablespoon lemon juice

1 clove garlic, minced

¼ teaspoon finely ground sea salt

Pinch of ground black pepper

SAMMIES:

1 small head iceberg lettuce

4 slices deli turkey

4 slices deli ham

1 medium Hass avocado, peeled, pitted, and sliced (about 4 oz/110 g of flesh)

1. Place the ingredients for the basil mayo in a small bowl and whisk to combine.

2. Cut the head of lettuce in half, then cut each half in half again so you have 4 wedges.

3. Set a lettuce wedge on its side on a plate and layer on 2 slices of turkey, 2 slices of ham, and half of the avocado slices. Top with half of the basil mayo, then set a second lettuce wedge on top, placing it so that the thick edge of the top wedge is aligned with the thin edge of the bottom wedge. (This will give your sandwich an even thickness, making it much easier to eat!)

4. Repeat with the remaining lettuce wedges, sandwich fixings, and basil mayo and enjoy.

MAKE IT AT HOME

Replace store-bought mayonnaise with my homemade version.

104

Mayonnaise

STORE IT: *Keep in an airtight container in the fridge for up to 3 days.*

PREP AHEAD: *Make the basil mayo up to 3 days ahead of time. The only concern here is that the basil in it can go bad, so if you're prepping it ahead, enjoy the sandwiches on the third day at the latest.*

make it EGG-FREE:
Use egg-free mayonnaise (see recipe on page 102) or replace the basil mayo with Basil Vinaigrette & Marinade (page 88).

Per sandwich, made with homemade mayonnaise:

calories: **653**	calories from fat: **514**	total fat: **57.1g**	saturated fat: **10g**	cholesterol: **78mg**	FAT:	CARBS:	PROTEIN:
sodium: **1921mg**	carbs: **16g**	dietary fiber: **6.4g**	net carbs: **9.6g**	sugars: **5.4g**	protein: **18.8g**	79%	10%	12%

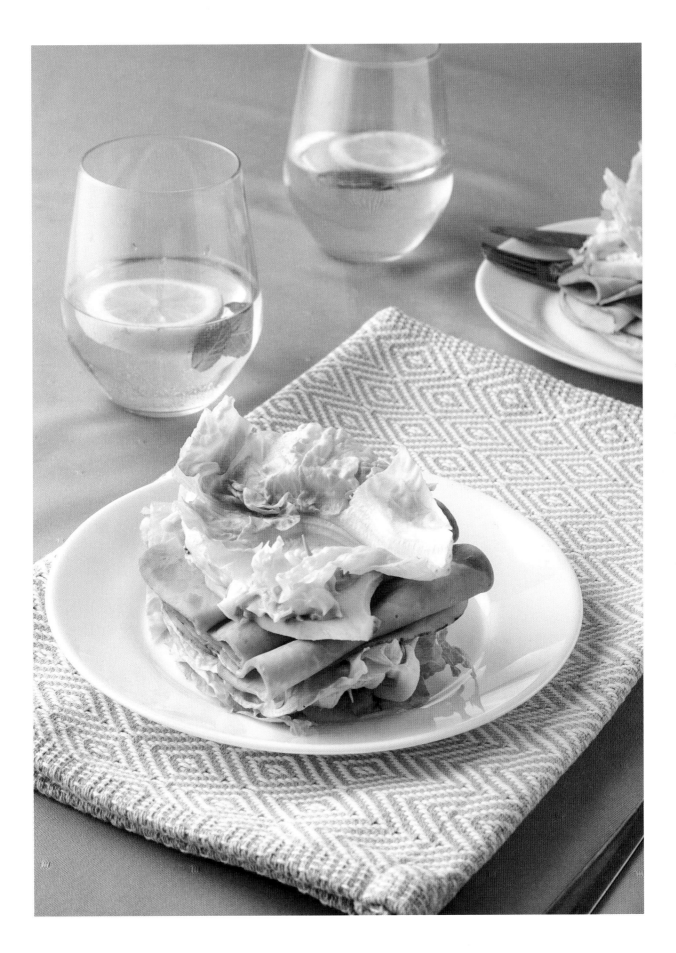

CREAM CHEESE MEAT BAGELS

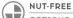 NUT-FREE

OPTIONS: COCONUT-FREE • DAIRY-FREE • LOW-FODMAP • NIGHTSHADE-FREE

MAKES 6 bagel sandwiches (1 per serving)

PREP TIME: 10 minutes

COOK TIME: 35 minutes

Meat bagels have become quite popular over the years, and I've eaten my fair share. The thing I don't like about the classic recipe is that you have to cut the bagel in half just perfectly to make a sandwich—and ground meat doesn't like to be cut evenly. Having to cut anything in half perfectly always makes me a little nervous, especially when failure means a broken sandwich. My solution? Make two thinner bagels for each sandwich rather than one fat one that requires slicing.

If dairy is part of your keto diet, feel free to use an equal amount of shredded cheddar or Parmesan cheese in place of the nutritional yeast.

If you don't want to make or buy cream cheese for this recipe, swap out the cream cheese for mayonnaise (page 104).

BAGELS:

2 tablespoons coconut oil, avocado oil, or ghee

2 small white onions, minced

2 cloves garlic, minced

2 pounds (910 g) ground pork

2 large eggs

½ cup (120 ml) tomato sauce

½ cup (35 g) nutritional yeast

2 teaspoons paprika

1½ teaspoons finely ground sea salt

½ teaspoon ground black pepper

SANDWICH FILLINGS:

¾ cup (6 oz/205 g) chive and onion cream cheese (dairy-free or regular)

½ cucumber, thinly sliced

6 ounces (170 g) sliced deli ham, chicken, or turkey

1 cup (50 g) alfalfa sprouts

MAKE IT AT HOME

Replace store-bought chive and onion cream cheese with my homemade dairy-free version.

Chive & Onion Cream Cheese

1. Heat the oil in a small frying pan over medium heat. Add the onions and garlic and sauté for 10 minutes, or until fragrant.

2. Preheat the oven to 400°F (205°C). Line 2 rimmed baking sheets with parchment paper or silicone baking mats.

3. Place the ground pork, eggs, tomato sauce, nutritional yeast, paprika, salt, and pepper in a large bowl. When the onions are cooked, add them to the bowl and mix with your hands until fully incorporated.

4. Divide the meat mixture into 12 equal portions. Taking one portion at a time, roll it into a ball between your hands and press onto the lined baking sheet. Use your fingers to shape the meat mixture into a circle, keeping the thickness to about ½ inch (1.25 cm), then use your pointer finger to create a 1½-inch (4-cm) hole in the middle of the patty. Repeat with remaining meat mixture to make a total of 12 bagels, placing 6 bagels on each baking sheet.

5. Bake the bagels for 20 to 25 minutes, until the internal temperature reaches 160°F (71°C).

6. Remove from the oven and allow to cool on the pans for 30 minutes before assembling the sandwiches.

7. To assemble, spread 2 tablespoons of the cream cheese on one of the bagels. Layer on one-sixth of the cucumber slices, followed by 1 ounce (28 g) of deli meat, finishing with one-sixth of the sprouts. Top with a second bagel and repeat with remaining ingredients to make a total of 6 bagel sandwiches.

Per bagel sandwich, made with coconut oil and homemade Chive & Onion Cream Cheese:

calories: **670** | calories from fat: **365** | total fat: **41g** | saturated fat: **14.7g** | cholesterol: **266mg**
sodium: **1134mg** | carbs: **14.7g** | dietary fiber: **3.7g** | net carbs: **11g** | sugars: **3g** | protein: **60.7g**

FAT:	CARBS:	PROTEIN:
55%	9%	36%

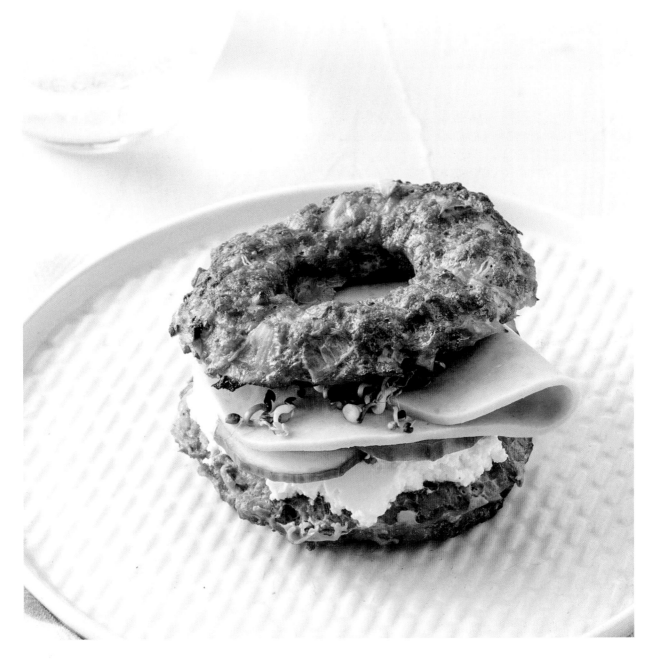

make it COCONUT-FREE:
Use avocado oil or ghee.

make it DAIRY-FREE:
Do not use ghee. Use dairy-free cream cheese.

make it LOW-FODMAP:
Omit the sautéed onions and garlic.

make it NIGHTSHADE-FREE:
Replace the tomato sauce with your favorite creamy salad dressing or ¼ cup (55 g) mayonnaise. Omit the paprika.

STORE IT: *Keep in an airtight container in the fridge for up to 3 days. The bagels can be frozen for up to 1 month.*

THAW IT: *Place the bagels in the fridge and allow to defrost completely before using.*

BLT-STUFFED AVOCADOS

COCONUT-FREE • DAIRY-FREE • EGG-FREE • NUT-FREE

OPTIONS: AIP • NIGHTSHADE-FREE

SERVES 4

PREP TIME: 10 minutes (not including time to cook bacon)

COOK TIME: –

This recipe is filled with all the favorites, but you can have fun with it and stuff the avocados with whatever you have kicking around. I add rotisserie chicken to my BLT mix to make it extra hearty. If you don't have rotisserie chicken, any leftover cooked chicken will do the trick. You can use any salad dressing you like, creamy or vinaigrette style, store-bought or homemade. My favorite homemade dressings for this recipe are Herby Vinaigrette & Marinade (page 98), Lemon Turmeric Dressing & Marinade (page 86), and Ranch Dressing (page 76).

1 (1½-lb/680-g) rotisserie chicken

4 lettuce leaves, chopped

4 strips bacon (about 4 oz/112 g), cooked until crispy and crumbled

1 small tomato, diced

¼ teaspoon ground black pepper

4 medium Hass avocados, peeled and pitted (about 16 oz/455 g of flesh)

½ cup (120 ml) salad dressing of choice

1. Remove the chicken skin and meat from the bones, then chop or tear the meat and skin into bite-sized pieces. Put the pieces of chicken and skin in a medium-sized bowl. Add the lettuce, bacon, tomato, and pepper and toss to combine.

2. Cut the avocados in half horizontally, remove the pits, and place on a clean plate. Open them up like burger buns, leaving 8 exposed avocado halves ready to be filled.

3. Stuff the avocado halves with the filling mixture. Drizzle each stuffed avocado with 1 tablespoon of dressing and enjoy immediately.

make it AIP:
Omit the tomato and black pepper.

make it NIGHTSHADE-FREE:
Omit the tomato.

STORE IT: *Keep in an airtight container in the fridge for up to 3 days. Do not stuff the avocados with the BLT filling mixture or drizzle with the dressing until ready to serve.*

Per serving, made with Herby Vinaigrette & Marinade:

calories: **675** | calories from fat: **394** | total fat: **44g** | saturated fat: **9.8g** | cholesterol: **155mg** | sodium: **1360mg** | carbs: **15.6g** | dietary fiber: **8.2g** | net carbs: **7.4g** | sugars: **1.3g** | protein: **54.2g**

FAT:	CARBS:	PROTEIN:
59%	9%	32%

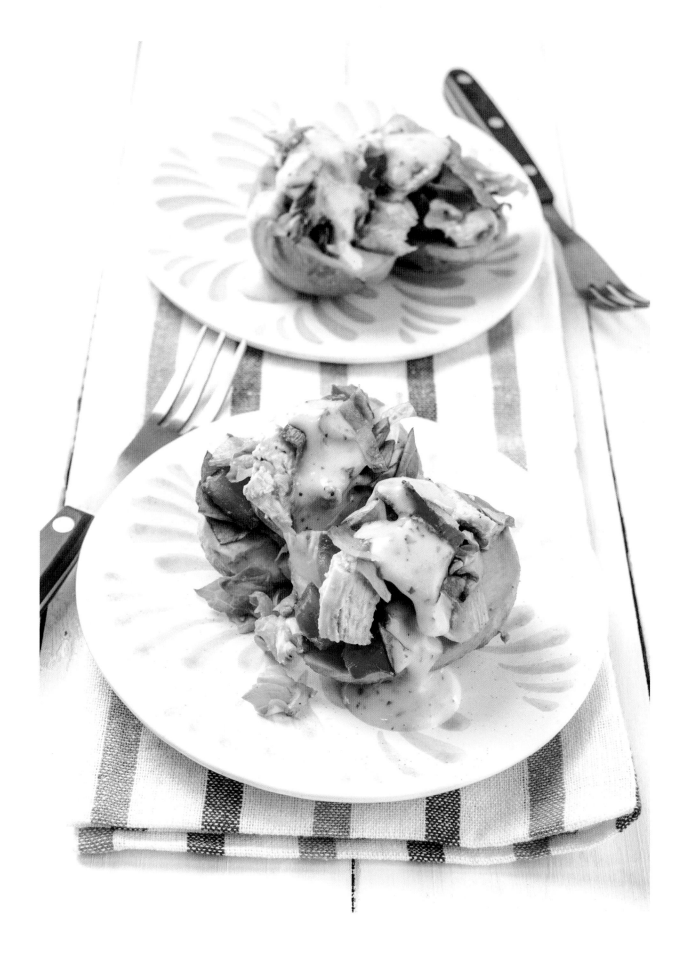

BROCCOLI TABBOULEH WITH GREEK CHICKEN THIGHS

 COCONUT-FREE • DAIRY-FREE • EGG-FREE • NUT-FREE
OPTIONS: AIP • NIGHTSHADE-FREE

SERVES 6

PREP TIME: 15 minutes, plus 4 hours to marinate chicken

COOK TIME: 30 minutes

Chopping the broccoli in two batches ensures that the florets are broken down perfectly for this quick salad. Serve it with the Greek chicken or go without. Either way, you'll love it!

If you have a batch of Herby Vinaigrette & Marinade (page 98) in the fridge, you can marinate the chicken in ½ cup (120 ml) of that instead.

GREEK CHICKEN THIGHS:

6 bone-in, skin-on chicken thighs (about 2½ lbs/1.2 kg)

¼ cup (60 ml) avocado oil

2 tablespoons lemon juice

2 cloves garlic, minced

2 teaspoons chopped fresh rosemary

2 teaspoons dried thyme leaves

1 teaspoon dried oregano leaves

TABBOULEH:

½ cup (120 ml) avocado oil

¼ cup (60 ml) lemon juice

4 cloves garlic, minced

4 green onions, finely chopped

3 tablespoons finely chopped fresh mint leaves

½ teaspoon finely ground sea salt

6 cups (425 g) broccoli florets

3 medium tomatoes, diced

1 cucumber, seeded and diced

1 bunch fresh parsley, finely chopped

make it AIP/NIGHTSHADE-FREE: Replace the tomatoes with 1 large zucchini, diced.

1. Place the chicken thighs, oil, lemon juice, garlic, rosemary, thyme, and oregano in a dish. Turn the thighs in the mixture to coat, then cover and place in the refrigerator to marinate for 4 hours or overnight.

2. When ready to cook the chicken, preheat the oven to 350°F (177°C). Line a rimmed baking sheet with parchment paper.

3. Place the chicken on the lined baking sheet and bake for 25 to 30 minutes, until the internal temperature reaches 165°F (74°C) and the juices run clear.

4. Meanwhile, make the tabbouleh: Place the oil, lemon juice, garlic, green onions, mint, and salt in a large mixing bowl. Mix until incorporated.

5. Place half of the broccoli florets in a blender or food processor. Pulse until the pieces are ⅛ inch (3 mm) in size. Transfer the pieces to the large mixing bowl and repeat with the remaining broccoli florets.

6. Add the tomatoes, cucumber, and parsley to the bowl with the other tabbouleh ingredients and toss until fully incorporated.

7. Serve the tabbouleh with the chicken thighs.

STORE IT: *Keep in an airtight container in the fridge for up to 3 days. The chicken can be frozen for up to 1 month.*

REHEAT IT: *Place a single serving of the chicken in a microwave-safe dish, cover, and microwave for 2 minutes, or place in a frying pan with a drop of oil, cover, and reheat over medium heat for 5 minutes. Serve with the cold tabbouleh.*

THAW IT: *Place the chicken in the fridge and allow to defrost completely, then follow the reheating instructions above.*

Per serving:

calories: **779** | calories from fat: **592** | total fat: **65.8g** | saturated fat: **14.3g** | cholesterol: **196mg**
sodium: **300mg** | carbs: **11.2g** | dietary fiber: **4.1g** | net carbs: **7.1g** | sugars: **4.1g** | protein: **35.5g**

FAT:	CARBS:	PROTEIN:
76%	**6%**	**18%**

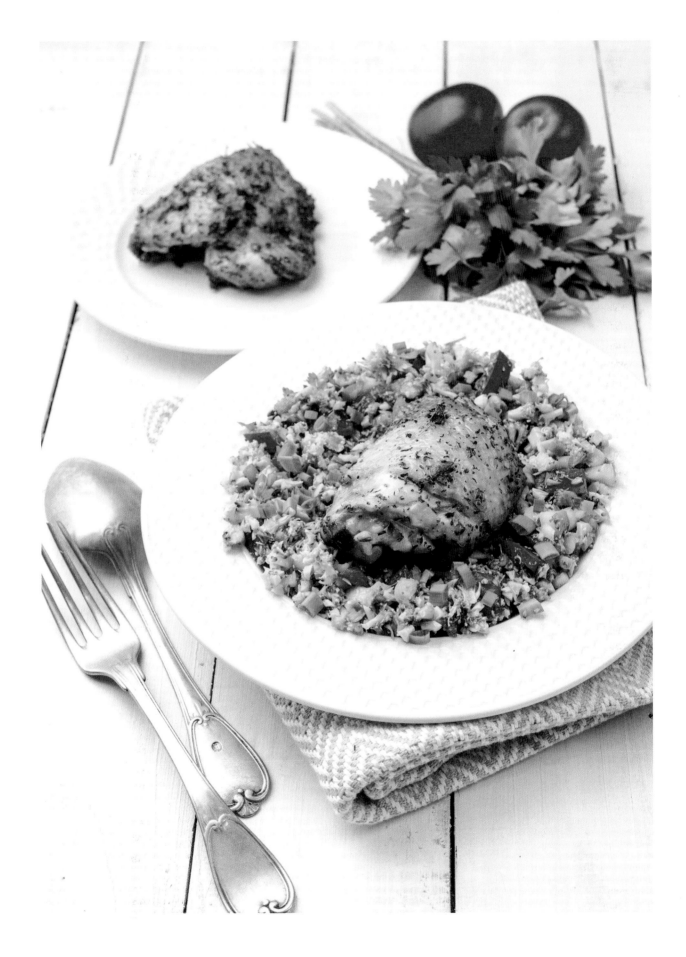

PAPRIKA CHICKEN SANDWICHES

DAIRY-FREE • NUT-FREE

OPTIONS: COCONUT-FREE • EGG-FREE • NIGHTSHADE-FREE

MAKES 4 sandwiches
(1 per serving)

PREP TIME: 5 minutes

COOK TIME: 20 minutes

The concept here is pounded chicken thighs used as "bread" for sandwiches. If you don't like the fillings, switch them up! You could also try swapping out the sauce for ¼ cup (60 ml) of Green Speckled Dressing (page 80) or Ranch Dressing (page 76).

BUNS:

2 pounds (910 g) boneless, skinless chicken thighs

¼ cup (55 g) coconut oil, or ¼ cup (60 ml) avocado oil

SAUCE:

⅓ cup (70 g) mayonnaise

2 teaspoons lemon juice

1 clove garlic, minced

¾ teaspoon paprika

¼ teaspoon ground black pepper

SANDWICH FILLINGS:

½ cup (35 g) fresh spinach

8 fresh basil leaves

4 ounces (115 g) salami, sliced

1. Place the chicken thighs on a sheet of parchment paper. (*Note:* If your package of chicken thighs did not give you 8 thighs, cut the largest thigh[s] in half until you have 8 pieces.) Using a meat mallet, pound the thighs until they're ¼ inch (6 mm) thick.

2. Heat the oil in a large frying pan over medium-low heat. Add the chicken and cook for 10 minutes, then turn the chicken over and cook for another 10 minutes, or until both sides are golden and the internal temperature reaches 165°F (74°C).

3. Meanwhile, make the sauce: Place the mayonnaise, lemon juice, garlic, paprika, and pepper in a small bowl. Whisk to combine.

4. When the chicken is done, divide evenly among 4 plates, 2 pieces per plate.

5. To assemble, spread one-quarter of the sauce on one piece of chicken on each plate, then top each sauced chicken piece with one-quarter of the spinach, 2 basil leaves, and 1 ounce (28 g) of salami. Top with the second chicken piece to make sandwiches.

make it **COCONUT-FREE:**
Use avocado oil.

make it **EGG-FREE:**
Use egg-free mayonnaise (see recipe on page 102).

make it **NIGHTSHADE-FREE:**
Omit the paprika.

STORE IT: *Keep in an airtight container in the fridge for up to 3 days.*

PREP AHEAD: *Prepare the chicken "buns" a couple of days ahead and put your sandwiches together when ready to enjoy.*

MAKE IT AT HOME

Replace store-bought mayonnaise with my homemade version.

104

Mayonnaise

Per sandwich, made with coconut oil and homemade mayonnaise:

| calories: **870** | calories from fat: **649** | total fat: **72.1g** | saturated fat: **35.8g** | cholesterol: **243mg** | FAT: | CARBS: | PROTEIN: |
| sodium: **1022mg** | carbs: **3g** | dietary fiber: **0.8g** | net carbs: **2.2g** | sugars: **1.1g** | protein: **52.3g** | **75%** | **1%** | **24%** |

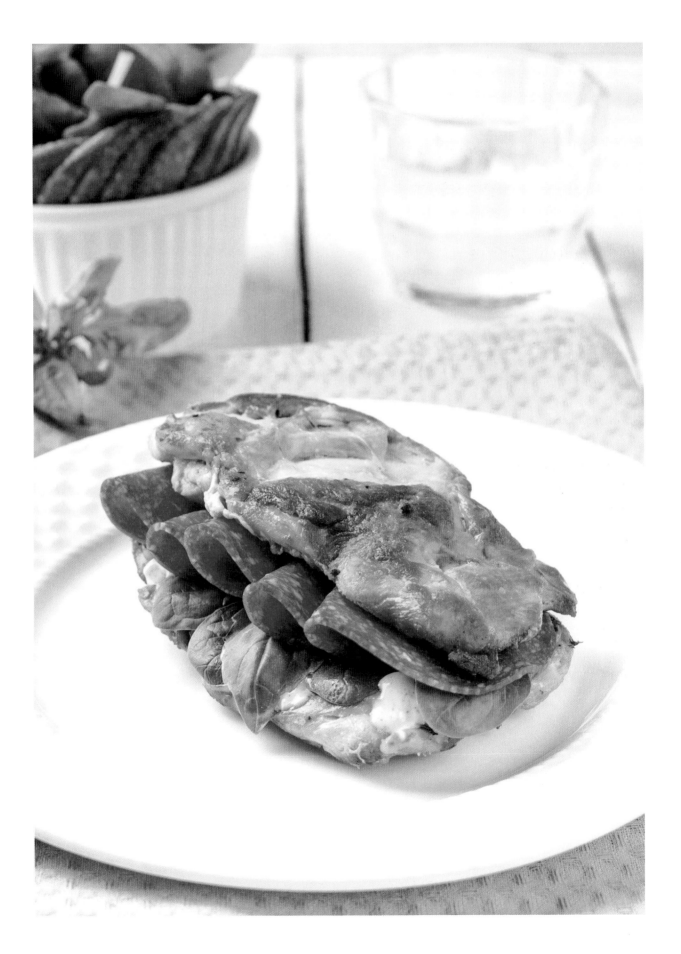

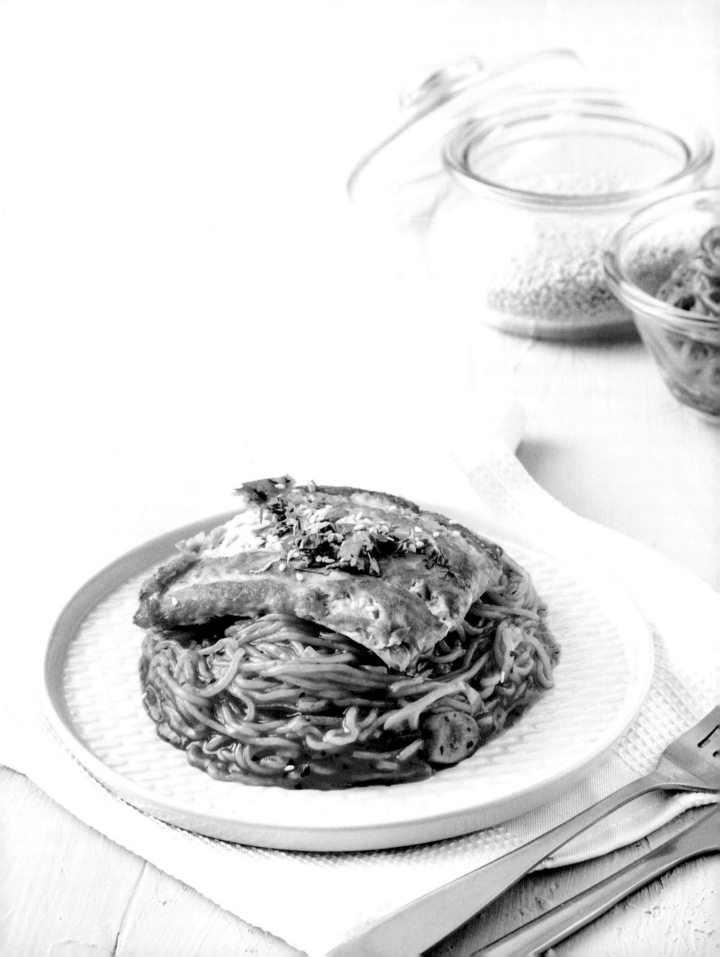

7.

DINNER

CRISPY THIGHS & MASH

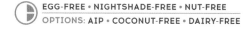

EGG-FREE • NIGHTSHADE-FREE • NUT-FREE

OPTIONS: AIP • COCONUT-FREE • DAIRY-FREE

SERVES 6

PREP TIME: 15 minutes

COOK TIME: 30 minutes

I love making this dish whenever we're in need of that stick-to-the-ribs feeling after a meal. Why the two different types of oil in this recipe? The chicken thighs will crisp up nicely because avocado oil has a higher smoke point than other oil choices. And the butternut mash will taste better if made with a butter-like oil, such as ghee or coconut oil—preferably butter-flavored coconut oil. If you can do butter, swap it in! If you have only one type of oil, use it and chow down.

This dish is awesome drizzled with Ranch Dressing (page 76).

CRISPY CHICKEN:

6 small or 3 large boneless, skinless chicken thighs (about 1 lb/455 g)

¼ cup (60 ml) melted coconut oil or avocado oil

1 teaspoon garlic powder

½ teaspoon onion powder

¼ teaspoon finely ground sea salt

¼ teaspoon ground black pepper

BUTTERNUT MASH:

1 medium butternut squash (about 1¼ lbs/570 g)

2 tablespoons coconut oil or ghee

½ teaspoon finely ground sea salt

⅛ teaspoon ground black pepper

⅓ cup (80 ml) milk (nondairy or regular)

1½ tablespoons chicken bone broth

1. Cook the chicken: Preheat the oven to 400°F (205°C). If using large chicken thighs, cut them in half to make 6 pieces. Place the chicken on a rimmed baking sheet. Pour the oil over the thighs and dust them with the spices. Turn the thighs until they're fully coated in the oil and spices. Bake for 25 to 30 minutes, until the internal temperature of the chicken reaches 165°F (74°C). Cut the chicken into ½-inch (1.25-cm) slices.

2. Meanwhile, make the mash: Peel and seed the squash, then cut the flesh into cubes. Measure 3 cups (455 g) of the cubes for the mash; store any remaining squash in the fridge for another use.

3. Heat the oil in a large frying pan over medium heat. Add the squash, salt, and pepper. Cover and cook for 10 to 15 minutes, until the squash is lightly browned. Add the milk and broth, cover, and continue to cook for 15 minutes, or until the squash is soft enough to mash easily. When the squash is done, mash it with the back of a fork right there in the pan.

4. To serve, divide the mash among 6 dinner plates. Top each portion with an equal amount of the sliced chicken thighs and enjoy!

make it **AIP:**
Omit the black pepper. Do not use ghee.

make it **COCONUT-FREE:**
Do not use coconut oil.

make it **DAIRY-FREE:**
Do not use ghee. Use a nondairy milk.

STORE IT: *Keep in an airtight container in the fridge for up to 3 days or in the freezer for up to 1 month.*

REHEAT IT: *Transfer a single serving to a microwave-safe dish, cover, and microwave for 3½ minutes, or place in an oven-safe dish, cover, and reheat in a preheated 350°F (177°C) oven for 15 minutes.*

THAW IT: *Place in the fridge and allow to defrost completely, then follow the reheating instructions above.*

Per serving, made with coconut oil and full-fat coconut milk:

| calories: **331** | calories from fat: **239** | total fat: **26.5g** | saturated fat: **13.1g** | cholesterol: **91mg** | | FAT: | CARBS: | PROTEIN: |
| sodium: **613mg** | carbs: **9.9g** | dietary fiber: **1.6g** | net carbs: **8.3g** | sugars: **1.8g** | protein: **16.2g** | **70%** | **11%** | **19%** |

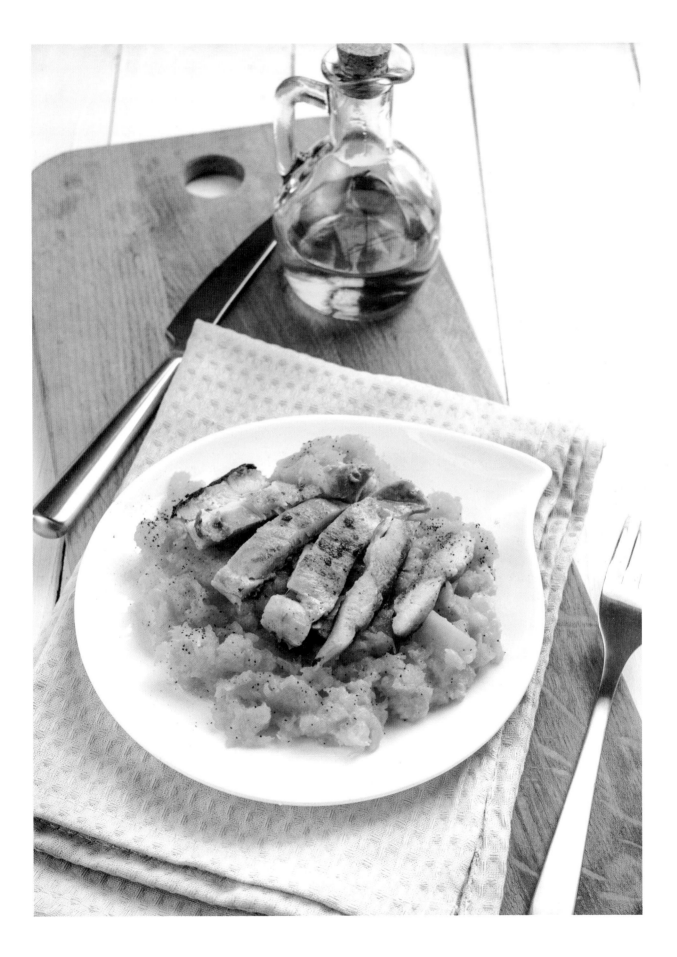

NOODLES & GLAZED SALMON

 DAIRY-FREE · EGG-FREE · NUT-FREE

OPTIONS: AIP · COCONUT-FREE · LOW-FODMAP · NIGHTSHADE-FREE

SERVES 4

PREP TIME: 5 minutes

COOK TIME: 20 minutes

It's no secret that I'm obsessed with adding various spiral-sliced veggie noodles to my keto dishes. And then there's riced cauliflower, a tried-and-true replacement for rice in just about any dish. While your carb replacements on keto can start and end with these two strategies, there is another option, and that's konjac. Konjac is a gluten-free herb from Asia with a stem that is rich in dietary fiber.

You may have heard of products like NuPasta, Miracle Noodles, and Miracle Rice, which transform this fiber into an awesome replacement for rice and noodles. These products are great, not only for the keto diet, but also for those looking to boost their dietary fiber intake while keeping noodles and rice in their life. If you're feeling a bit adventurous, you can use these products to replace spiral-sliced veggies or riced cauliflower in any keto recipe. I order them from Thrive Market, but you can also find them in health food stores and on Amazon.

I've used konjac noodles in this recipe, but they can be replaced with spiral-sliced vegetable noodles—my favorites are zucchini, daikon, and broccoli stalks—or cooked spaghetti squash. (Note: I like vegetable noodles raw, for the crunch, but you can lightly cook them if you prefer.) Or you could look for kelp noodles; I don't particularly enjoy them, but a lot of people love them, and they're a bit higher in nutrients than konjac noodles.

¼ cup plus 2 tablespoons (75 ml) avocado oil, divided

¼ cup (60 ml) coconut aminos

2 tablespoons plus 2 teaspoons tomato paste

2 tablespoons apple cider vinegar

1 (2-in/5-cm) piece fresh ginger root, grated

4 cloves garlic, minced

½ teaspoon finely ground sea salt

1 pound (455 g) salmon fillets, cut into 4 equal portions

2 (7-oz/198-g) packages konjac noodles or equivalent amount of other low-carb noodles of choice

2 green onions, sliced

Handful of fresh cilantro leaves, roughly chopped

1 teaspoon sesame seeds

1. Heat 2 tablespoons of the oil in a large frying pan over medium heat.

2. While the oil is heating, make the sauce: In a small bowl, whisk together the remaining ¼ cup of oil, the coconut aminos, tomato paste, vinegar, ginger, garlic, and salt.

3. Place the salmon in the hot pan, reduce the heat to low, and slather with the sauce. Drizzle any remaining sauce directly into the pan. Cover and cook on low for 15 minutes, until seared and lightly cooked through.

4. Once the salmon is done, pile the salmon up on one side of the pan, leaving enough space for the noodles. Add the noodles and green onions to the pan and toss to coat in the remaining sauce. Then place the cooked salmon on top of the noodles. Cook for another 3 to 5 minutes, just long enough to heat the noodles.

5. Sprinkle the cilantro and sesame seeds over the top of the salmon. Divide the noodles and salmon among 4 dinner plates, drizzling each portion with the leftover pan sauce, and enjoy.

Per serving, made with konjac noodles:

calories: **333** | calories from fat: **202** | total fat: **22.4g** | saturated fat: **2.5g** | cholesterol: **45mg**
sodium: **287mg** | carbs: **8.2g** | dietary fiber: **3.6g** | net carbs: **4.6g** | sugars: **0.9g** | protein: **24.7g**

FAT:	CARBS:	PROTEIN:
61%	10%	30%

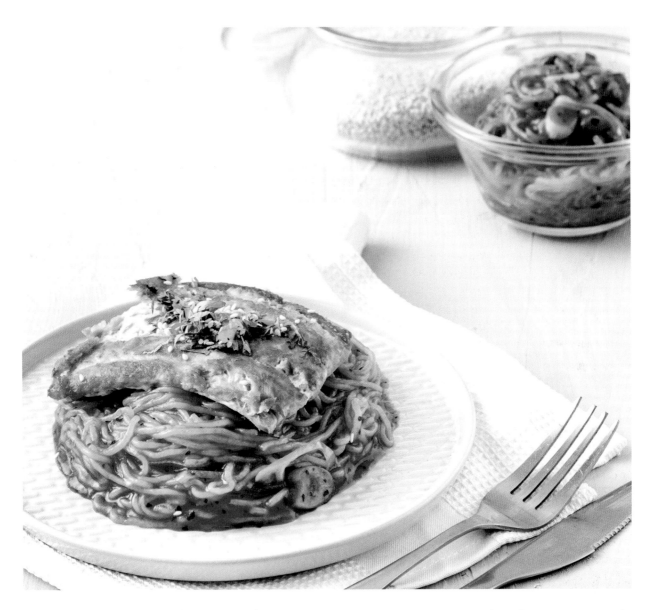

make it AIP:
Omit the tomato paste and add an additional teaspoon of coconut aminos. Skip the sesame seeds.

make it COCONUT-FREE:
Replace the coconut aminos with soy sauce and omit the salt.

make it LOW-FODMAP:
Replace 2 tablespoons of the avocado oil in the sauce with garlic-infused oil and omit the minced garlic. Use only the green parts of the green onions.

make it NIGHTSHADE-FREE:
Omit the tomato paste and add an additional teaspoon of coconut aminos.

STORE IT: *Keep in an airtight container in the fridge for up to 3 days or in the freezer for up to 1 month.*

REHEAT IT: *Transfer a single serving to a microwave-safe dish, cover, and microwave for 2½ minutes. Alternatively, to remove as much liquid as possible, place in a frying pan over medium heat and reheat, uncovered, for 5 minutes.*

THAW IT: *Place in the fridge and allow to defrost completely, then follow the reheating instructions above.*

PREP AHEAD: *Make the sauce as far ahead of time as you'd like. You can store it in the fridge for up to 3 days or in the freezer for up to 1 month.*

SCALLOPS & MOZZA BROCCOLI MASH

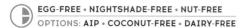
EGG-FREE · NIGHTSHADE-FREE · NUT-FREE
OPTIONS: AIP · COCONUT-FREE · DAIRY-FREE

SERVES 4
PREP TIME: 5 minutes
COOK TIME: 35 minutes

Was your childhood filled with cheese-covered broccoli? Mine was. For a while there, it was the only way I'd eat vegetables. This is a fun and exciting new way to prepare cheesy broccoli that I think you're really going to like!

MOZZA BROCCOLI MASH:

¼ cup (55 g) coconut oil or ghee, or ¼ cup (60 ml) avocado oil

6 cups (570 g) broccoli florets

4 cloves garlic, minced

1 (2-in/5-cm) piece fresh ginger root, grated

⅔ cup (160 ml) chicken bone broth

½ cup (70 g) shredded mozzarella cheese (dairy-free or regular)

SCALLOPS:

1 pound (455 g) sea scallops

¼ teaspoon finely ground sea salt

¼ teaspoon ground black pepper

2 tablespoons coconut oil, avocado oil, or ghee

Lemon wedges, for serving

1. Prepare the mash: Heat the oil in a large frying pan over low heat. Add the broccoli, garlic, and ginger and cook, uncovered, for 5 minutes, or until the garlic is fragrant.

2. Pour in the broth, then cover and cook on low for 25 minutes, or until the broccoli is easily mashed.

3. About 5 minutes before the broccoli is ready, prepare the scallops: Pat the scallops dry and season them on both sides with the salt and pepper. Heat the oil in a medium-sized frying pan over medium heat. When the oil is hot, add the scallops. Cook for 2 minutes per side, or until lightly golden.

4. When the broccoli is done, add the cheese and mash with a fork. Divide the mash among 4 dinner plates and top with the scallops. Serve with lemon wedges and enjoy!

make it AIP:
Do not use ghee. Omit the cheese and black pepper.

make it COCONUT-FREE:
Use avocado oil or ghee. If using dairy-free cheese, make sure it's also coconut-free.

make it DAIRY-FREE:
Do not use ghee. Use dairy-free cheese.

STORE IT: *Keep in an airtight container in the fridge for up to 3 days or in the freezer for up to 1 month.*

REHEAT IT: *Transfer a single serving to a microwave-safe dish, cover, and microwave for 2 minutes; or place in a small frying pan, cover, and reheat over medium heat for 5 minutes. Note: The scallops will get chewy if overcooked, so try to just warm the leftovers.*

THAW IT: *Place in the fridge and allow to defrost completely, then follow the reheating instructions above.*

Per serving, made with coconut oil and dairy-free cheese:

calories: **353** | calories from fat: **229** | total fat: **25.4g** | saturated fat: **19.9g** | cholesterol: **27mg**	FAT: **65%**
sodium: **768mg** | carbs: **12g** | dietary fiber: **7g** | net carbs: **5g** | sugars: **1g** | protein: **19.2g**	CARBS: **14%** | PROTEIN: **22%**

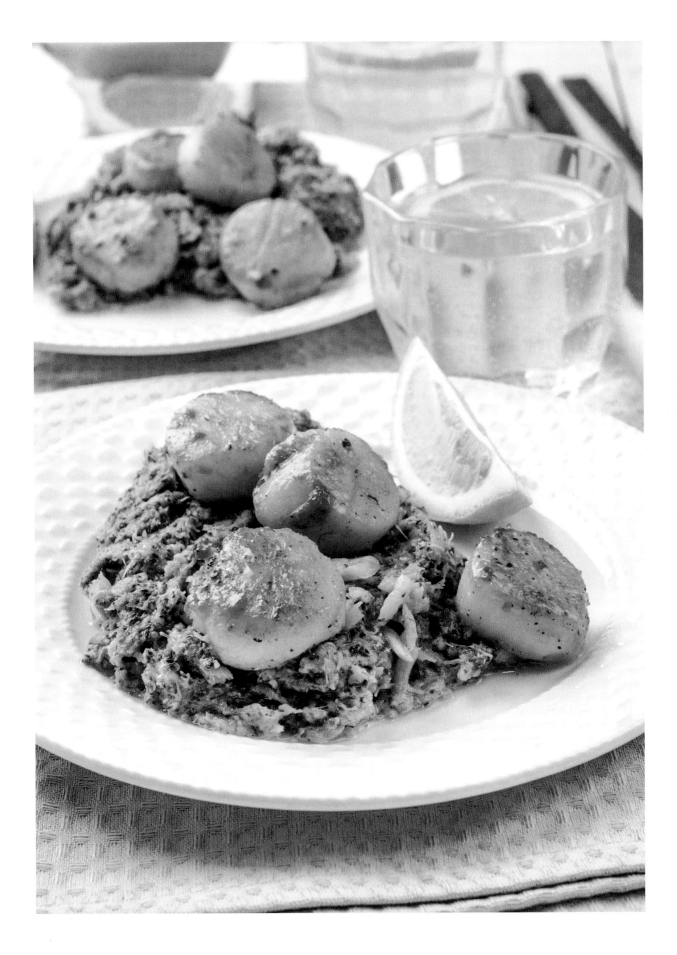

BBQ BEEF & SLAW

COCONUT-FREE • DAIRY-FREE • EGG-FREE • NUT-FREE
OPTIONS: AIP • NIGHTSHADE-FREE

SERVES 4

PREP TIME: 10 minutes

COOK TIME: 45 minutes or 4 to 6 hours, depending on method

A classic meal everyone should know how to make keto! You can make the BBQ beef in a slow cooker or a pressure cooker. For the slaw, any creamy dressing will do, though my favorite is poppy seed dressing—especially my homemade version. If you don't have poppy seed dressing on hand or don't care for it, use whatever you have (or check out the Sauces & Spreads chapter on pages 68 to 105 for other creamy dressing recipes).

BBQ BEEF:

1 pound (455 g) boneless beef chuck roast

1 cup (240 ml) beef bone broth

½ teaspoon finely ground sea salt

½ cup (80 g) sugar-free barbecue sauce

SLAW:

9 ounces (255 g) coleslaw mix

½ cup (120 ml) sugar-free poppy seed dressing

1. Place the chuck roast, broth, and salt in a pressure cooker or slow cooker. If using a pressure cooker, seal the lid and cook on high pressure for 45 minutes. When complete, allow the pressure to release naturally before removing the lid. If using a slow cooker, cook on high for 4 hours or on low for 6 hours.

2. When the meat is done, drain it almost completely, leaving ¼ cup (60 ml) of the cooking liquid in the cooker. Shred the meat with two forks, then add the barbecue sauce and toss to coat.

3. Place the coleslaw mix and dressing in a salad bowl and toss to coat.

4. Divide the BBQ beef and coleslaw among 4 dinner plates, placing the beef first and then the slaw on top, and enjoy.

MAKE IT AT HOME

Replace store-bought barbecue sauce and/or poppy seed dressing with my homemade version(s).

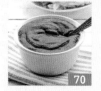

Quick 'n' Easy Barbecue Sauce

Poppy Seed Dressing

STORE IT: Keep the BBQ beef and slaw in separate airtight containers in the fridge for up to 3 days. The beef can be frozen for up to 1 month.

REHEAT IT: Place a single serving of the BBQ beef in a microwave-safe dish, cover, and microwave for 2 minutes, or place in a frying pan with a drop of oil, cover, and reheat over medium heat for 5 minutes.

THAW IT: Place the beef in the fridge and allow to defrost completely, then follow the reheating instructions above.

PREP AHEAD: Always have a jar of store-bought barbecue sauce in your pantry or homemade barbecue sauce in the freezer, ready for action!

make it AIP:
Replace the barbecue sauce with Bacon Dressing (page 82) and use Honey Mustard Dressing & Marinade (page 78) in the slaw.

make it NIGHTSHADE-FREE:
Replace the barbecue sauce with ½ cup (120 ml) Lemon Turmeric Dressing & Marinade (page 86) or another dressing of your choice, or omit it completely.

Per serving, made with Quick 'n' Easy Barbecue Sauce and homemade poppy seed dressing: ——

| calories: **354** | calories from fat: **240** | total fat: **26.7g** | saturated fat: **4.7g** | cholesterol: **70mg** | | FAT: | CARBS: | PROTEIN: |
| sodium: **566mg** | carbs: **4.6g** | dietary fiber: **1.7g** | net carbs: **2.9g** | sugars: **2.5g** | protein: **23.9g** | | **68%** | **5%** | **27%** |

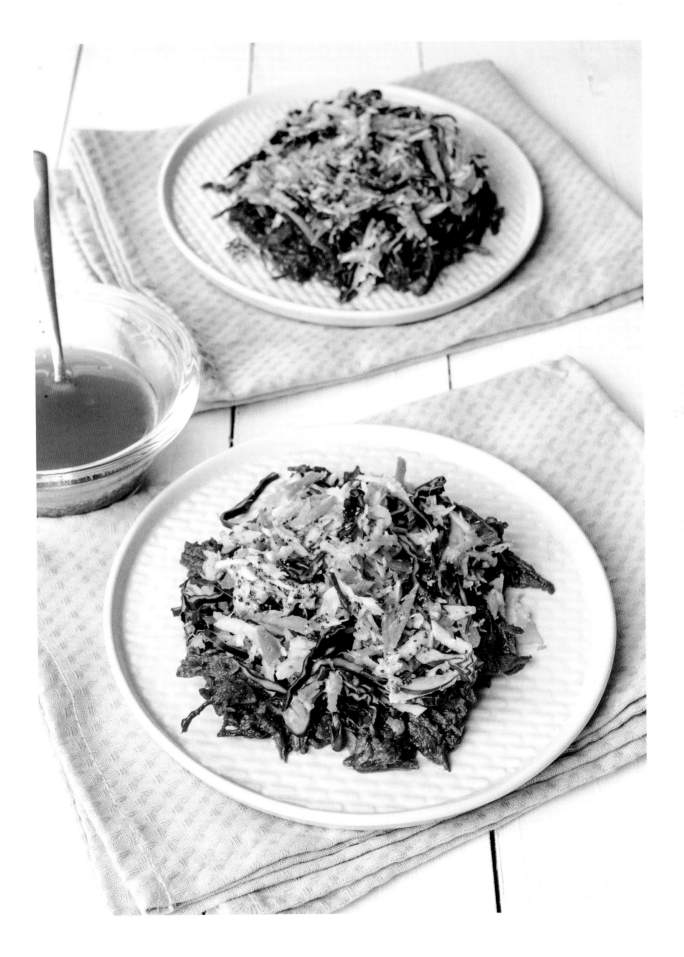

CREAM OF MUSHROOM-STUFFED CHICKEN

EGG-FREE • NIGHTSHADE-FREE • NUT-FREE

OPTIONS: AIP • COCONUT-FREE • DAIRY-FREE

SERVES 4

PREP TIME: 10 minutes

COOK TIME: 45 minutes

I could eat this meal every day for the rest of my life and be perfectly happy. It's that delicious! And it's pretty easy as far as dinner recipes go. If you can eat dairy or you have a favorite dairy-free shredded mozzarella cheese, filling the breasts with a little cheese is a tasty addition. Also, I chose full-fat coconut milk for the pan, but any full-fat milk (dairy-free or regular) is fair game.

3 tablespoons coconut oil, avocado oil, or ghee

7 ounces (200 g) cremini mushrooms, chopped

4 cloves garlic, minced

3 teaspoons dried parsley, divided

¾ teaspoon finely ground sea salt, divided

¼ teaspoon ground black pepper

1 pound (455 g) boneless, skin-on chicken breasts

1 teaspoon onion powder

1 teaspoon garlic powder

½ cup (120 ml) milk (nondairy or regular)

4 cups (280 g) spinach, for serving

make it AIP:
Omit the black pepper and do not use ghee.

make it COCONUT-FREE:
Do not use coconut oil or coconut milk.

make it DAIRY-FREE:
Do not use ghee. Use a nondairy milk.

1. Preheat the oven to 400°F (205°C). Line a rimmed baking sheet with parchment paper or a silicone baking mat.

2. Heat the oil in a large frying pan over medium heat. Add the mushrooms, garlic, 2 teaspoons of the parsley, ¼ teaspoon of the salt, and the pepper. Toss to coat and sauté for 10 minutes.

3. Meanwhile, slice each chicken breast horizontally, stopping the knife about ½ inch (1.25 cm) from the opposite side, so that it opens like a book; be careful not to slice the breasts all the way through. The best way to do this is to use a sharp knife and place your palm on the top of the breast to hold it steady.

4. Place the chicken breasts on the lined baking sheet and open them up. Place one-quarter of the mushroom mixture in the middle of each opened breast. If there is leftover mushroom mixture, simply drop it into the pan, around the chicken.

5. Fold over the chicken breasts to cover the filling. Dust the stuffed breasts with the garlic powder, onion powder, remaining 1 teaspoon of parsley, and remaining ½ teaspoon of salt.

6. Pour the milk between the chicken breasts, directly into the pan.

7. Bake for 30 to 35 minutes, until the internal temperature of the chicken reaches 165°F (74°C).

8. Divide the spinach among 4 dinner plates. Divide the stuffed chicken breasts among the plates, drizzle the spinach with the creamy pan juices, and enjoy! (*Note:* If you did not end up with one breast half per person in the package, cut the stuffed breasts into portions and divide them equally among the plates.)

Per serving, made with coconut oil and full-fat coconut milk:

| calories: **388** | calories from fat: **219** | total fat: **24.3g** | saturated fat: **11.4g** | cholesterol: **96mg** | | FAT: | CARBS: | PROTEIN: |
| sodium: **492mg** | carbs: **6.6g** | dietary fiber: **2.3g** | net carbs: **4.3g** | sugars: **1.6g** | protein: **38.2g** | **55%** | **7%** | **38%** |

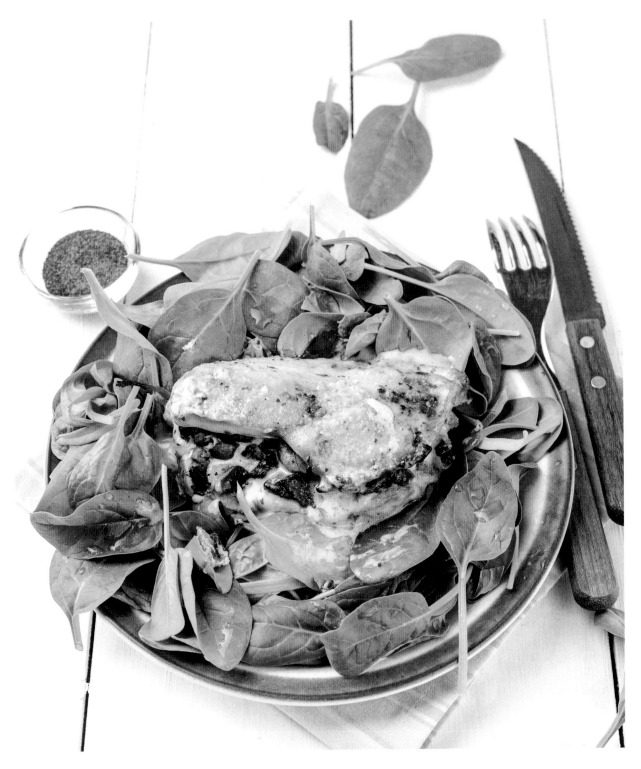

STORE IT: *Keep the chicken and pan juices in an airtight container in the fridge for up to 3 days or in the freezer for up to 1 month.*

REHEAT IT: *Place a single serving of the chicken and pan juices in a microwave-safe dish, cover, and microwave for 2 minutes; or place in a frying pan, cover, and reheat over medium heat for 5 to 7 minutes.*

THAW IT: *Place the chicken in the fridge and allow to defrost completely, then follow the reheating instructions above.*

CRISPY PORK WITH LEMON-THYME CAULI RICE

EGG-FREE · NIGHTSHADE-FREE · NUT-FREE
OPTIONS: **AIP · COCONUT-FREE · DAIRY-FREE**

SERVES 4
PREP TIME: 5 minutes
COOK TIME: 40 minutes

This recipe is impressive and, while a little lengthy, really straightforward. Just think, instead of rushing through dinner, you can get it going on the stove, pour yourself a glass of wine, and get caught up with the family happenings of the day. To speed things up a bit, you can use pre-riced cauliflower. I tend to rice cauliflower myself because it's less expensive.

CRISPY PORK:

¼ cup (55 g) coconut oil or ghee, or ¼ cup (60 ml) avocado oil

½ cup (38 g) crushed pork rinds

1 teaspoon garlic powder

1 teaspoon dried oregano leaves

1 teaspoon dried thyme leaves

½ teaspoon finely ground sea salt

¼ teaspoon ground black pepper

1 pound (455 g) boneless pork chops (about 1 in/2.5 cm thick)

LEMON-THYME CAULI RICE:

1 medium head cauliflower (about 1½ lbs/680 g), or 3 cups (375 g) pre-riced cauliflower

1 small white onion, diced

4 cloves garlic, minced

¼ cup (60 ml) chicken bone broth

2 tablespoons lemon juice

½ teaspoon finely ground sea salt

Leaves from 6 sprigs fresh thyme

1. Heat the oil in a large frying pan over medium-low heat.

2. While the oil is heating, place the crushed pork rinds, garlic powder, oregano, thyme, salt, and pepper in a medium-sized bowl. Stir to blend, then add the pork chops, one at a time, and coat in the mixture. When the chops are well coated, transfer to the frying pan.

3. Cook the pork chops for 10 minutes per side, until well seared.

4. If you're using pre-riced cauliflower, skip ahead to Step 5. Otherwise, cut the base off the head of cauliflower and remove the florets. Transfer the florets to a food processor or blender and pulse 3 or 4 times to break them up into small (¼-inch/6-mm) pieces.

5. Once the pork has cooked for a total of 20 minutes, transfer the chops to a clean plate, leaving the cooking oil in the pan. Add the riced cauliflower, onion, garlic, broth, lemon juice, and salt. Cover and cook until the cauli rice is soft but not mushy, about 15 minutes, stirring a couple of times during cooking.

6. Meanwhile, cut the pork chops into ½-inch (1.25-cm) slices. When the cauli rice is done, add the sliced pork to the pan. If the pork is not cooked through, continue cooking, uncovered, for another 5 minutes, just to cook it through.

7. Divide the pork and cauli rice among 4 dinner plates, sprinkle with the thyme leaves, and enjoy!

make it AIP:
Omit the black pepper. Do not use ghee.

make it COCONUT-FREE:
Use avocado oil or ghee.

make it DAIRY-FREE:
Do not use ghee.

STORE IT: *Keep in an airtight container in the fridge for up to 3 days or in the freezer for up to 1 month.*

REHEAT IT: *Transfer a single serving to a microwave-safe dish, cover, and microwave for 2½ minutes.*

THAW IT: *Place in the fridge and allow to defrost completely, then follow the reheating instructions above.*

Per serving, made with coconut oil:

calories: **419** | calories from fat: **244** | total fat: **27.7g** | saturated fat: **16.3g** | cholesterol: **104mg**
sodium: **728mg** | carbs: **9g** | dietary fiber: **3g** | net carbs: **6g** | sugars: **3g** | protein: **34g**

FAT:	CARBS:	PROTEIN:
58%	8%	34%

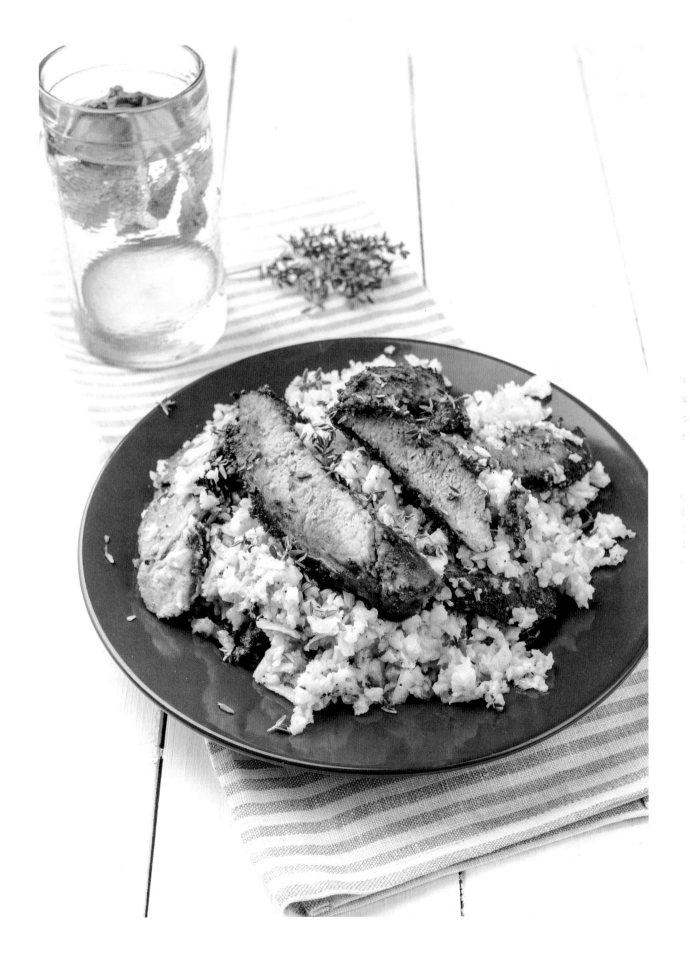

ONE-POT PORKY KALE

NUT-FREE

OPTIONS: AIP • COCONUT-FREE • DAIRY-FREE • EGG-FREE • NIGHTSHADE-FREE

SERVES 4
PREP TIME: 5 minutes
COOK TIME: 35 minutes

There's nothing quite like a one-pot meal. Not only is there less stress when cooking and less cleanup, but the flavors meld all up in each other's business, making the dish scrumptious without all the hassle. Don't have kale? You could use any kind of greens in its place—spinach, bok choy, mustard greens, or whatever you can find. If the idea of making a batch of homemade dressing has you stressed, use whatever creamy dressing you have on hand.

3 tablespoons coconut oil, avocado oil, or ghee

1 teaspoon paprika

½ teaspoon finely ground sea salt

¼ teaspoon ground black pepper

1 pound (455 g) boneless pork chops (about 1 in/2.5 cm thick)

1 small yellow onion, sliced

6 cloves garlic, minced

4 cups (240 g) destemmed kale leaves

⅓ cup (80 ml) creamy Italian dressing or other creamy salad dressing of choice

¼ cup (17 g) chopped fresh parsley, for serving

1. Heat the oil in a large frying pan over medium-low heat.

2. While the oil is heating, place the paprika, salt, and pepper in a medium-sized bowl. Stir to blend, then add the pork chops, one at a time, and coat with the paprika mixture.

3. Cook the coated pork chops for 10 minutes per side, until well seared.

4. Once the chops have cooked for a total of 20 minutes, transfer them to a clean plate, leaving the cooking oil in the pan. Add the onion and garlic and cook for 5 minutes, or until fragrant.

5. Add the kale and dressing to the pan and continue to cook for 2 minutes; do not allow the kale to wilt. Remove from the heat.

6. Cut the pork chops into ½-inch (1.25-cm) slices. If the meat is not cooked through, place the slices in the pan and cook, uncovered, for another 5 minutes, just to cook through.

7. Divide among 4 dinner plates, sprinkle with the parsley, and enjoy!

make it AIP:
Do not use ghee, omit the paprika and black pepper, and use a compliant dressing.

make it COCONUT-FREE:
Do not use coconut oil.

make it DAIRY-FREE:
Do not use ghee.

make it EGG-FREE:
Use an egg-free dressing.

make it NIGHTSHADE-FREE:
Omit the paprika and use a nightshade-free dressing.

STORE IT: *Keep in an airtight container in the fridge for up to 3 days or in the freezer for up to 1 month.*

REHEAT IT: *Transfer a single serving to a microwave-safe dish, cover, and microwave for 2½ minutes.*

THAW IT: *Place in the fridge and allow to defrost completely, then follow the reheating instructions above.*

MAKE IT AT HOME

Replace store-bought creamy salad dressing with my homemade version.

Creamy Italian Dressing

Per serving, made with coconut oil and homemade creamy Italian dressing:

calories: **429**	calories from fat: **275**	total fat: **31g**	saturated fat: **13.3g**	cholesterol: **77mg**
sodium: **432mg**	carbs: **9.7g**	dietary fiber: **3.1g**	net carbs: **6.6g**	sugars: **2.1g**	protein: **28g**

FAT:	CARBS:	PROTEIN:
65%	9%	26%

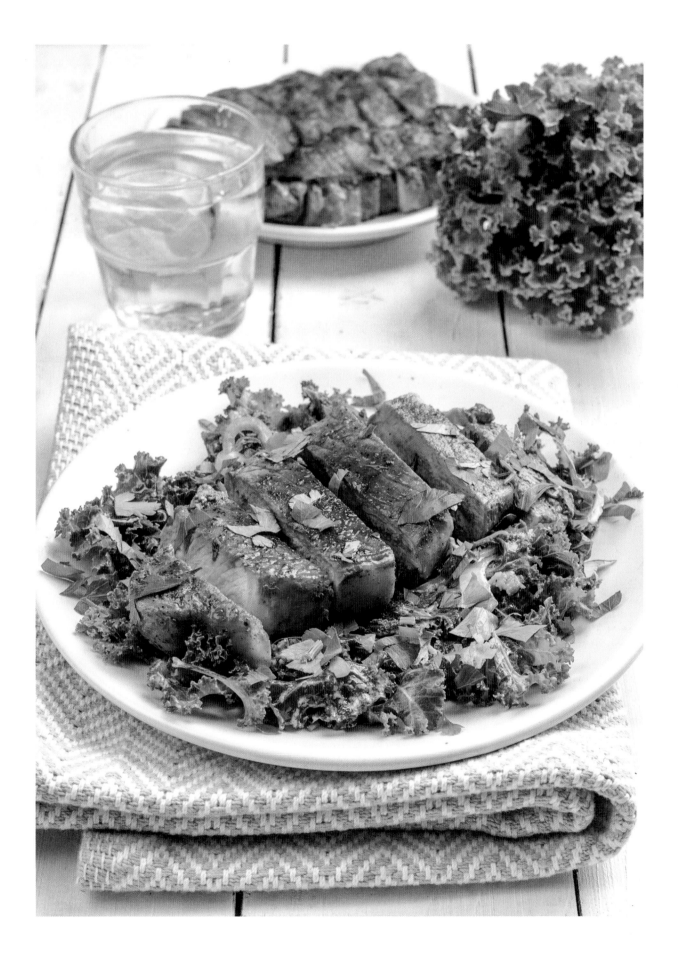

SALMON & KALE

COCONUT-FREE • DAIRY-FREE • EGG-FREE • NUT-FREE
OPTIONS: AIP • NIGHTSHADE-FREE

SERVES 4

PREP TIME: 5 minutes, plus 2 hours to marinate

COOK TIME: 15 minutes

Salmon is one of those easy proteins that's quick to make and scrumptious to eat. Just about any vinaigrette-style dressing works well as a marinade for salmon. I hope you enjoy this dish as much as Kevin and I do!

1 pound (455 g) salmon fillets, cut into 4 equal portions

¾ cup (180 ml) vinaigrette of choice

1 small red onion, sliced

4 cups (240 g) destemmed kale leaves

¼ teaspoon red pepper flakes

¼ teaspoon finely ground sea salt

make it AIP:
Follow the AIP instructions for the vinaigrette (or make sure the vinaigrette you're using is AIP). Omit the red pepper flakes.

make it NIGHTSHADE-FREE:
Omit the red pepper flakes.

1. Set the salmon in a shallow dish and pour the vinaigrette over the top. Cover and set in the fridge for 2 hours to marinate.

2. When ready to cook, transfer the salmon and all the marinade to a large frying pan. Distribute the onion slices around the fish, then turn the heat to medium-low. Continue cooking the salmon for 6 minutes per side, until seared.

3. Once the salmon has cooked for a total of 12 minutes, push the fish to the sides of the pan, making room for the kale. Add the kale, red pepper flakes, and salt and toss to coat the kale in the pan drippings. Cover and cook for 3 minutes, or until the kale is wilted.

4. Divide the salmon fillets and braised kale among 4 dinner plates and serve.

MAKE IT AT HOME

Replace store-bought vinaigrette with one of my homemade versions. My favorite for this recipe is the Basil Vinaigrette.

Basil Vinaigrette & Marinade

STORE IT: *Keep in an airtight container in the fridge for up to 3 days or in the freezer for up to 1 month.*

REHEAT IT: *Transfer a single serving to a microwave-safe dish, cover, and microwave for 2 minutes; or place in a small frying pan, cover, and reheat over medium heat for 5 minutes.*

THAW IT: *Place in the fridge and allow to defrost completely, then follow the reheating instructions above.*

Per serving, made with Basil Vinaigrette & Marinade:

					FAT:	CARBS:	PROTEIN:
calories: **438**	calories from fat: **296**	total fat: **33g**	saturated fat: **4.3g**	cholesterol: **52mg**	**68%**	**8%**	**24%**
sodium: **374mg**	carbs: **9.1g**	dietary fiber: **3.3g**	net carbs: **5.8g**	sugars: **3.8g**			

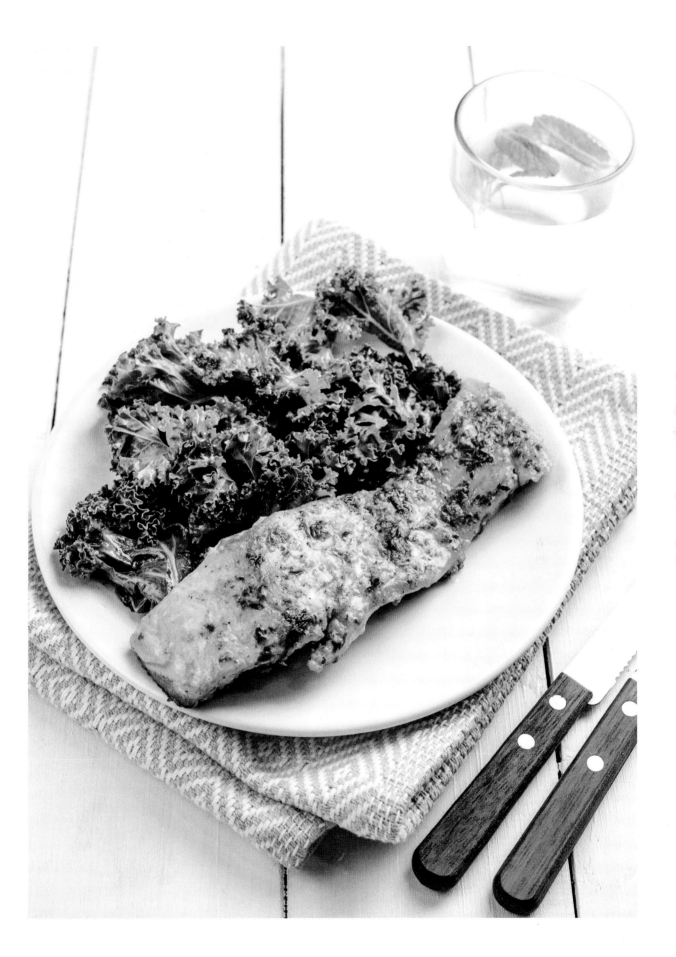

CREAMY SPINACH ZUCCHINI BOATS

DAIRY-FREE • NUT-FREE

OPTIONS: EGG-FREE • NIGHTSHADE-FREE

MAKES 8 boats (2 per serving)

PREP TIME: 15 minutes

COOK TIME: 30 minutes

Even though there's no muscle or organ meat in this dish, there's plenty of protein in each serving thanks to the pork rinds and collagen. Don't have collagen? Omitting it won't change the structure of this recipe; it'll just lower the overall protein count.

If you can't live without cheese and it's part of your keto diet, you could top the boats with 1 cup (140 g) of shredded dairy-free or regular mozzarella cheese after adding the pork rinds.

4 medium zucchinis

1 cup (250 g) coconut cream

½ cup (105 g) mayonnaise

⅓ cup (55 g) collagen peptides (optional)

1 tablespoon onion powder

2 teaspoons garlic powder

½ teaspoon finely ground sea salt

¼ teaspoon paprika

¼ teaspoon red pepper flakes

1 packed cup (70 g) spinach, finely chopped

1¼ cups (95 g) crushed pork rinds

1. Preheat the oven to 400°F (205°C). Line a 13 by 9-inch (33 by 23-cm) baking pan with parchment paper for easier cleanup.

2. Slice the zucchinis in half lengthwise, keeping the stems intact. Then, with a small spoon, scoop out the insides, leaving the sides at least ¼ to ½ inch (6 to 12 mm) thick. Be careful not to crack the zucchinis in half—take it slow!

3. Lay the zucchinis hollowed-out side up in the lined baking pan.

4. Place the remaining ingredients, except the spinach and pork rinds, in a blender or food processor. Blend until smooth, then add the spinach and stir by hand just to mix it in.

5. Spoon the spinach mixture into the zucchini boats, filling them to the top. Pile the pork crushed rinds on top of the boats.

6. Bake for 30 minutes, until the tops are lightly golden. Let cool for 10 minutes before serving.

make it EGG-FREE:
Use egg-free mayonnaise (see recipe on page 102).

make it NIGHTSHADE-FREE:
Omit the paprika and red pepper flakes.

STORE IT: *Keep in an airtight container in the fridge for up to 5 days.*

REHEAT IT: *Transfer a single serving to a microwave-safe dish, cover, and microwave for 2½ minutes; or place in an oven-safe dish and reheat in a preheated 400°F (205°C) oven for 15 minutes.*

MAKE IT AT HOME

Replace store-bought mayonnaise with my homemade version.

104

Mayonnaise

Per serving, made with homemade mayonnaise and collagen:

calories: **453**	calories from fat: **288**	total fat: **32g**	saturated fat: **17.4g**	cholesterol: **40mg**		FAT:	CARBS:	PROTEIN:
sodium: **1061mg**	carbs: **9.4g**	dietary fiber: **4.2g**	net carbs: **5.2g**	sugars: **2.1g**	protein: **32g**	64%	8%	28%

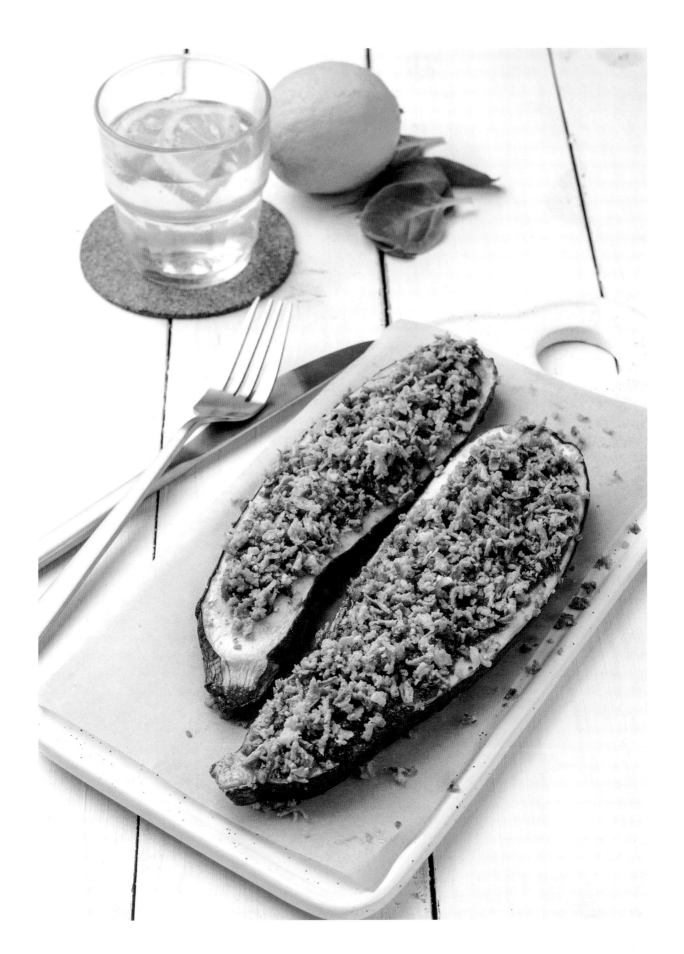

MY FAVORITE CREAMY PESTO CHICKEN

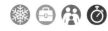

 DAIRY-FREE · EGG-FREE

OPTIONS: COCONUT-FREE · LOW-FODMAP · NIGHTSHADE-FREE · NUT-FREE

SERVES 4

PREP TIME: 10 minutes

COOK TIME: 20 minutes

The title reads like I've had so many pesto chicken dishes in my life and this is my favorite one of all, when in reality, this recipe could very well be my favorite recipe in the whole book. Wait, in all the books I've ever created. Yes, it's that bold of a statement. Gosh, if you don't like this recipe, we may have a problem.

Here is where I struggle with this recipe—it's so, so, so good that I have a hard time deciding what I like most with it. So I'll leave that up to you: try raw or cooked spiral-sliced zucchini or daikon noodles (I like them raw!), or perhaps some heated konjac noodles, cooked cauliflower rice, or cooked spaghetti squash; or enjoy the chicken on its own. It's all good!

CHICKEN:

¼ cup (60 ml) avocado oil

1 pound (455 g) boneless, skinless chicken breasts, thinly sliced

1 small white onion, thinly sliced

½ cup (105 g) sun-dried tomatoes, drained and chopped

¾ teaspoon dried oregano leaves

½ teaspoon dried thyme leaves

⅛ teaspoon red pepper flakes

PESTO CREAM SAUCE:

2 cloves garlic

¼ cup (37 g) pine nuts

¼ cup (17 g) nutritional yeast

½ cup (120 ml) chicken bone broth

½ cup (120 ml) full-fat coconut milk

½ teaspoon finely ground sea salt

½ teaspoon ground black pepper

½ ounce (14 g) fresh basil leaves and stems

2 medium zucchinis, spiral sliced, raw or cooked, for serving

1. Heat the oil in a large frying pan over medium heat. When hot, add the chicken, onion, sun-dried tomatoes, oregano, thyme, and red pepper flakes. Sauté for 5 minutes, or until fragrant.

2. Meanwhile, place all the ingredients for the pesto cream sauce, except the basil, in a food processor or blender. Blend on high until smooth, about 30 seconds. Add the basil and pulse to break it up slightly, but before the sauce turns a bright green color—don't pulverize the basil!

3. Pour the sauce into the pan and toss the chicken to coat. Reduce the heat to low, cover, and cook for 15 minutes, stirring every couple of minutes, until the chicken is cooked through.

4. Divide the spiral-sliced zucchini among 4 dinner plates and top with equal portions of the chicken and sauce. Dig in!

STORE IT: *Keep in an airtight container in the fridge for up to 3 days or in the freezer for up to 1 month.*

REHEAT IT: *Transfer a single serving to a microwave-safe dish, cover, and microwave for 2½ minutes. Alternatively, to remove as much liquid as possible, place in a frying pan and reheat over medium heat, uncovered, for 5 minutes.*

THAW IT: *Place in the fridge and allow to defrost completely, then follow the reheating instructions above.*

PREP AHEAD: *Make the sauce as far ahead of time as you'd like. You can store it in the fridge for up to 3 days or in the freezer for up to 1 month.*

Per serving:

calories: **455** | calories from fat: **264** | total fat: **29.3g** | saturated fat: **2.2g** | cholesterol: **74mg**

sodium: **437mg** | carbs: **15.8g** | dietary fiber: **4.4g** | net carbs: **11.4g** | sugars: **3.3g** | protein: **32.2g**

FAT:	CARBS:	PROTEIN:
58%	**14%**	**28%**

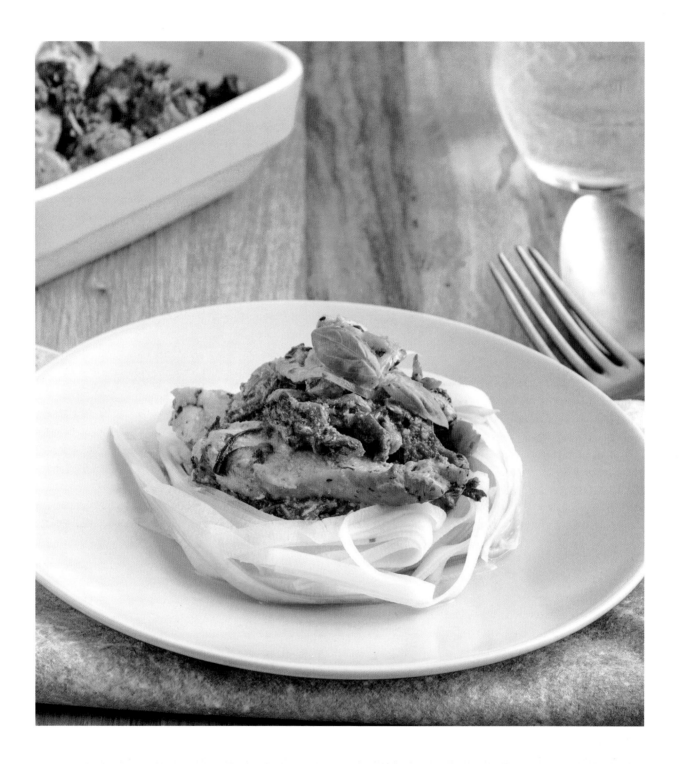

make it COCONUT-FREE:
Replace the coconut milk with a coconut-free option like cashew milk or macadamia nut milk. If you can eat dairy, heavy cream would work, too!

make it LOW-FODMAP:
Replace the white onion with ½ cup (40 g) sliced green onions (green parts only). For the sauce, omit the garlic, add 1 tablespoon garlic-infused oil, and use just 2 tablespoons pine nuts.

make it NIGHTSHADE-FREE:
Omit the sun-dried tomatoes and red pepper flakes.

make it NUT-FREE:
Replace the pine nuts with hulled sunflower seeds.

CHICKEN LAKSA

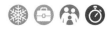

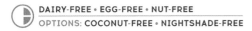

DAIRY-FREE · EGG-FREE · NUT-FREE

OPTIONS: COCONUT-FREE · NIGHTSHADE-FREE

SERVES 4

PREP TIME: 5 minutes

COOK TIME: 25 minutes

Laksa is traditionally served with noodles, and you're free to add spiral-sliced vegetables, kelp noodles, or konjac noodles to this recipe. I opted to use bean sprouts in place of noodles for a quick-and-easy solution, but anything goes here!

⅓ cup (70 g) coconut oil or ghee, or ⅓ cup (80 ml) avocado oil

¼ cup (40 g) diced white onions

4 stalks lemongrass, cut lengthwise to fit in the pan

1 fresh green chili pepper, diced

1 (2-in/5-cm) piece fresh ginger root, minced

4 cloves garlic, minced

2 teaspoons ground coriander

2 teaspoons curry powder

1 teaspoon ground cumin

½ teaspoon finely ground sea salt

1 pound (455 g) boneless, skinless chicken thighs, sliced

1 (13½-oz/400-ml) can lite coconut milk

2 cups (475 ml) chicken bone broth

FOR SERVING:

8 ounces (240 g) bean sprouts

4 lime wedges

8 fresh mint leaves

1. Heat the oil in a large saucepan over medium heat. Add the onions, lemongrass, chili pepper, ginger, garlic, coriander, curry powder, cumin, and salt and sauté for 10 minutes, or until fragrant.

2. Add the sliced chicken thighs, coconut milk, and broth. Cover and bring to a boil over high heat. Reduce the heat to low and simmer for 15 minutes, or until the chicken is cooked through.

3. Before serving, remove and discard the pieces of lemongrass. Divide the laksa among 4 large soup bowls. Top each bowl with 2 ounces (60 g) of bean sprouts, then squeeze a lime wedge over each bowl and drop the wedges into the bowls. Garnish each bowl with 2 mint leaves and serve!

STORE IT: *Keep in an airtight container in the fridge for up to 3 days or in the freezer for up to 1 month. The bean sprouts, mint leaves, and lime juice (but not the wedges) can be added to the soup before storing if you wish.*

REHEAT IT: *Transfer a single serving to a microwave-safe dish, cover, and microwave for 2½ minutes; or pour into a small saucepan, cover, and reheat over medium heat for 5 minutes.*

THAW IT: *Place in the fridge and allow to defrost completely, then follow the reheating instructions above.*

make it COCONUT-FREE:

Do not use coconut oil. Replace the coconut milk with the milk of your choice. Macadamia nut milk is great in this dish; make your own using the recipe on page 346 or purchase unsweetened macadamia nut milk from the store.

make it NIGHTSHADE-FREE:

Check the ingredients in the curry powder to ensure it is nightshade-free.

Per serving, made with coconut oil:

calories: **480**	calories from fat: **296**	total fat: **32.9g**	saturated fat: **22.6g**	cholesterol: **101mg**	
sodium: **745mg**	carbs: **8.9g**	dietary fiber: **0.6g**	net carbs: **8.3g**	sugars: **0.7g**	protein: **37.3g**

FAT:	CARBS:	PROTEIN:
62%	7%	31%

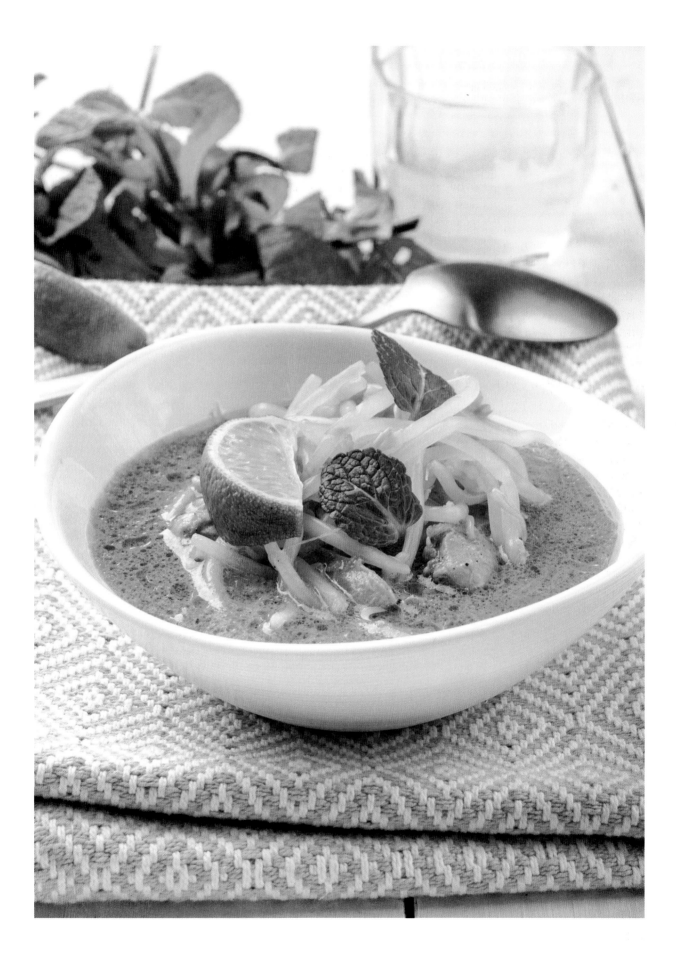

SUPER CHEESY SALMON ZOODLES

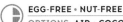
EGG-FREE · NUT-FREE

OPTIONS: **AIP · COCONUT-FREE · DAIRY-FREE · LOW-FODMAP · NIGHTSHADE-FREE**

SERVES 4

PREP TIME: 5 minutes (not including time to cook bacon)

COOK TIME: 35 minutes

If you can eat cheese, use the real stuff in this recipe. If you can't, use dairy-free cheese, the next best thing. Or, if you're living your keto life without cheese and feeling fine, simply omit it altogether! I prefer this dish without cheese, but I'm weird like that. In that case, this recipe would just be called Salmon Zoodles, but I'm okay with that if you are.

2 tablespoons avocado oil, coconut oil, or ghee

1 teaspoon paprika

1 teaspoon dried thyme leaves

½ teaspoon dried basil

½ teaspoon dried oregano leaves

¾ teaspoon finely ground sea salt, divided

¼ teaspoon ground black pepper

1 pound (455 g) salmon fillets, cut into 4 equal portions

2 large tomatoes, diced

½ cup (120 ml) chicken bone broth

½ cup (120 ml) full-fat coconut milk

3 cloves garlic, minced

½ teaspoon red pepper flakes

2 medium zucchinis, spiral sliced

1 cup (70 g) spinach, chopped

4 strips bacon (about 4 oz/112 g), cooked until crispy and crumbled

¾ cup (105 g) shredded mozzarella cheese (dairy-free or regular)

1. Heat the oil in a large frying pan over medium-low heat.

2. While the oil is heating, place the paprika, thyme, basil, oregano, ¼ teaspoon of the salt, and the pepper in a medium-sized bowl. Stir to blend, then dredge the salmon fillets, one at a time, in the mixture. When all the fillets are coated, place in the frying pan.

3. Cook the salmon for 6 minutes per side, until seared.

4. Once the salmon has cooked for a total of 12 minutes, transfer to a clean plate, leaving the cooking oil in the pan. Add the diced tomatoes, broth, coconut milk, garlic, red pepper flakes, and remaining ½ teaspoon of salt to the pan. Cook over medium heat, stirring often, for 15 minutes, until the sauce has thickened slightly.

5. Add the spiral-sliced zucchini and chopped spinach to the pan and toss to coat in the creamy tomato sauce. Set the cooked salmon on top of the zucchini mixture, then top with the bacon pieces and cheese. Cover, reduce the heat to low, and cook for another 5 minutes, or until the cheese has melted.

6. Divide the zoodles and cheese-topped salmon among 4 dinner plates and enjoy.

> **STORE IT:** *Keep in an airtight container in the fridge for up to 3 days or in the freezer for up to 1 month.*
>
> **REHEAT IT:** *Transfer a single serving to a microwave-safe dish, cover, and microwave for 2½ minutes.*
>
> **THAW IT:** *Place in the fridge and allow to defrost completely, then follow the reheating instructions above.*

Per serving, made with avocado oil and dairy-free cheese:

calories: **485** | calories from fat: **307** | total fat: **35g** | saturated fat: **19g** | cholesterol: **71mg**
sodium: **829mg** | carbs: **12.5g** | dietary fiber: **6.5g** | net carbs: **6g** | sugars: **3g** | protein: **30g**

FAT:	CARBS:	PROTEIN:
65%	**10%**	**25%**

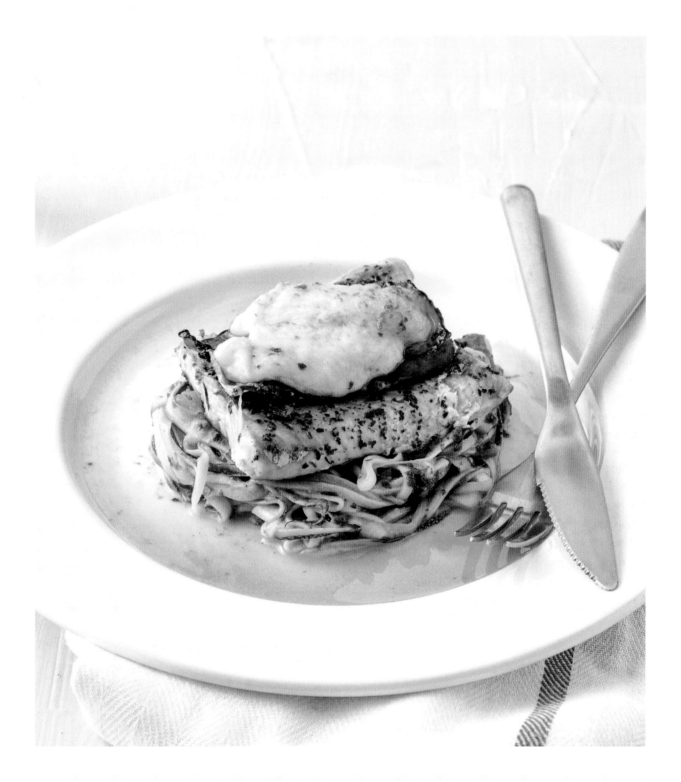

make it AIP:
Do not use ghee. Use chopped summer squash in place of the tomatoes and omit the paprika, black pepper, red pepper flakes, and cheese.

make it COCONUT-FREE:
Use avocado oil or ghee. If using dairy-free cheese, make sure it's also coconut-free.

make it DAIRY-FREE:
Do not use ghee. Use dairy-free cheese.

make it LOW-FODMAP:
Omit the garlic.

make it NIGHTSHADE-FREE:
Use chopped summer squash in place of the tomatoes and omit the paprika and red pepper flakes.

EPIC CAULIFLOWER NACHO PLATE

NUT-FREE

OPTIONS: COCONUT-FREE • DAIRY-FREE • EGG-FREE

SERVES 4

PREP TIME: 10 minutes

COOK TIME: 25 minutes

My sister introduced me to the concept of using roasted cauliflower "chips" as a base for nacho toppings. Good call, Christina! This is tasty! I like pairing my nachos with an avocado sauce as a replacement for sour cream. If your keto diet does not include dairy, go hog wild with the avocado sauce, or try Avocado Lime Dressing (page 84) instead. If you can eat sour cream, feel free to use it.

"CHIPS" AND MEAT TOPPING:

1 tablespoon chili powder

1 teaspoon ground cumin

1 teaspoon onion powder

¾ teaspoon finely ground sea salt

1 medium head cauliflower (about 1½ lbs/680 g), florets removed

¼ cup (60 ml) avocado oil, melted coconut oil, or melted ghee

1 pound (455 g) ground pork

AVOCADO SAUCE:

1 medium Hass avocado, peeled and pitted (about 4 oz/110 g of flesh)

2 cloves garlic

2 green onions

¼ cup (52 g) mayonnaise

1 tablespoon lime juice

¼ teaspoon ground black pepper

1 small tomato, diced

¼ cup (15 g) fresh cilantro leaves, chopped

1. Preheat the oven to 400°F (205°C). Line a rimmed baking sheet with parchment paper or a silicone baking mat.

2. Place the seasonings for the "chips" in a small bowl and stir to combine.

3. Using a sharp knife, thinly slice the cauliflower florets lengthwise through the stem, making sure that every piece has a bit of stem attached.

4. Place the cauliflower chips on the lined baking sheet. Drizzle with the oil and sprinkle with 2 teaspoons of the seasoning mixture. Gently toss to coat, then lay the chips flat on the baking sheet. Roast for 20 minutes, until the chips are fork-tender and lightly golden on the corners.

5. Place the ground pork in a large frying pan. Sprinkle with the remaining seasoning mixture and cook over medium heat until no longer pink, stirring occasionally to break up the meat, 5 to 7 minutes.

6. Meanwhile, place all the ingredients for the avocado sauce in a blender or food processor and blend until smooth.

7. To serve, place the roasted cauliflower chips on a large serving plate, then top with the seasoned meat, diced tomato, chopped cilantro, and avocado sauce.

make it COCONUT-FREE:
Do not use coconut oil.

make it DAIRY-FREE:
Do not use ghee.

make it EGG-FREE:
Use egg-free mayonnaise (see recipe on page 102).

MAKE IT AT HOME

Replace store-bought mayonnaise with my homemade version.

104

Mayonnaise

Per serving, made with avocado oil and homemade mayonnaise:

calories: **488**	calories from fat: **296**	total fat: **32.9g**	saturated fat: **5.2g**	cholesterol: **88mg**		FAT:	CARBS:	PROTEIN:
sodium: **576mg**	carbs: **14g**	dietary fiber: **6.9g**	net carbs: **7.1g**	sugars: **4.7g**	protein: **34.1g**	61%	11%	28%

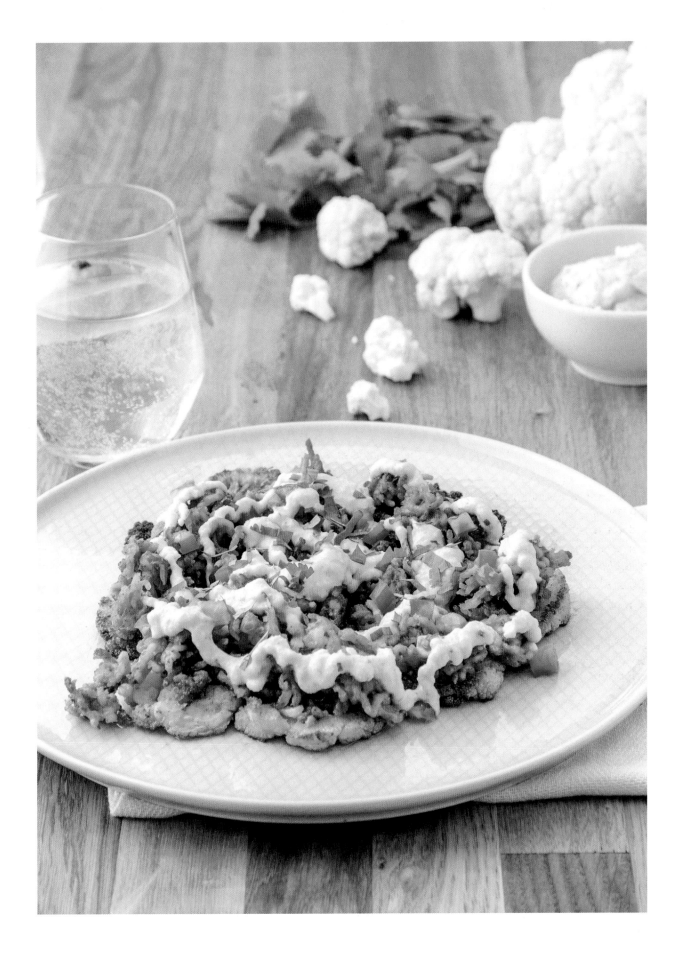

SHHH SLIDERS

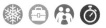

MAKES 16 sliders (4 per serving)

PREP TIME: 9 minutes

COOK TIME: 6 minutes

Sardines aren't something many of us gravitate toward when we're hungry, but these mini burgers might change your mind! Sardines are rich in omega-3, vitamin B12, calcium, and many of the minerals we need on keto to balance our electrolytes. This recipe is so good that I made it multiple times while writing the book. It's my go-to meal when we're hungry and I have very little time to create something fancy. Even my sardine-hating husband asks for it!

Don't want to make the mayo-based sauce? Replace it with ⅓ cup (80 ml) of Creamy Italian Dressing (page 94) or Ranch Dressing (page 76).

2 (3-oz/85-g) cans sardines

⅔ cup (140 g) mayonnaise, divided

½ cup (38 g) crushed pork rinds

2 teaspoons dried chives

1 teaspoon garlic powder

¾ teaspoon finely ground sea salt, divided

½ teaspoon paprika

½ teaspoon onion powder

½ teaspoon dried thyme leaves

3 tablespoons avocado oil

SAUCE:

1 tablespoon Dijon mustard

1 tablespoon pickle or caper brine

⅛ teaspoon cayenne pepper

7 to 10 lettuce leaves, torn into 4-inch (10-cm) pieces

14 cucumber slices

1. Place the sardines in a medium-sized bowl and mash with the back of a fork. Add ⅓ cup (70 g) of the mayonnaise, the crushed pork rinds, chives, garlic powder, ½ teaspoon of the salt, the paprika, onion powder, and thyme. Stir to combine.

2. Heat the oil in a large frying pan over medium heat.

3. Scoop up 1 tablespoon of the sardine mixture and roll it between your palms, then flatten to a ½-inch (2.5-cm) patty and place in the pan. Repeat with the remaining mixture, making a total of 16 patties. Cook the patties for 3 minutes per side, or until golden and a touch crispy. By the time you've finished forming the patties, the first patty you made should be ready to flip. Once done, remove the patties from the pan.

4. Meanwhile, make the sauce: Place the remaining ⅓ cup (70 g) of mayonnaise and remaining ¼ teaspoon of salt in a small dish along with the mustard, pickle brine, and cayenne pepper. Stir to incorporate.

5. To assemble the sliders, place the lettuce pieces on a large serving plate. Spoon a bit of sauce on a piece of lettuce, then place a sardine patty on top, followed by a cucumber slice and another dollop of sauce. Top with a second piece of lettuce. Repeat with the remaining lettuce, sauce, patties, and cucumber slices and serve.

make it LOW-FODMAP:
Omit the garlic and onion powder.

make it NIGHTSHADE-FREE:
Omit the paprika and cayenne.

STORE IT: *Keep the patties in an airtight container in the fridge for up to 3 days or in the freezer for up to 1 month. The sauce, lettuce, and cucumbers are best kept in the fridge for up to 5 days.*

REHEAT IT: *Transfer a single serving of the patties to a microwave-safe dish, cover, and microwave for 1 minute; or place in a frying pan with a tablespoon of oil and reheat over medium heat for 1 to 2 minutes.*

THAW IT: *Place the patties in the fridge and allow to thaw completely, then follow the reheating instructions above.*

PREP AHEAD: *Make the sauce ahead; it will keep in the fridge for up to 5 days.*

Per serving of 4 sliders:

calories: **488** | calories from fat: **413** | total fat: **45.9g** | saturated fat: **7.6g** | cholesterol: **87mg** | sodium: **949mg** | carbs: **1.8g** | dietary fiber: **0.5g** | net carbs: **1.3g** | sugars: **0.6g** | protein: **17.1g**

FAT: **85%** | CARBS: **1%** | PROTEIN: **15%**

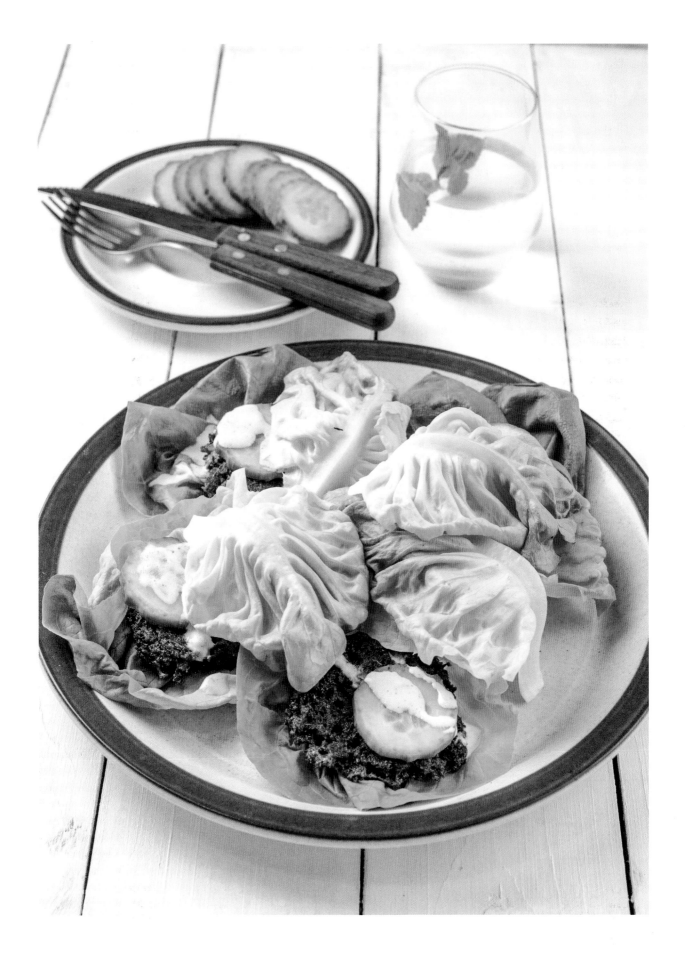

SHRIMP CURRY

DAIRY-FREE • EGG-FREE • NUT-FREE
OPTION: **COCONUT-FREE**

SERVES 4

PREP TIME: 15 minutes

COOK TIME: 30 minutes

Shave some time off this recipe by not pureeing the onion mixture. Simply skip Step 2 and, instead, add the coconut milk directly to the pan, then cook as instructed in Step 3. One less thing to clean!

You can save even more time by using store-bought riced cauliflower. I tend to rice my own because it's less expensive; the florets from one small to medium-sized head of cauliflower should give you the quantity of rice you need for this recipe. To prepare your own riced cauliflower, follow Step 4 of the Crispy Pork with Lemon-Thyme Cauli Rice recipe on page 208. To get 2 cups of riced cauliflower, you'll need about 5 cups/480 g of florets.

⅓ cup (70 g) coconut oil or ghee, or ⅓ cup (80 ml) avocado oil

1 small white onion, sliced

1 small fennel bulb, sliced

3 tablespoons red curry paste

1 (2-in/5-cm) piece fresh ginger root, minced

¾ teaspoon finely ground sea salt

1 (13½-oz/400-ml) can lite coconut milk

1 pound (455 g) medium shrimp, peeled, deveined, and tails removed

2 cups (250 g) riced cauliflower

½ cup (35 g) fresh cilantro leaves and stems, for serving

1. Heat the oil in a large saucepan over medium heat. Add the onion, fennel, curry paste, ginger, and salt. Sauté for 10 minutes, or until fragrant.

2. Transfer the sautéed onion mixture to a blender or food processor. Add the coconut milk and blend until smooth.

3. Return the mixture to the saucepan and add the shrimp and riced cauliflower. Cover and bring to a light boil over medium-high heat. Once lightly boiling, reduce the heat to medium-low and simmer for 20 minutes, until the cauliflower is soft.

4. Divide the curry among 4 bowls. Top with the cilantro and serve.

make it COCONUT-FREE:
Use avocado oil or ghee. Replace the coconut milk with the milk of your choice.

PRESSURE COOK IT: *Use the sauté mode for Step 1. After completing Step 2, return the pureed mixture to the cooker. Add the shrimp and riced cauliflower, seal the lid, and cook on high pressure for 15 minutes. Allow the pressure to release naturally before removing the lid. Continue with Step 4.*

STORE IT: *Keep in an airtight container in the fridge for up to 3 days or in the freezer for up to 1 month.*

REHEAT IT: *Place in a saucepan, cover, and reheat over medium-low heat for 5 minutes.*

THAW IT: *Place in the fridge and allow to defrost completely, then follow the reheating instructions above.*

Per serving, made with coconut oil:

calories: **499** | calories from fat: **334** | total fat: **37.1g** | saturated fat: **29.8g** | cholesterol: **222mg**
sodium: **1259mg** | carbs: **14.2g** | dietary fiber: **3.4g** | net carbs: **10.8g** | sugars: **2.3g** | protein: **27.2g**

FAT:	CARBS:	PROTEIN:
67%	11%	22%

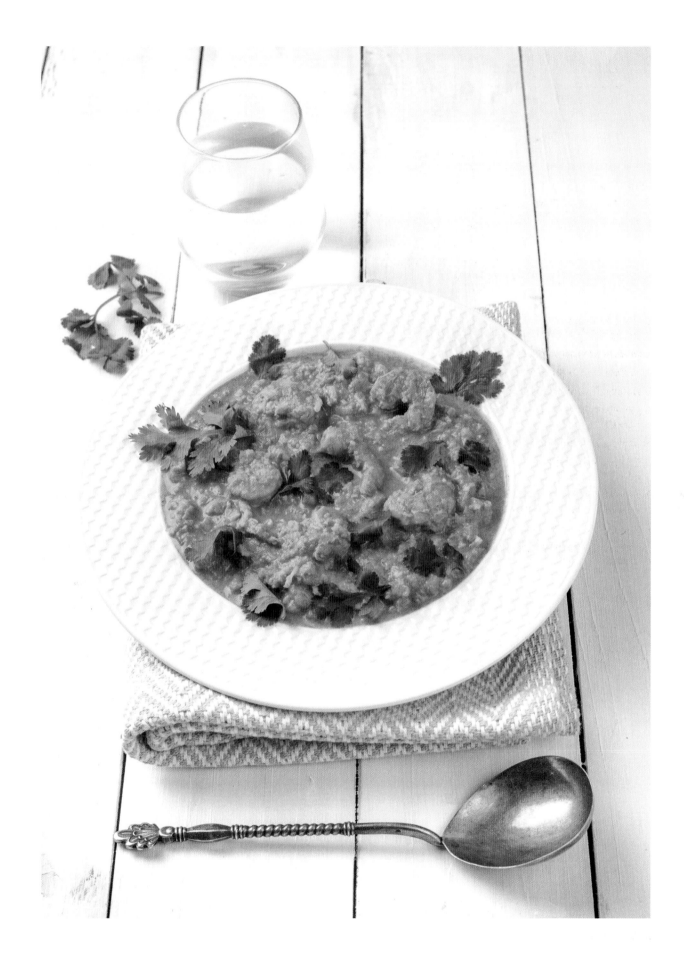

CABBAGE & SAUSAGE WITH BACON

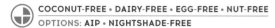

COCONUT-FREE • DAIRY-FREE • EGG-FREE • NUT-FREE
OPTIONS: AIP • NIGHTSHADE-FREE

SERVES 4
PREP TIME: 10 minutes
COOK TIME: 25 minutes

Mexican-style chorizo is one of my favorites for this recipe, but you can use any type of sausage you like. If you go with chorizo, look for the fresh stuff, not the dry-cured Spanish style.

6 strips bacon (about 6 oz/170 g), diced

1 small red onion, diced

4 cloves garlic, minced

1 small head green cabbage (about 1⅓ lbs/600 g), cored and thinly sliced

12 ounces (340 g) Mexican-style fresh (raw) chorizo, thinly sliced

¼ cup (60 ml) beef bone broth

1. Place the bacon, onion, and garlic in a large frying pan and sauté over medium heat until the bacon begins to crisp, about 10 minutes.

2. Add the cabbage, sausage slices, and broth. Cover and cook for 15 minutes, until the cabbage is fork-tender and the sausage is cooked through.

3. Remove the lid, divide among 4 dinner plates, and enjoy!

make it AIP/NIGHTSHADE-FREE:
Use a nightshade-free sausage.

PRESSURE COOK IT: *Use the sauté mode for Step 1. In Step 2, seal the lid and cook on high pressure for 5 minutes. Allow the pressure to release naturally before removing the lid, then serve.*

STORE IT: *Keep in an airtight container in the fridge for up to 3 days or in the freezer for up to 1 month.*

REHEAT IT: *Place a single serving in a microwave-safe dish, cover, and microwave for 2 minutes; or place in a small frying pan, cover, and reheat over medium heat for 5 minutes.*

THAW IT: *Place in the fridge and allow to defrost completely, then follow the reheating instructions above.*

Per serving:

calories: **523**	calories from fat: **395**	total fat: **43.8g**	saturated fat: **15.3g**	cholesterol: **93mg**	FAT:	CARBS:	PROTEIN:
sodium: **980mg**	carbs: **12g**	dietary fiber: **4g**	net carbs: **8g**	sugars: **6g**	protein: **20g**	76%	9%	16%

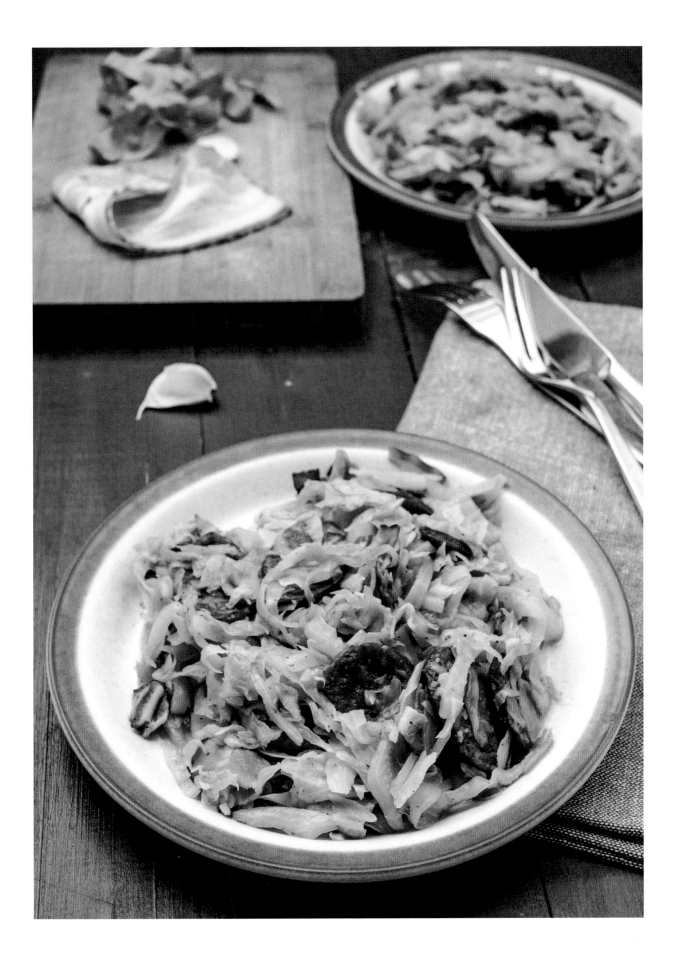

SECRET STUFFED PEPPERS

COCONUT-FREE • EGG-FREE • NUT-FREE

OPTIONS: AIP • DAIRY-FREE • LOW-FODMAP • NIGHTSHADE-FREE

MAKES 4 stuffed peppers (1 per serving)

PREP TIME: 10 minutes, plus 24 hours to soak livers

COOK TIME: 45 minutes

What's the secret? That there's liver in here! But you can't taste it, so eat on! That said, there is one trick: for the best flavor and texture, the livers should be soaked before cooking, so don't skip Step 1.

You can prepare your own riced cauliflower by following Step 4 of the Crispy Pork with Lemon-Thyme Cauli Rice recipe on page 208. (To get 1 cup of riced cauliflower, you'll need about 2½ cups/240 g of florets.) Or you can purchase pre-riced cauliflower, which you can find at Costco, Trader Joe's, and many other grocery and health food stores.

4 ounces (115 g) chicken livers

1 tablespoon apple cider vinegar

1 pound (455 g) ground beef

¼ cup (60 ml) avocado oil, or ¼ cup (55 g) coconut oil or ghee

1 small red onion, diced

6 cloves garlic, minced

1½ teaspoons ground black pepper

1 teaspoon dried oregano leaves

½ teaspoon finely ground sea salt

4 medium bell peppers, any color

1 cup (125 g) riced cauliflower

1 cup (140 g) shredded cheddar cheese (dairy-free or regular), divided

1. Soak the livers: Place the livers in a medium-sized bowl and cover with water. Add the vinegar. Cover and place in the fridge to soak for 24 to 48 hours.

2. After at least 24 hours, rinse and drain the soaked livers, then chop them into very small pieces with either a knife or a sharp pair of scissors.

3. Place the livers in a large frying pan along with the ground beef, oil, onion, garlic, black pepper, oregano, and salt. Sauté over medium heat until no longer pink, about 15 minutes, stirring often to crumble the meat as it cooks.

4. Meanwhile, cut the tops off the bell peppers, then core them, being sure to remove all the seeds and white membranes.

5. Place the peppers right side up in an 8-inch (20-cm) square baking pan and preheat the oven to 350°F (177°C).

6. After the meat mixture has cooked for 15 minutes, toss in the riced cauliflower and ¾ cup (105 g) of the cheese and stir to combine. Spoon the mixture into the peppers, dividing it evenly. Then sprinkle the tops with the remaining cheese, 1 tablespoon per pepper.

7. Bake for 25 to 30 minutes, until the peppers have softened and the cheese has melted. Enjoy!

PRESSURE COOK IT: *Complete Steps 1 through 4, then place the peppers in a pressure cooker. Complete Step 6, then pour ¼ cup (60 ml) water into the cooker. Seal the lid and set to the steam mode for 15 minutes. Allow the pressure to release naturally before removing the lid, then serve.*

STORE IT: *Keep in an airtight container in the fridge for up to 5 days or in the freezer for up to 1 month.*

REHEAT IT: *Place a single serving in a microwave-safe dish, cover, and microwave for 2 minutes; or place in a small frying pan, cover, and reheat over medium heat for 5 minutes.*

THAW IT: *Place in the fridge and allow to defrost completely, then follow the reheating instructions above.*

Per serving, made with avocado oil and dairy-free cheese:

calories: **573**	calories from fat: **373**	total fat: **41g**	saturated fat: **13.9g**	cholesterol: **263mg**	FAT:	CARBS:	PROTEIN:
sodium: **371mg**	carbs: **11.8g**	dietary fiber: **7.6g**	net carbs: **4.2g**	sugars: **1.6g**	protein: **39.4g**	**65%**	**8%**	**27%**

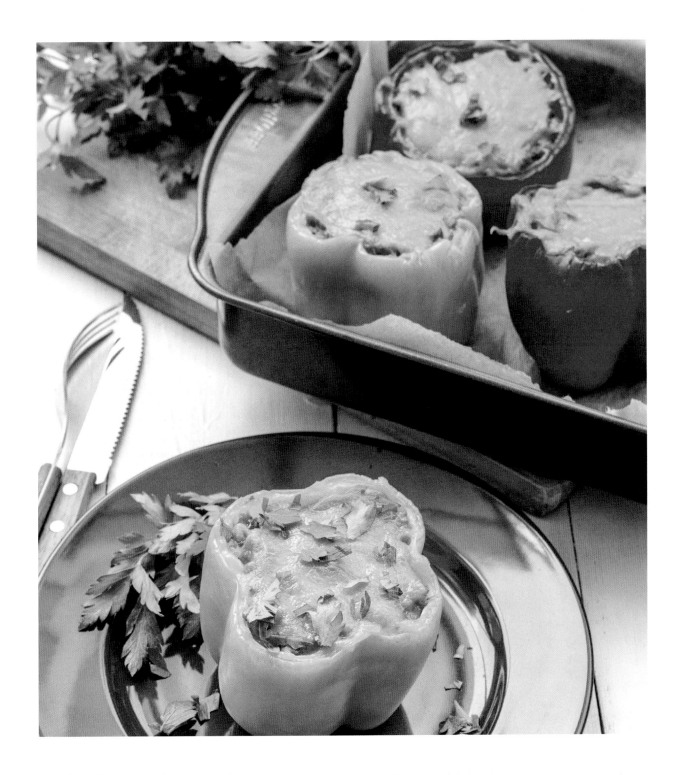

make it AIP/NIGHTSHADE-FREE:
Stuff zucchinis instead of bell peppers. Cut 4 medium zucchinis in half lengthwise, remove the seeds with a spoon, and fill the zucchini boats. Reduce the baking time to 15 minutes. For AIP, also omit the black pepper and cheese and opt for coconut oil or avocado oil.

make it DAIRY-FREE:
Do not use ghee. Use dairy-free cheese.

make it LOW-FODMAP:
Omit the red onion. Replace the garlic with 1 cup (80 g) sliced green onions (green parts only) and add 1 tablespoon garlic-infused oil to the meat mixture. Replace the riced cauliflower with riced broccoli.

SHRIMP FRY

 DAIRY-FREE • EGG-FREE • NUT-FREE

OPTIONS: AIP • COCONUT-FREE • LOW-FODMAP • NIGHTSHADE-FREE

SERVES 4

PREP TIME: 5 minutes

COOK TIME: 20 minutes

This is one of my favorite recipes when I'm at home and want to snuggle up on the couch with one (or all) of our pups!

¼ cup (55 g) coconut oil

1 pound (455 g) medium shrimp, peeled, deveined, and tails removed

12 ounces (340 g) smoked sausage (chicken, pork, beef—anything goes), cubed

5 asparagus spears, woody ends snapped off, thinly sliced

4 ounces (115 g) cremini mushrooms, sliced

1 medium zucchini, cubed

1 tablespoon paprika

2 teaspoons garlic powder

1 teaspoon onion powder

1 teaspoon dried thyme leaves

½ teaspoon finely ground sea salt

¼ teaspoon ground black pepper

Pinch of cayenne pepper (optional)

Handful of fresh parsley leaves, chopped, for serving

1. Melt the oil in a large frying pan over medium heat.

2. Add the remaining ingredients, except the parsley. Toss to coat in the oil, then cover and cook for 15 to 20 minutes, until the asparagus is tender and the shrimp has turned pink.

3. Divide the mixture among 4 serving plates, sprinkle with parsley, and serve.

STORE IT: *Keep in an airtight container in the fridge for up to 3 days or in the freezer for up to 1 month.*

REHEAT IT: *Transfer a single serving to a microwave-safe dish, cover, and microwave for 2 minutes; or place in a frying pan, cover, and reheat over medium heat for 5 minutes.*

THAW IT: *Place in the fridge and allow to defrost completely, then follow the reheating instructions above.*

make it AIP:
Omit the black pepper and paprika.

make it COCONUT-FREE:
Replace the coconut oil with avocado oil or ghee.

make it LOW-FODMAP:
Replace 2 tablespoons of the coconut oil with garlic-infused oil; check the ingredients in the sausage to ensure they're safe; double the amount of zucchini and omit the asparagus; replace the mushrooms with 1 cup (60 g) destemmed kale leaves, added in the last 10 minutes of cooking; and omit the garlic and onion powder.

make it NIGHTSHADE-FREE:
Omit the paprika.

Per serving, made with beef sausage:

calories: **574** | calories from fat: **361** | total fat: **40.1g** | saturated fat: **20.2g** | cholesterol: **311mg**
sodium: **1157mg** | carbs: **8.4g** | dietary fiber: **2.3g** | net carbs: **6.1g** | sugars: **2.6g** | protein: **45g**

FAT:	CARBS:	PROTEIN:
63%	6%	31%

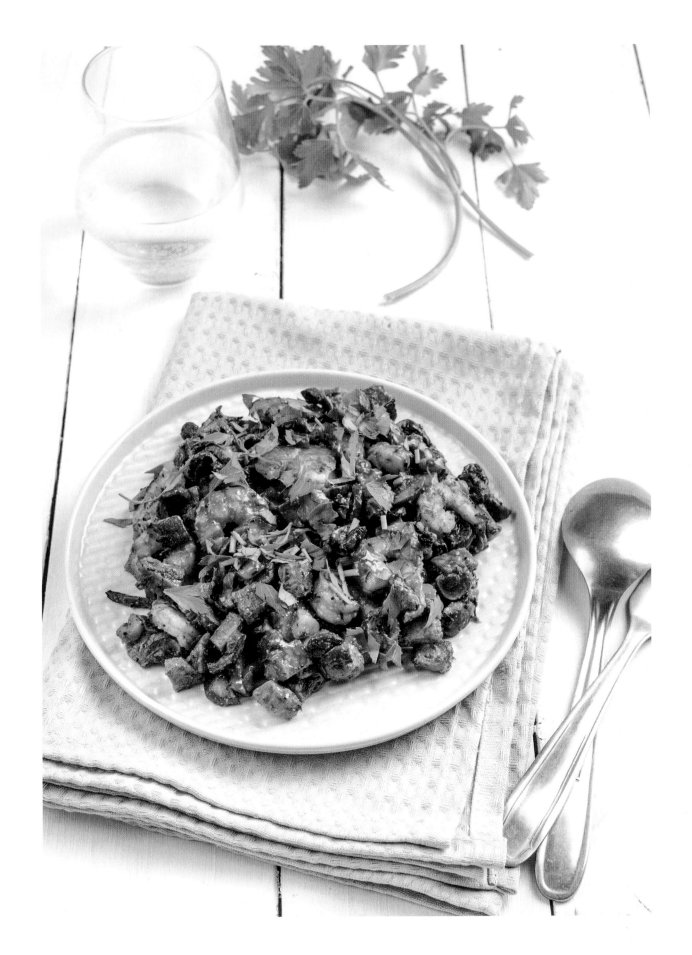

ROASTED BROCCOLI & MEAT SAUCE

 COCONUT-FREE • DAIRY-FREE • EGG-FREE • NUT-FREE
OPTION: LOW-FODMAP

SERVES 4
PREP TIME: 10 minutes
COOK TIME: 35 minutes

During a recent sailing trip, I realized that I'd forgotten to purchase zucchini for the noodle bowls I was planning to prepare for the crew on the night before heading home. We were low on food, had been sailing all day, and were totally wiped out. I had all the ingredients for meat sauce but no noodles to put it on. Instead of transforming the meat sauce into chili, I decided to serve the sauce over roasted broccoli, and it was delicious! The crew was happy, and I discovered a new way to enjoy meat sauce.

If you can eat dairy, Parmesan cheese would be amazing grated over the top of this dish. If you can't, nutritional yeast is a great alternative.

MEAT SAUCE:

¼ cup (60 ml) avocado oil
1 pound (455 g) ground turkey
1 cup (240 g) canned diced tomatoes
1 cup (250 g) tomato sauce
1 tablespoon tomato paste
2 teaspoons onion powder
2 teaspoons dried oregano leaves
1½ teaspoons dried basil
1 teaspoon garlic powder
½ teaspoon finely ground sea salt
⅛ teaspoon ground black pepper

ROASTED BROCCOLI:

1½ pounds (680 g) broccoli florets
¼ cup (60 ml) avocado oil
2 teaspoons lemon juice
¼ teaspoon finely ground sea salt
Pinch of ground black pepper

make it LOW-FODMAP:
For the meat sauce, omit the onion powder and garlic powder and replace 1 tablespoon of the avocado oil with garlic-infused oil.

1. Preheat the oven to 400°F (205°C). Line a rimmed baking sheet with parchment paper or a silicone baking mat.

2. Start the meat sauce: Heat the oil in a large frying pan over medium heat for 1 minute, then add the turkey. Cook, stirring frequently, until no longer pink, about 10 minutes.

3. Meanwhile, roast the broccoli: Place the broccoli florets on the lined baking sheet, sprinkle with the oil, lemon juice, salt, and pepper, and toss to coat. Bake for 20 to 25 minutes, until the broccoli is fork-tender and a little crispy on the edges.

4. When the turkey is fully cooked, add the remaining ingredients for the meat sauce to the pan. Cover and bring to a simmer over medium-high heat, then reduce the heat to medium-low to maintain a light simmer. Continue cooking, stirring frequently, until the broccoli is finished roasting.

5. Divide the roasted broccoli among 4 dinner plates. Pile the meat sauce on top and dig in!

PRESSURE COOK IT: *You can prepare the meat sauce in a pressure cooker. Use the sauté mode for Step 2. Then add the rest of the sauce ingredients to the cooker, seal the lid, and cook on high pressure for 15 minutes. Allow the pressure to release naturally before removing the lid, then serve the meat sauce with the roasted broccoli.*

STORE IT: *Keep in an airtight container in the fridge for up to 3 days. The meat sauce can be frozen for up to 1 month.*

REHEAT IT: *Transfer a single serving to a microwave-safe dish, cover, and microwave for 2½ minutes; or place in a frying pan, cover, and reheat over medium heat for 5 minutes.*

THAW IT: *Place in the fridge and allow to defrost completely, then follow the reheating instructions above.*

Per serving:

calories: **585**	calories from fat: **359**	total fat: **39.9g**	saturated fat: **5.5g**	cholesterol: **116mg**	
sodium: **644mg**	carbs: **18.9g**	dietary fiber: **6.3g**	net carbs: **12.6g**	sugars: **7.4g**	protein: **37.6g**

FAT:	CARBS:	PROTEIN:
61%	13%	26%

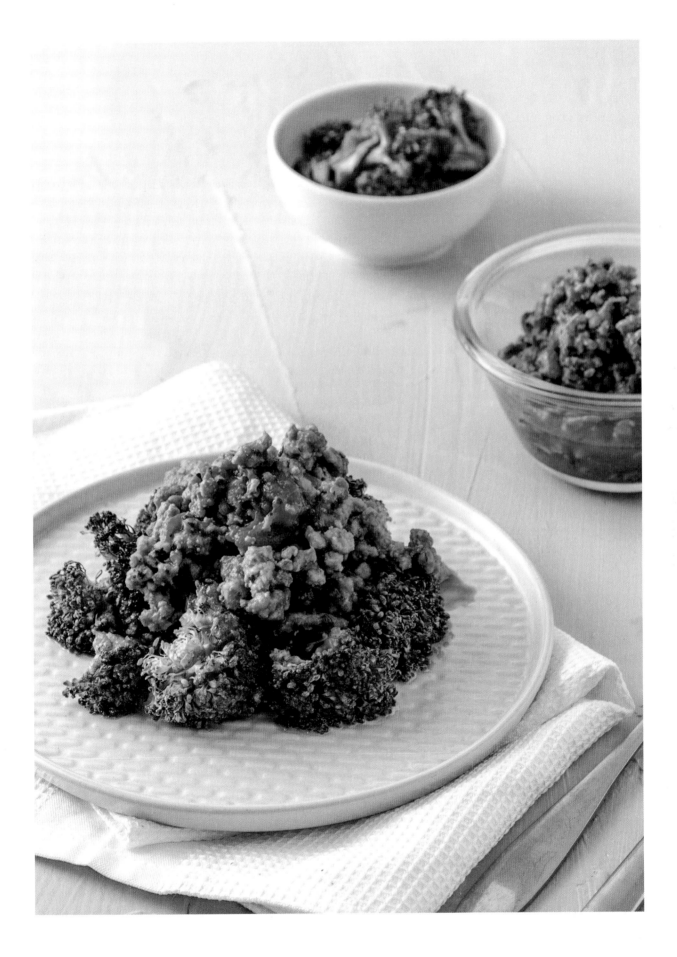

CHEESY MEATBALLS & NOODLES

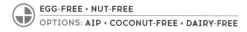

EGG-FREE • NUT-FREE

OPTIONS: **AIP • COCONUT-FREE • DAIRY-FREE**

SERVES 6

PREP TIME: 10 minutes

COOK TIME: 20 minutes

If you can eat dairy, swap out the dairy-free shredded cheese for the real thing. If you can't eat dairy, any dairy-free cheese option would do great; one of my favorites is from a company called Daiya. If all this cheese talk has you confused, just omit it from the recipe completely.

MEATBALLS:

1 pound (455 g) ground turkey

1 pound (455 g) ground pork

½ cup (70 g) shredded mozzarella cheese (dairy-free or regular)

2 tablespoons hot sauce

2 teaspoons dried oregano leaves

1½ teaspoons dried basil

1¼ teaspoons garlic powder

1 teaspoon onion powder

¾ teaspoon finely ground sea salt

½ teaspoon dried rosemary leaves

3 tablespoons avocado oil or coconut oil

4 medium zucchinis, spiral sliced

1 tablespoon lemon juice

1. Place the turkey, pork, cheese, hot sauce, oregano, basil, garlic powder, onion powder, salt, and rosemary in a large mixing bowl and combine with your hands until fully incorporated.

2. Heat the oil in a large frying pan over medium heat. While the oil is heating, form the meatballs: Take 3 tablespoons of the meat mixture, roll it into a ball between your palms, and place it in the frying pan. Repeat with the remaining meat mixture, placing the meatballs as close together as possible so that they all fit in the pan at one time. You should get about 18 meatballs.

3. Cover the pan and cook the meatballs for 15 minutes, or until fully cooked.

4. Add the spiral-sliced zucchini and lemon juice to the pan with the cooked meatballs. Cover and cook for another 5 minutes.

5. Divide the noodles and meatballs among 6 dinner plates and dig in.

make it AIP:
Omit the hot sauce. Ensure that the cheese you use is AIP or omit the cheese.

make it COCONUT-FREE:
If using dairy-free cheese, make sure it's also coconut-free.

make it DAIRY-FREE:
Use dairy-free cheese.

STORE IT: *Keep in an airtight container in the fridge for up to 3 days or in the freezer for up to 1 month.*

REHEAT IT: *Transfer a single serving to a microwave-safe dish, cover, and microwave for 2 minutes; or place in a frying pan, cover, and reheat over medium-low heat for 5 minutes.*

THAW IT: *Place in the fridge and allow to defrost completely, then follow the reheating instructions above.*

Per serving, made with dairy-free cheese and avocado oil:

calories: **595**	calories from fat: **407**	total fat: **45.2g**	saturated fat: **20.9g**	cholesterol: **163mg**
sodium: **670mg**	carbs: **3.6g**	dietary fiber: **1g**	net carbs: **2.6g**	sugars: **0.9g**	protein: **43.8g**

FAT:	CARBS:	PROTEIN:
68%	2%	30%

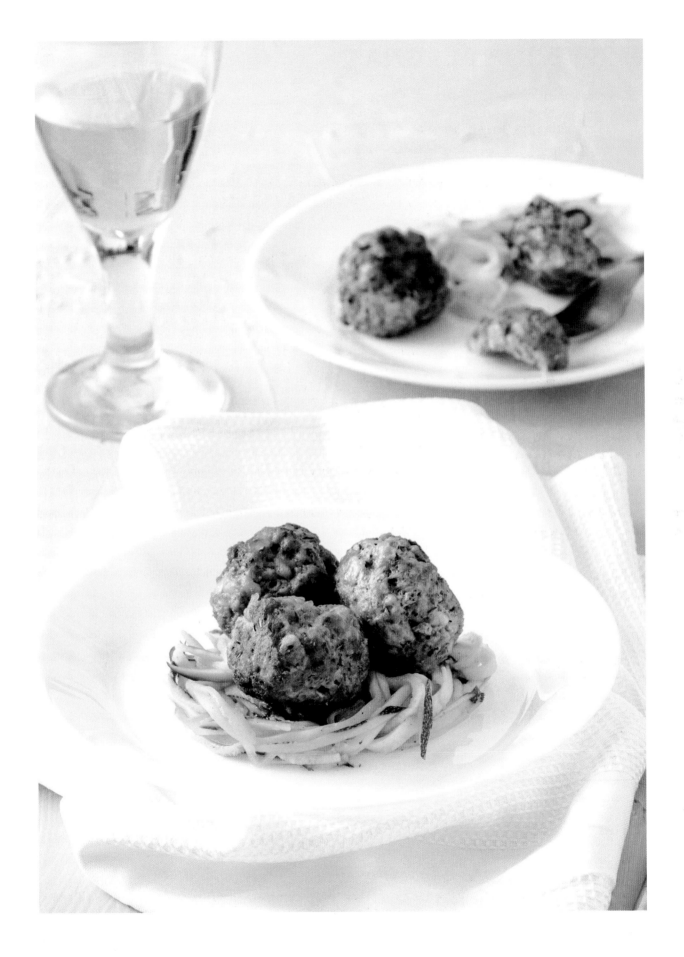

ZUCCHINI LASAGNA

NUT-FREE

OPTIONS: COCONUT-FREE • DAIRY-FREE

SERVES 6

PREP TIME: 10 minutes, plus 20 minutes to rest

COOK TIME: 55 minutes

Not feeling the cheese in this recipe? Use the Melty "Cheese" on page 243 instead.

2 teaspoons dried basil

1 teaspoon dried oregano leaves

1 teaspoon dried rosemary leaves

½ teaspoon dried thyme leaves

¾ teaspoon finely ground sea salt

½ cup (120 ml) avocado oil, or ½ cup (105 g) ghee

1 pound (455 g) ground turkey

1 small yellow onion, diced

2 cloves garlic, minced

2 cups (280 g) shredded mozzarella cheese (dairy-free or regular), divided

2 large eggs, beaten

3 medium zucchinis, sliced lengthwise into thin sheets

2 cups (475 ml) marinara sauce

1. Preheat the oven to 400°F (205°C).

2. Place the dried herbs and salt in a small bowl. Pinch with your fingers to mix.

3. Heat the oil in a medium-sized frying pan over medium heat. Add the turkey, onion, garlic, and 2 teaspoons of the herb mixture and sauté until the turkey is no longer pink, about 10 minutes.

4. Meanwhile, place 1 cup (140 g) of the cheese and the beaten eggs in a medium-sized bowl along with the remaining herb mixture; stir to combine.

5. When the meat is cooked, assemble the lasagna: Place half of the zucchini slices in a 13 by 9-inch (33 by 23-cm) baking dish, followed by the turkey mixture, the cheese mixture, half of the sauce, the rest of the zucchini slices, and the remaining sauce. Top with the remaining 1 cup (140 g) of shredded cheese.

6. Bake for 45 minutes, until bubbly and the cheese has melted. Allow to sit for 20 minutes before serving.

make it COCONUT-FREE:
If using dairy-free cheese, make sure it's also coconut-free.

make it DAIRY-FREE:
Use avocado oil and dairy-free cheese.

STORE IT: *Keep in an airtight container in the fridge for up to 3 days or in the freezer for up to 1 month.*

REHEAT IT: *Transfer a single serving to a microwave-safe dish, cover, and microwave for 2 minutes.*

THAW IT: *Place in the fridge and allow to defrost completely, then follow the reheating instructions above.*

Per serving, made with avocado oil and dairy-free cheese:

				FAT:	CARBS:	PROTEIN:
calories: **600** | calories from fat: **405** | total fat: **45g** | saturated fat: **12.6g** | cholesterol: **134mg**				**68%**	**15%**	**17%**
sodium: **688mg** | carbs: **22.6g** | dietary fiber: **15.8g** | net carbs: **6.8g** | sugars: **3.7g** | protein: **26.3g**						

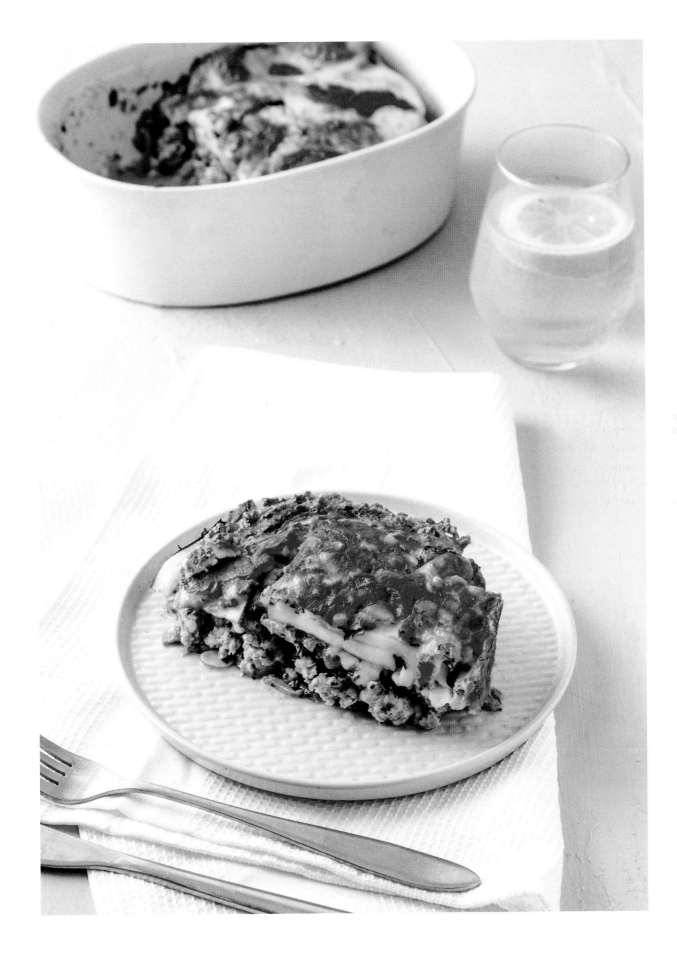

MEXICAN MEATZZA

EGG-FREE

OPTIONS: COCONUT-FREE · DAIRY-FREE · NUT-FREE

SERVES 4

PREP TIME: 10 minutes

COOK TIME: 45 minutes

I love, love this recipe, and the cilantro cream that goes with it is to die for! Either drizzle it on top of the meatzza or use as a dipping sauce; you won't be disappointed.

If you don't want to use dairy-free or regular shredded cheese, there's another option that I think you'll like: Walnut "Cheese." I use the recipe all the time. It's a great finishing touch for anything that needs a cheesy flavor, but you shouldn't cook or bake with it because of the walnuts. Another plus is that it adds fiber and fat, which is never a bad thing! If you decide to make it, just remember that you'll need to give the walnuts a 24-hour soak beforehand.

Don't want to make the cilantro cream? Try serving the meatzza with ⅔ cup (160 ml) of Avocado Lime Dressing (page 84) instead.

MEATZZA CRUST:

1 pound (455 g) ground beef

1 cup (75 g) crushed pork rinds

½ cup (75 g) finely diced white onions

1 tablespoon chili powder

2 teaspoons garlic powder

1 teaspoon ground cumin

1 teaspoon finely ground sea salt

½ teaspoon ground black pepper

½ medium bell pepper, any color, thinly sliced

1 cup (140 g) shredded cheddar cheese (dairy-free or regular), or 1 batch Walnut "Cheese" (see recipe, opposite)

CILANTRO CREAM:

½ cup (125 g) coconut cream

⅓ cup (20 g) fresh cilantro leaves and stems, finely chopped

1 tablespoon lime juice

1 clove garlic

¼ teaspoon finely ground sea salt

make it COCONUT-FREE:
Omit the cilantro cream.

make it DAIRY-FREE:
Use dairy-free cheddar cheese or Walnut "Cheese."

make it NUT-FREE:
Use dairy-free or regular cheese.

1. Preheat the oven to 350°F (177°C). Line a rimmed baking sheet with parchment paper or a silicone baking mat.

2. Make the crust: Place the ground beef, crushed pork rinds, onions, chili powder, garlic powder, cumin, salt, and black pepper in a large bowl and stir to combine. Press the mixture into the lined baking sheet, shaping it into a ½-inch (1.25-cm)-thick rectangle.

3. Bake the crust for 30 minutes, or until the internal temperature reaches 160°F (71°C).

4. Remove the baking sheet from the oven and top the crust with the sliced bell pepper, followed by the cheddar cheese, if using. Return the baking sheet to the oven and continue to cook for 15 minutes, or until the peppers have softened and the cheese has melted.

5. Meanwhile, place the cilantro cream ingredients in a medium-sized bowl and whisk until smooth.

6. Remove the meatzza from the oven. If using Walnut "Cheese," sprinkle it on the meatzza. Cut the meatzza into 8 equal slices and serve with the cilantro cream, either drizzled over the slices or alongside as a dipping sauce. Enjoy!

STORE IT: *Keep the meatzza and cilantro cream in separate airtight containers in the fridge for up to 5 days. When ready to serve, allow the cilantro cream to sit out on the counter for 5 to 10 minutes to soften up. You can speed up the process by whipping it with a fork until smooth.*

REHEAT IT: *Transfer a single serving of meatzza to a microwave-safe dish, cover, and microwave for 2 minutes; or place in a large frying pan, cover, and reheat over medium heat for 5 minutes. Then drizzle with cilantro cream.*

Per serving, made with dairy-free cheddar cheese:

calories: **603**	calories from fat: **369**	total fat: **41.1g**	saturated fat: **20.6g**	cholesterol: **128mg**
sodium: **1077mg**	carbs: **13.3g**	dietary fiber: **8.3g**	net carbs: **5g**	sugars: **0g**	protein: **44.9g**

FAT:	CARBS:	PROTEIN:
61%	**9%**	**30%**

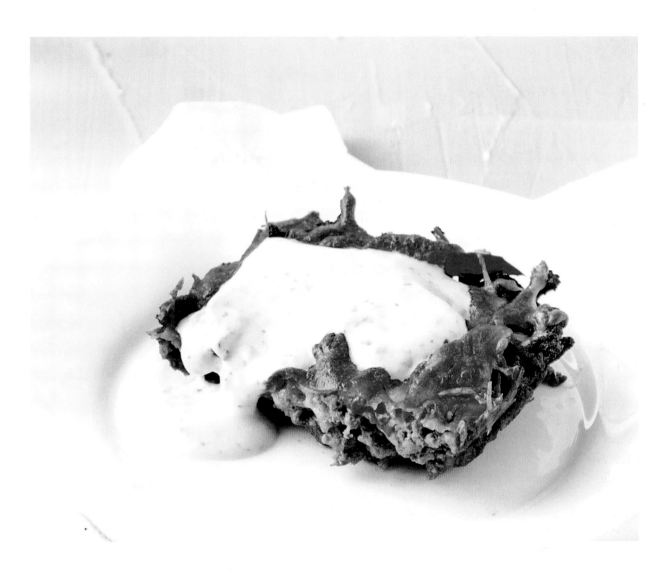

HOW TO MAKE WALNUT "CHEESE"

¾ cup (85 g) raw walnut pieces, soaked for 24 hours, then drained, rinsed, and finely chopped

3 tablespoons olive oil or avocado oil

⅓ cup (22 g) nutritional yeast

2 teaspoons lemon juice

½ teaspoon Dijon mustard

¼ teaspoon garlic powder

¼ teaspoon onion powder

Pinch of finely ground sea salt

Pinch of ground black pepper

Use this in place of shredded cheddar cheese; it will taste just as good! Unlike the cheddar, this is added to the meatzza after it comes out of the oven, instead of before.

Place all the ingredients in a large bowl and stir to combine.

Per serving, made with Walnut "Cheese":

calories: **737**	calories from fat: **485**	total fat: **53.9g**	saturated fat: **18.3g**	cholesterol: **128mg**
sodium: **1081mg**	carbs: **11.5g**	dietary fiber: **4.9g**	net carbs: **6.6g**	sugars: **3.3g**	protein: **51.7g**

FAT:	CARBS:	PROTEIN:
66%	**6%**	**28%**

NOODLE BAKE

EGG-FREE • NUT-FREE

OPTIONS: AIP • COCONUT-FREE • DAIRY-FREE • NIGHTSHADE-FREE

SERVES 6

PREP TIME: 10 minutes

COOK TIME: 55 minutes

If you don't want to use shredded cheese in this recipe, check out the Melty "Cheese" on the opposite page. It's 100 percent dairy-free and delicious in this dish.

Not sure how to spiral-slice a jicama? It's easy! Simply peel the jicama, then slice it in half from the top down. You'll be left with two moon-shaped pieces. Cut the ends off the pieces at the pointiest part to give you a flat space to use in a spiral slicer.

⅓ cup (80 ml) avocado oil, or ⅓ cup (70 g) coconut oil or ghee

1¾ pounds (785 g) bulk/ground Italian sausage

1 large jicama (about 25 oz/700 g), peeled and spiral sliced

1 small red onion, sliced

1 tomato, diced

3 cloves garlic, minced

2 teaspoons dried basil

1 teaspoon dried oregano leaves

1 teaspoon dried thyme leaves

1 teaspoon finely ground sea salt

½ teaspoon dried rosemary leaves

¼ teaspoon ground black pepper

2 cups (280 g) shredded cheddar cheese (dairy-free or regular), or 1 batch Melty "Cheese" (see recipe, opposite)

1. Preheat the oven to 400°F (205°C).

2. Heat the oil in a large frying pan over medium heat. Add the sausage and sauté until no longer pink, about 10 minutes.

3. Meanwhile, place the remaining ingredients, except the cheese, in a 13 by 9-inch (33 by 23-cm) baking pan. Toss to combine.

4. When the sausage is done, transfer it to the baking pan along with the fat in the pan. Toss to coat, then top the entire dish with the shredded cheese or Melty "Cheese."

5. Bake for 45 minutes, until the jicama noodles are fork-tender and the cheese has melted.

make it AIP:
Omit the tomato and black pepper. Do not use ghee.

make it COCONUT-FREE:
Do not use coconut oil. If using dairy-free cheese, make sure it's also coconut-free.

make it DAIRY-FREE:
Do not use ghee. Use dairy-free cheddar cheese or Melty "Cheese."

make it NIGHTSHADE-FREE:
Omit the tomato.

STORE IT: *Keep in an airtight container in the fridge for up to 5 days.*

REHEAT IT: *Transfer a single serving to a microwave-safe dish, cover, and microwave for 2 minutes; or place in a frying pan, cover, and reheat over medium heat for 5 minutes.*

Per serving, made with avocado oil and dairy-free cheddar cheese:

calories: **607** | calories from fat: **436** | total fat: **48g** | saturated fat: **15g** | cholesterol: **93mg**

sodium: **1438mg** | carbs: **19g** | dietary fiber: **10g** | net carbs: **9g** | sugars: **5g** | protein: **24.8g**

FAT:	CARBS:	PROTEIN:
71%	13%	16%

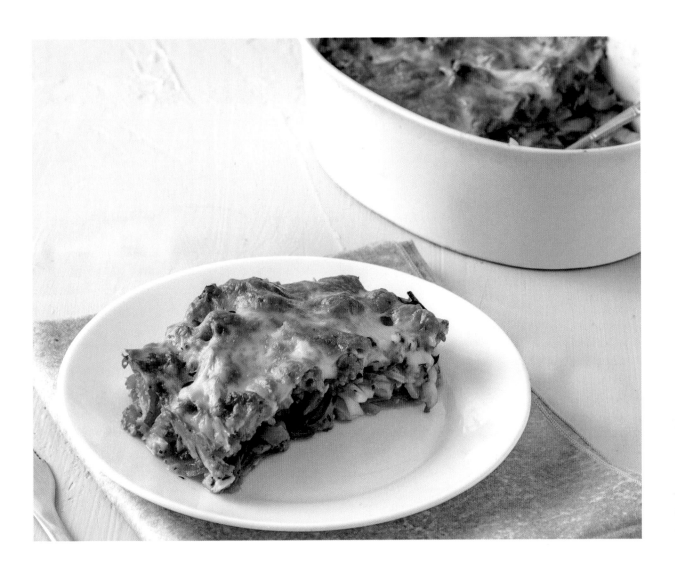

HOW TO MAKE MELTY "CHEESE"

¼ cup (55 g) coconut oil or lard

2 cups (475 ml) nondairy milk

1½ teaspoons finely ground sea salt

1 teaspoon lemon juice

½ teaspoon garlic powder

½ teaspoon onion powder

3 tablespoons arrowroot starch or
tapioca starch

3 large eggs

This is a great dairy-free cheese alternative for lasagna and other similar casseroles. For the nondairy milk, I like to use almond milk or coconut milk.

Melt the oil in a small saucepan over medium heat. Meanwhile, place the milk, salt, lemon juice, garlic powder, and onion powder in a small bowl; stir to combine. Whisk the starch into the melted oil. When the starch is fully incorporated, slowly pour the milk mixture into the starch mixture, whisking to combine. Continue to whisk until smooth, then remove the pan from the heat and allow to cool for 15 minutes.

Meanwhile, beat the eggs in a small bowl. Once the milk mixture has cooled, slowly whisk in the eggs. Adding the eggs will make the sauce thinner. Do not worry! The sauce will thicken up when it's baked. Pour the Melty "Cheese" over the top of the casserole and bake as you normally would.

Use the Melty "Cheese" immediately; it does not keep well.

Per serving, made with "Melty Cheese":

calories: **599**	calories from fat: **401**	total fat: **44.6g**	saturated fat: **19.5g**	cholesterol: **175mg**
sodium: **1998mg**	carbs: **18.4g**	dietary fiber: **7g**	net carbs: **11.4g**	sugars: **5.5g**	protein: **27.8g**

FAT:	CARBS:	PROTEIN:
68%	**13%**	**19%**

BACON-WRAPPED STUFFED CHICKEN

COCONUT-FREE • DAIRY-FREE • EGG-FREE • NIGHTSHADE-FREE • NUT-FREE
OPTION: **AIP**

SERVES 4
PREP TIME: 15 minutes
COOK TIME: 45 minutes

A keto cookbook wouldn't be complete without a bacon-wrapped dinner option. I always look out for sales on nitrate-free bacon and stock the freezer when I can.

Also, note the sodium level in this recipe—it's off the charts! This is because I go for the most common ingredient options when I calculate the nutrition information. So the sodium level per serving assumes that you are using conventionally produced bacon. You can lower the amount of sodium by opting for a better-quality bacon.

4 boneless, skinless chicken thighs (about 1 lb/455 g)

¾ cup (130 g) canned artichoke hearts

2 tablespoons avocado oil

Handful of fresh basil leaves and stems

2 cloves garlic

¼ teaspoon finely ground sea salt

¼ teaspoon ground black pepper

12 strips bacon (about 12 oz/340 g)

8 cups (160 g) arugula, divided

1. Preheat the oven to 400°F (205°C). Line a rimmed baking sheet with parchment paper or a silicone baking mat.

2. Place the chicken thighs on a sheet of parchment paper. Using a meat mallet, pound the thighs until they're ¼ inch (6 mm) thick. Place on the lined baking sheet.

3. Place the artichoke hearts, oil, basil, garlic, salt, and pepper in a blender or food processor. Pulse until chopped but not smooth.

4. Spread one-quarter of the artichoke mixture on a chicken thigh, starting at the shortest end, about 1 inch (5 cm) from the edge of the thigh. Roll the thigh in on itself and wrap tightly with 3 strips of bacon. Set the bacon-wrapped thigh, ends down, on the lined baking sheet. Repeat with the remaining thighs, artichoke mixture, and bacon.

5. Bake the stuffed thighs for 45 minutes, or until the internal temperature reaches 165°F (74°C) and the bacon is crisp.

6. To serve, place 1 thigh and 2 cups (40 g) of arugula on each plate, then drizzle the arugula with the leftover cooking juices.

make it AIP:
Omit the black pepper.

STORE IT: *Keep the arugula and the chicken and cooking juices in separate airtight containers in the fridge for up to 3 days, or wrap and freeze the chicken for up to 1 month.*

REHEAT IT: *Transfer a single serving of chicken to a microwave-safe dish, cover, and microwave for 2½ minutes; or place in a frying pan and reheat over medium heat for 5 minutes, flipping it as it cooks to recrisp the bacon on both sides.*

THAW IT: *Place in the fridge and allow to defrost completely, then follow the reheating instructions above.*

Per serving:

calories: **666** | calories from fat: **427** | total fat: **47.4g** | saturated fat: **13.5g** | cholesterol: **189mg**
sodium: **2223mg** | carbs: **6.8g** | dietary fiber: **2.5g** | net carbs: **4.3g** | sugars: **1.2g** | protein: **53.1g**

FAT:	CARBS:	PROTEIN:
64%	4%	32%

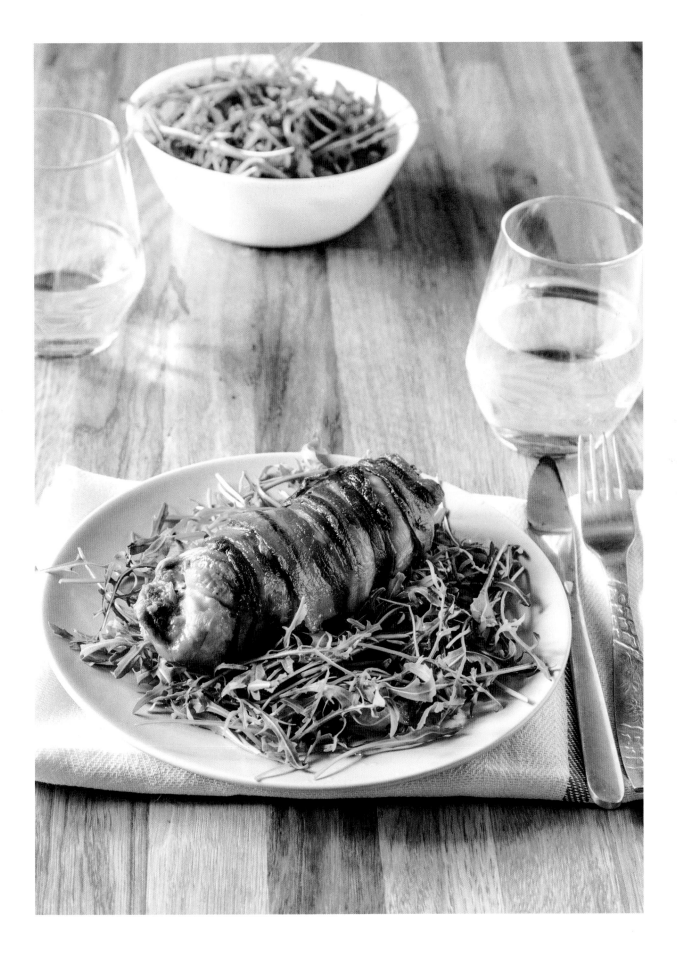

ONE-POT STUFFIN'

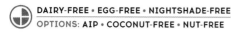 **DAIRY-FREE • EGG-FREE • NIGHTSHADE-FREE**
OPTIONS: AIP • COCONUT-FREE • NUT-FREE

SERVES 4
PREP TIME: 10 minutes
COOK TIME: 25 minutes

It tastes like holiday stuffing, but without all the work! When Kevin and I are in the mood for shovel food (you know, the type of meal that you just shovel into your mouth—glamorous, I know), this dish is a top pick!

¼ cup (55 g) coconut oil, or ¼ cup (60 ml) avocado oil

2 (7-oz/198-g) packages precooked breakfast sausage, roughly chopped

2 medium carrots (about 4 oz/110 g), diced

1 small rutabaga (about 4½ oz/130 g), peeled and diced

1 small white onion, diced

1 leek, white part only, thinly sliced

1 clove garlic, minced

½ cup (120 ml) chicken bone broth

½ teaspoon finely ground sea salt

¼ teaspoon ground black pepper

¼ cup (17 g) fresh parsley leaves, finely chopped

2 teaspoons fresh thyme leaves

6 fresh savory or sage leaves, finely chopped

¾ cup (110 g) shelled raw or roasted pistachios

1. Heat the oil in a large frying pan over medium heat. Add the sausage, carrots, rutabaga, onion, leek, garlic, broth, salt, and pepper. Stir, cover, and cook for 15 minutes, until the carrots and rutabaga are fork-tender.

2. Remove the lid and add the herbs. Continue to cook for 10 minutes, until fragrant.

3. Toss in the pistachios, divide among 4 dinner plates, and enjoy.

PRESSURE COOK IT: *Place all the ingredients listed in Step 1 in a pressure cooker. Seal the lid and cook on high pressure for 10 minutes. Allow the pressure to release naturally before removing the lid, then follow Step 2, using the sauté mode for the last 10 minutes of cooking. Continue with Step 3.*

STORE IT: *Keep in an airtight container in the fridge for up to 3 days or in the freezer for up to 1 month.*

REHEAT IT: *Transfer a single serving to a microwave-safe dish, cover, and microwave for 2½ minutes.*

THAW IT: *Place in the fridge and allow to defrost completely, then follow the reheating instructions above.*

make it AIP:
Omit the black pepper and pistachios.

make it COCONUT-FREE:
Use avocado oil.

make it NUT-FREE:
Use ½ cup (75 g) hulled sunflower seeds instead of the pistachios.

Per serving, made with coconut oil:

calories: **681** | calories from fat: **509** | total fat: **57.9g** | saturated fat: **24.7g** | cholesterol: **76mg**
sodium: **1165mg** | carbs: **22g** | dietary fiber: **6g** | net carbs: **16g** | sugars: **8g** | protein: **22g**

FAT: **75%** | CARBS: **12%** | PROTEIN: **13%**

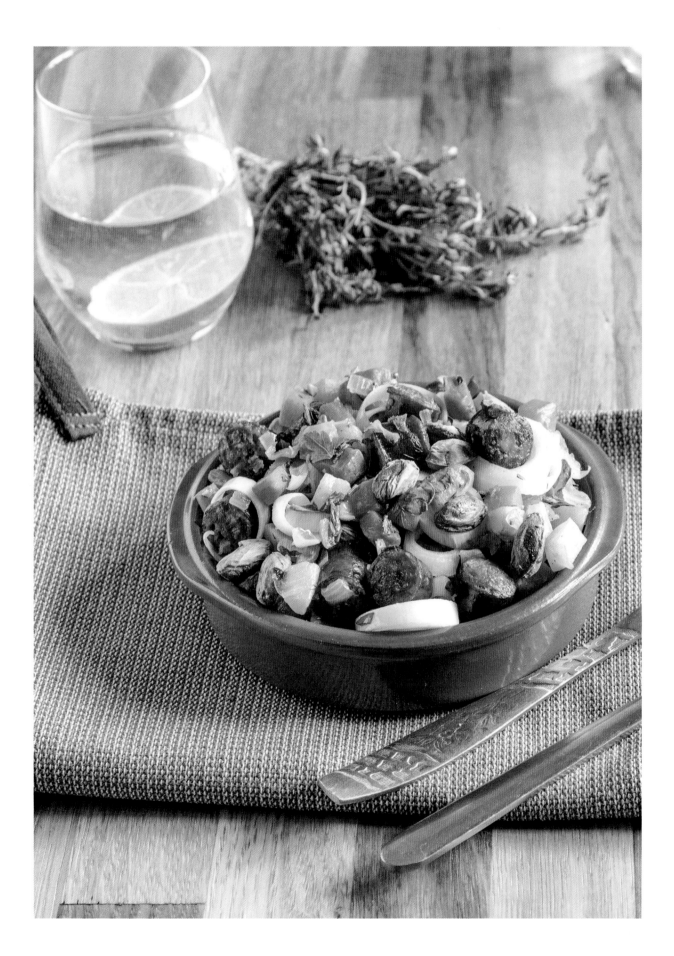

SOUTHERN PULLED PORK "SPAGHETTI"

 COCONUT-FREE • DAIRY-FREE • EGG-FREE • NUT-FREE

SERVES 6

PREP TIME: 10 minutes

COOK TIME: 45 minutes or 4 to 6 hours, depending on method

Meat on top of meat with more meat is the story of this recipe! My previous vegan self is shaming me right now, but my body's always happy when I eat this dish. Think of the shredded pork as the "spaghetti" and the barbecue pork sauce as the meat sauce.

Don't love pork? Swap out the pork shoulder for an equal amount of chicken thighs and the ground pork for ground chicken. You could do the same with turkey or beef.

PORK "SPAGHETTI":

2 pounds (910 g) boneless pork shoulder

1 cup (240 ml) chicken bone broth

1 teaspoon finely ground sea salt

BARBECUE PORK SAUCE:

2 tablespoons avocado oil

1 red bell pepper, diced

1 small white onion, diced

8 cremini mushrooms, diced

1 pound (455 g) ground pork

¾ cup (120 g) sugar-free barbecue sauce

½ cup (120 ml) reserved pork shoulder cooking liquid (from above)

1. Make the "spaghetti": Place all the ingredients for the spaghetti in a pressure cooker or slow cooker.

2. If using a pressure cooker, seal the lid and cook on high pressure for 45 minutes. Allow the pressure to release naturally before removing the lid. Remove ½ cup (120 ml) of the cooking liquid and set aside for the sauce. Drain the meat almost completely, leaving ¼ cup (60 ml) of the cooking liquid in the cooker.

If using a slow cooker, cook on high for 4 hours or low for 6 hours. When the meat is done, remove ½ cup (120 ml) of the cooking liquid and set aside for the sauce. Drain the meat almost completely, leaving ⅓ cup (80 ml) of the cooking liquid in the cooker.

3. Meanwhile, make the sauce: Heat the oil in a large frying pan over medium heat. Add the bell pepper, onion, and mushrooms and sauté for 5 minutes, until softened. Add the ground pork and cook until no longer pink, 5 to 7 minutes, stirring to break up the meat as it cooks. Add the barbecue sauce and the reserved cooking liquid. Stir to combine, then cover and cook for another 3 minutes, just to heat through.

4. Shred the meat with two forks. Divide the shredded pork among 6 dinner plates, top with the barbecue pork sauce, and dig in!

MAKE IT AT HOME

Replace store-bought barbecue sauce with my homemade version.

Quick 'n' Easy Barbecue Sauce

STORE IT: *Keep in an airtight container in the fridge for up to 5 days or in the freezer for up to 1 month.*

REHEAT IT: *Transfer a single serving to a microwave-safe dish, cover, and microwave for 2 minutes; or place in a small frying pan, cover, and reheat over medium heat for 5 minutes.*

THAW IT: *Place in the fridge and allow to defrost completely, then follow the reheating instructions above.*

PREP AHEAD: *Prep and freeze the barbecue pork sauce until ready to use!*

Per serving, made with Quick 'n' Easy Barbecue Sauce:

			FAT:	CARBS:	PROTEIN:
calories: **683**	calories from fat: **413**	total fat: **46g**	saturated fat: **15.8g**	cholesterol: **211mg**	**62%**	**1%**	**36%**
sodium: **768mg**	carbs: **7.2g**	dietary fiber: **1.8g**	net carbs: **5.4g**	sugars: **3.2g**	protein: **57.8g**			

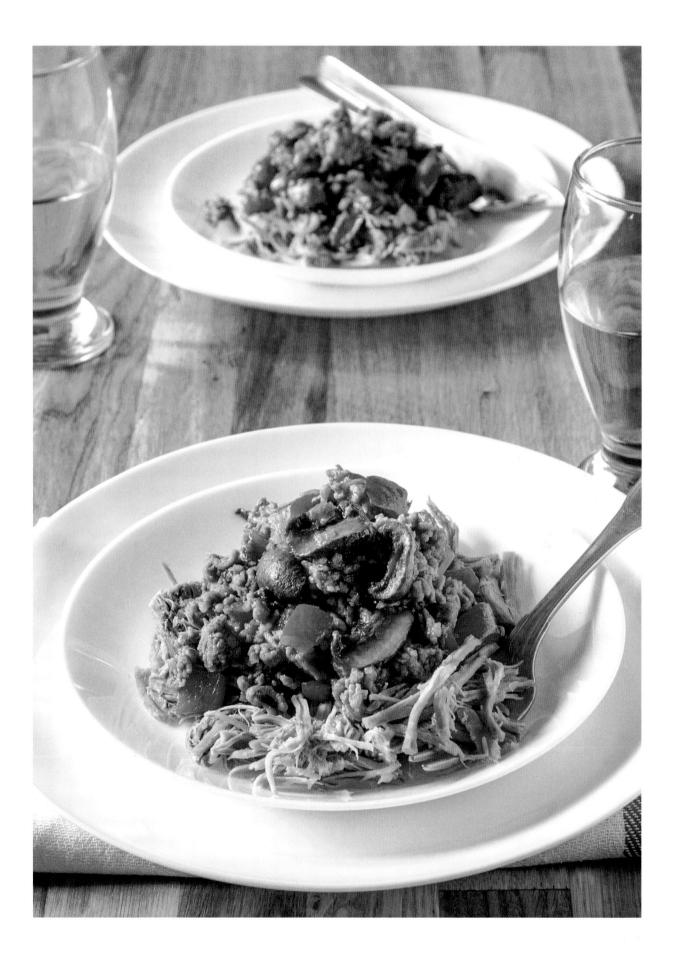

SWEET BEEF CURRY

DAIRY-FREE • EGG-FREE • NUT-FREE
OPTIONS: COCONUT-FREE • NIGHTSHADE-FREE

SERVES 4
PREP TIME: 10 minutes
COOK TIME: 30 minutes

The first time I ordered curry with apples, I thought it was a little weird, but I decided to try it anyway. And boy, am I happy I did! Now, you get to enjoy it, too, keto style. You can use any type of apple you like with this recipe; the sweeter the apple, the sweetener the end result. On the other side of things, tart apples like Granny Smith are also great here.

½ cup (105 g) coconut oil, or ½ cup (120 ml) avocado oil

1 small apple, peeled, cored, and diced

1 small yellow onion, sliced

2 cloves garlic, minced

1 (3-in/7.5-cm) piece fresh ginger root, minced

2 tablespoons curry powder

2 teaspoons garam masala

1 pound (455 g) boneless beef chuck roast, cut into ¾-inch (2-cm) cubes

1 small butternut squash (about 1 lb/ 455 g), cubed

1 cup (240 ml) beef bone broth

1 tablespoon coconut aminos

1. Heat the oil in a large saucepan over medium heat. Add the apple, onion, garlic, ginger, curry powder, and garam masala and toss to coat. Sauté for 10 minutes, or until fragrant.

2. Add the beef, squash, broth, and coconut aminos. Cover and bring to a boil over high heat. Reduce the heat to medium-low and simmer for 20 minutes, until the squash is fork-tender to soft.

3. Divide the curry among 4 bowls and enjoy.

make it COCONUT-FREE:
Use avocado oil or ghee. Replace the coconut aminos with soy sauce.

make it NIGHTSHADE-FREE:
Check the ingredients in the curry powder and garam masala to ensure they do not contain nightshades.

PRESSURE COOK IT: *Complete Step 1 using the sauté mode. In Step 2, seal the lid and either set to the soup mode or cook on high pressure for 20 minutes. Allow the pressure to release naturally before removing the lid, then serve.*

STORE IT: *Keep in an airtight container in the fridge for up to 3 days or in the freezer for up to 1 month.*

REHEAT IT: *Transfer a single serving to a microwave-safe dish, cover, and microwave for 2½ minutes; or place in a saucepan, cover, and reheat over medium heat for 5 minutes.*

THAW IT: *Place in the fridge to thaw completely, then follow the reheating instructions above.*

Per serving, made with coconut oil:

| calories: **698** | calories from fat: **504** | total fat: **56g** | saturated fat: **34.4g** | cholesterol: **118mg** | FAT: | CARBS: | PROTEIN: |
| sodium: **82mg** | carbs: **16.9g** | dietary fiber: **3.5g** | net carbs: **13.4g** | sugars: **5.8g** | protein: **31.8g** | **72%** | **10%** | **18%** |

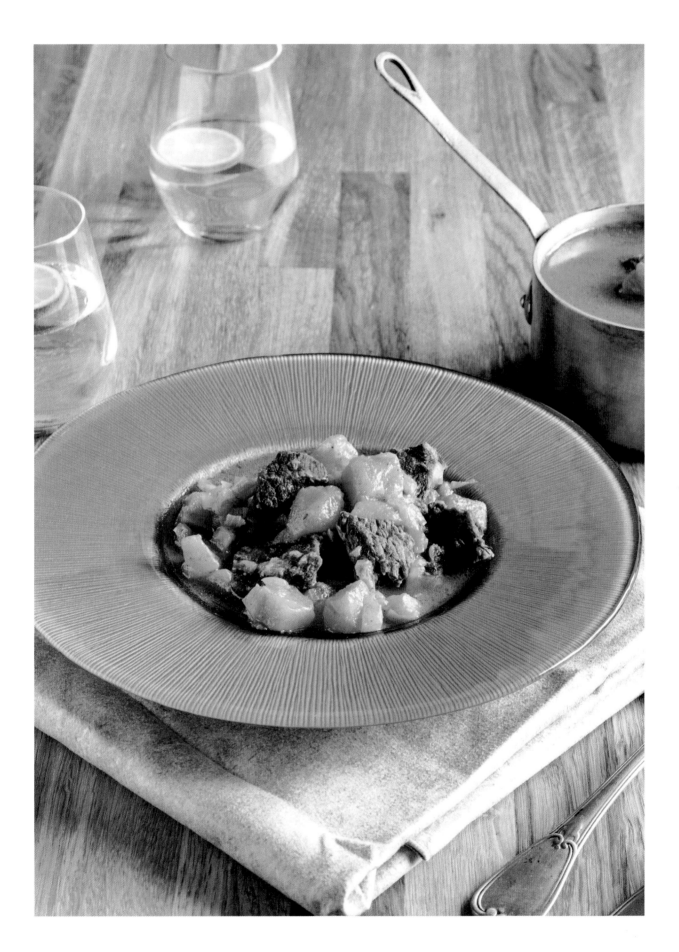

OPEN-FACED TACOS

EGG-FREE • NUT-FREE

OPTIONS: COCONUT-FREE • DAIRY-FREE • LOW-FODMAP

SERVES 4

PREP TIME: 10 minutes

COOK TIME: 20 minutes

As I was whacking away at a boneless chicken thigh for another recipe (the Paprika Chicken Sandwiches on page 194), I thought to myself, "If I hit this enough times, it'll be as thin as a tortilla." And then it hit me—chicken tortillas!

Seriously, though, everyone in the family is going to love this recipe. It's simple, delicious, and perfect for Taco Tuesday!

Also, if you can eat cheese, now's the time to pile it high on each and every taco. For everyone else, omit the cheese or use dairy-free cheese. So Delicious has the best dairy-free "cheddar cheese" around.

To make this recipe even more crazy awesome, drizzle some Avocado Lime Dressing (page 84) or Chimichurri (page 284) on each taco.

TORTILLAS:

2 pounds (910 g) boneless, skinless chicken thighs

⅓ cup (80 ml) avocado oil, or ⅓ cup (70 g) coconut oil

FILLING:

1 pound (455 g) ground beef

1 clove garlic, minced

1½ teaspoons chili powder

½ teaspoon ground cumin

½ teaspoon paprika

½ teaspoon finely ground sea salt

¼ teaspoon red pepper flakes

⅛ teaspoon ground black pepper

TOPPINGS:

⅔ cup (95 g) shredded cheddar cheese (dairy-free or regular)

1 small tomato, diced

4 leaves green leaf lettuce, chopped

1. Place the chicken thighs on a sheet of parchment paper. Using a meat mallet, pound the thighs until they're ¼ inch (6 mm) thick.

2. Heat the oil in a large frying pan over medium-high heat. Add the chicken and cook for 10 minutes, then flip and cook for another 10 minutes, or until each side is golden and the internal temperature reaches 165°F (74°C).

3. Meanwhile, place the ground beef, garlic, chili powder, cumin, paprika, salt, red pepper flakes, and black pepper in another large frying pan. Cook over medium heat until the meat is no longer pink, about 10 minutes, stirring to crumble it as it cooks.

4. To assemble, place the cooked chicken "tortillas" on serving plates and top with the ground beef filling, then the shredded cheese, diced tomato, and chopped lettuce. Dig in!

Per serving, made with avocado oil and dairy-free cheese:

calories: **832**	calories from fat: **540**	total fat: **60g**	saturated fat: **18.6g**	cholesterol: **255mg**	FAT: **65%**	CARBS: **2%**	PROTEIN: **33%**
sodium: **501mg**	carbs: **5g**	dietary fiber: **4g**	net carbs: **1g**	sugars: **1g**	protein: **68g**			

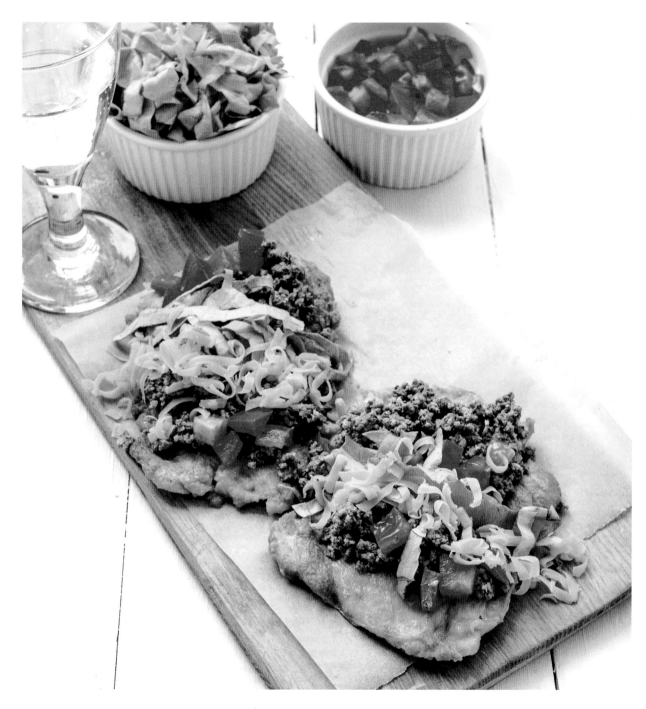

make it COCONUT-FREE:
Use avocado oil. If using dairy-free cheese, make sure it's also coconut-free.

make it DAIRY-FREE:
Use dairy-free cheese.

make it LOW-FODMAP:
Omit the garlic. Use a low-FODMAP dairy-free cheese or the real thing.

PRESSURE COOK IT: *The beef filling can be made in a pressure cooker. Use the sauté mode for Step 3, then seal the lid and cook on high pressure for 3 minutes. Allow the pressure to release naturally before removing the lid.*

STORE IT: *Keep the chicken tortillas, beef filling, and toppings in separate airtight containers in the fridge for up to 3 days. The tortillas and filling can be frozen for up to 1 month.*

REHEAT IT: *Serve the chicken tortillas cold. To reheat the beef filling, transfer a single serving to a microwave-safe dish, cover, and microwave for 2 minutes; or place in a frying pan and reheat over medium heat for 5 minutes. Then top with the cheese, tomato, and lettuce.*

THAW IT: *Place in the fridge and allow to defrost completely, then follow the reheating instructions above.*

BREADED SHRIMP SALAD

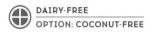
DAIRY-FREE
OPTION: COCONUT-FREE

SERVES 4

PREP TIME: 10 minutes

COOK TIME: 7 minutes

This salad couldn't be easier to whip up. And the combination of the almond flour coating, the coconut oil used for frying, and the chipotle mayo dressing makes for one heck of a fat-bomb salad! Before beginning the recipe, remember to place the skewers in water to soak.

If you're not in the mood for the chipotle mayo dressing, replace it with ⅔ cup (160 ml) of Thai Dressing (page 72) or Herby Vinaigrette & Marinade (page 98).

SHRIMP SKEWERS:

24 large shrimp (about 14 oz/400 g), peeled, deveined, and tails removed

¾ cup (85 g) blanched almond flour

¾ teaspoon finely ground sea salt

½ teaspoon garlic powder

¼ teaspoon ginger powder

¼ teaspoon ground black pepper

1 large egg

½ cup (210 g) coconut oil, for the pan

CHIPOTLE MAYO DRESSING:

⅔ cup (140 g) mayonnaise

2 teaspoons lime juice

1 teaspoon chipotle powder

SALAD:

4 cups (280 g) iceberg lettuce mix

SPECIAL EQUIPMENT:

8 (6-in/15-cm) bamboo skewers, soaked in water for 10 minutes

make it COCONUT-FREE:
Replace the coconut oil with avocado oil or ghee.

1. Skewer 3 shrimp per bamboo skewer. Place on a clean plate.

2. Combine the almond flour, salt, garlic powder, ginger powder, and pepper in a small shallow dish that is long enough to accommodate the skewers.

3. Beat the egg in another small shallow dish.

4. Dip a shrimp skewer into the beaten egg, then coat generously in the almond flour mixture. Once coated, set on one half of a wire cooling rack (keeping the other half of the rack clean for the cooked shrimp). Repeat with the remaining skewers.

5. Melt the oil in a large frying pan over medium-low heat. Once melted, wait 1 minute before carefully placing all the skewers in the hot oil. You may need to cook them in batches if your pan is not large enough to hold all of them at once.

6. Cook the skewers until lightly golden on the first side, up to 4 minutes. If, after 4 minutes, the coating hasn't turned a light golden color, turn the heat up to medium and continue cooking until they're lightly golden. Flip over and cook for another 2 to 3 minutes, until the shrimp are lightly golden on the other side. Transfer the finished skewers to the clean side of the wire rack.

7. While the shrimp skewers are cooking, prepare the chipotle mayo dressing: Combine all the ingredients in a small bowl.

8. Divide the lettuce mix evenly among 4 salad plates. Top with the cooked shrimp skewers and drizzle with the dressing.

STORE IT: *Keep in an airtight container in the fridge for up to 3 days.*

REHEAT IT: *Place the shrimp in a large frying pan and reheat over medium heat for 2 minutes, until heated through.*

PREP AHEAD: *Make the dressing up to 3 days before preparing the remainder of the recipe.*

Per serving:

calories: **883** | calories from fat: **753** | total fat: **83.7g** | saturated fat: **30.9g** | cholesterol: **167mg**
sodium: **911mg** | carbs: **7.7g** | dietary fiber: **4.3g** | net carbs: **3.4g** | sugars: **3.3g** | protein: **24.8g**

FAT:	CARBS:	PROTEIN:
86%	**3%**	**11%**

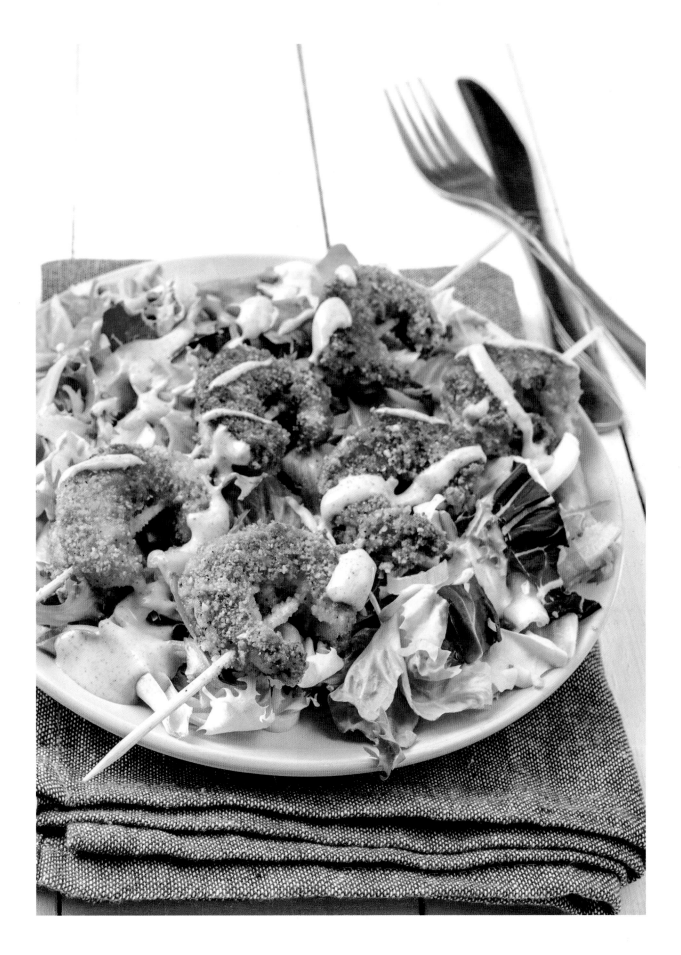

SHREDDED MOJO PORK WITH AVOCADO SALAD

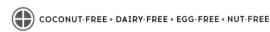 COCONUT-FREE · DAIRY-FREE · EGG-FREE · NUT-FREE

SERVES 4

PREP TIME: 10 minutes

COOK TIME: 45 minutes or 4 to 6 hours, depending on method

Generally, I just cook pork shoulder in vegetable broth and eat it plain. Yeah, I'm boring. But, with a little spice and a simple salad to accompany it, you can transform pork from drab to flavorful so easily! You can cook the pork in either a pressure cooker or a slow cooker.

SHREDDED PORK:

2 pounds (910 g) bone-in pork shoulder

1 cup (240 ml) vegetable broth

¼ cup (60 ml) lime juice

2 teaspoons ground cumin

2 teaspoons dried oregano leaves

4 cloves garlic, minced

2 teaspoons finely ground sea salt

2 bay leaves

¼ teaspoon ground black pepper

¼ teaspoon red pepper flakes

AVOCADO SALAD:

¼ cup (60 ml) avocado oil or olive oil

2 tablespoons lime juice

1½ teaspoons chili powder

¼ teaspoon finely ground sea salt

2 bunches (400 g) radishes, thinly sliced

2 medium Hass avocados, peeled and pitted (about 8 oz/220 g of flesh)

4 green onions, sliced

½ cup (112 g) hulled pumpkin seeds

1. Place all the ingredients for the shredded pork in a pressure cooker or slow cooker. If using a pressure cooker, seal the lid and cook on high pressure for 45 minutes. When complete, allow the pressure to release naturally before removing the lid. If using a slow cooker, cook on high for 4 hours or low for 6 hours.

2. When the meat is done, drain it almost completely, leaving ¼ cup (60 ml) of cooking liquid in the cooker. Shred the meat with two forks.

3. Prepare the salad: Place the oil, lime juice, chili powder, and salt in a medium-sized salad bowl. Whisk to combine, then add the remaining ingredients and toss to coat.

4. Divide the salad evenly among 4 plates or bowls, then top with the shredded pork.

> **STORE IT:** *Keep the shredded pork and salad in separate airtight containers in the fridge for up to 3 days. Do not add the avocado to the salad until you're ready to serve it. The pork can be frozen for up to 1 month.*
>
> **REHEAT IT:** *Place a serving of the shredded pork in a microwave-safe dish, cover, and reheat for 2 minutes; or place in a frying pan with a splash of oil, cover, and reheat over medium heat for 7 minutes.*
>
> **THAW IT:** *Place the shredded pork in the fridge to thaw completely, then follow the reheating instructions above.*

Per serving, made with avocado oil:

calories: **938** | calories from fat: **633** | total fat: **70.3g** | saturated fat: **19g** | cholesterol: **222mg**
sodium: **1502mg** | carbs: **14g** | dietary fiber: **6.8g** | net carbs: **7.2g** | sugars: **2.9g** | protein: **64g**

FAT:	CARBS:	PROTEIN:
66%	5%	29%

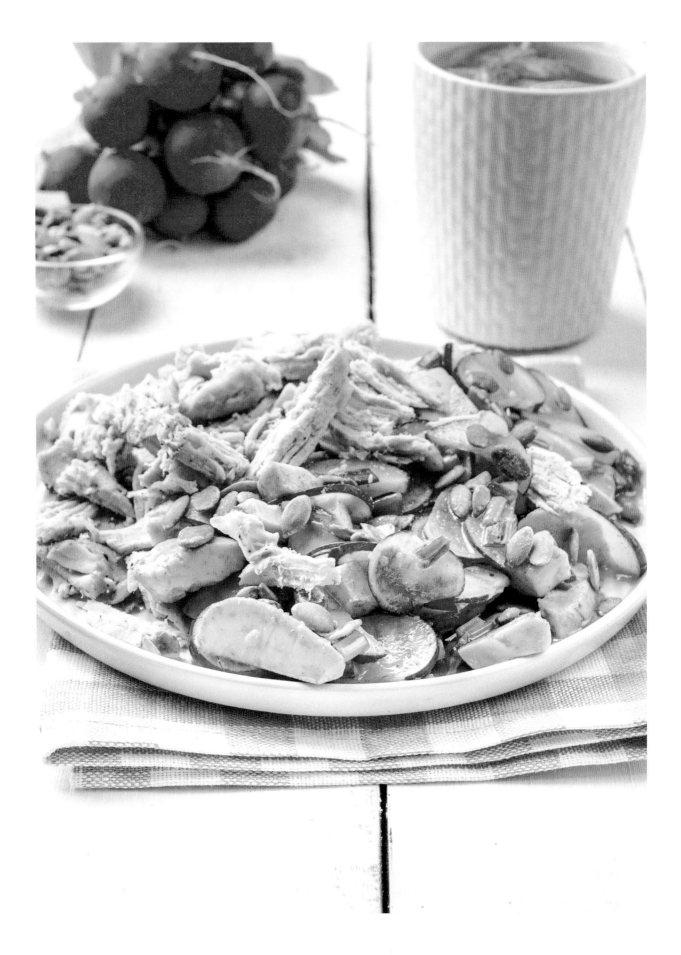

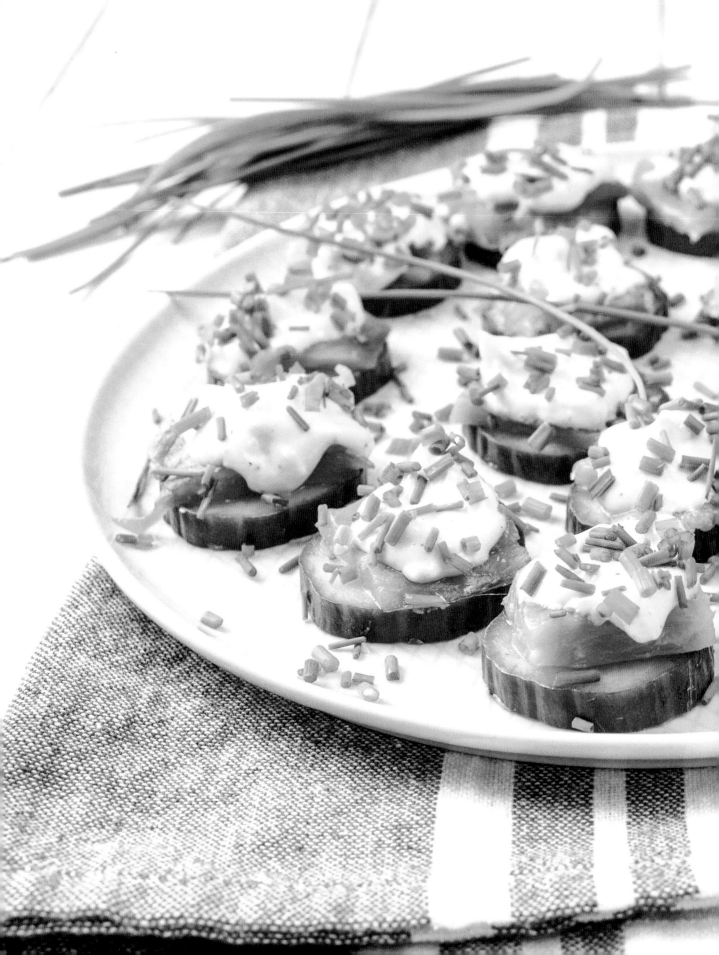

8.

SAVORY SNACKS

CRUNCHY JICAMA FRIES

COCONUT-FREE • DAIRY-FREE • NUT-FREE • VEGETARIAN
OPTIONS: AIP • EGG-FREE • NIGHTSHADE-FREE • VEGAN

SERVES 4
PREP TIME: 5 minutes
COOK TIME: 40 minutes

I was introduced to jicama during a special trip to Las Vegas, where Kevin proposed to me! After my nerves had calmed down a touch, we went out for a laid-back vegan dinner; I was vegan at the time, and I ordered jicama fries, a smoothie, and tempeh. Those fries were delicious! Ever since, when I make a batch of these fries, I'm reminded of those precious hours following our engagement and how wonderful it felt to be marrying my best friend.

I know, these are a bit heavier on the carbs and lighter on the fat than you may be used to, but when you look at the net carbohydrates and consider how great a replacement they are for potato fries, they're worth it! Serve with mayonnaise or sugar-free ketchup if you're into that sort of thing. My favorite sugar-free ketchup is from Primal Kitchen, a company that understands how important food quality is.

If you don't want to use mayonnaise or ketchup for serving, Creamy Italian Dressing (page 94), Green Speckled Dressing (page 80), and Honey Mustard Dressing & Marinade (page 78) are other great options.

1 medium jicama (about 1 lb/455 g), peeled and cut into fry-like pieces

2 tablespoons avocado oil

½ teaspoon paprika

Pinch of finely ground sea salt

1 teaspoon finely chopped fresh parsley

½ cup (105 g) mayonnaise or sugar-free ketchup, for serving (optional)

1. Preheat the oven to 400°F (205°C). Line a rimmed baking sheet with parchment paper or a silicone baking mat.

2. Place the jicama pieces on the baking sheet and toss with the oil and paprika. Bake for 40 minutes, flipping the fries over halfway through baking.

3. Remove from the oven, sprinkle the fries with the salt and parsley, and enjoy immediately. Serve with the mayonnaise on the side for dipping, if desired.

make it AIP:
Omit the paprika and serve with your favorite dressing instead of mayonnaise.

make it NIGHTSHADE-FREE:
Omit the paprika.

make it EGG-FREE/VEGAN:
Serve with ketchup or use egg-free mayonnaise (see recipe on page 102).

MAKE IT AT HOME

Replace store-bought mayonnaise with my homemade version.

Mayonnaise

Per serving, fries only:

calories: **96**	calories from fat: **33**	total fat: **3.7g**	saturated fat: **0.4g**	cholesterol: **0mg**
sodium: **65mg**	carbs: **14.7g**	dietary fiber: **8.2g**	net carbs: **6.5g**	sugars: **3g**	protein: **1.2g**

FAT:	CARBS:	PROTEIN:
34%	**61%**	**5%**

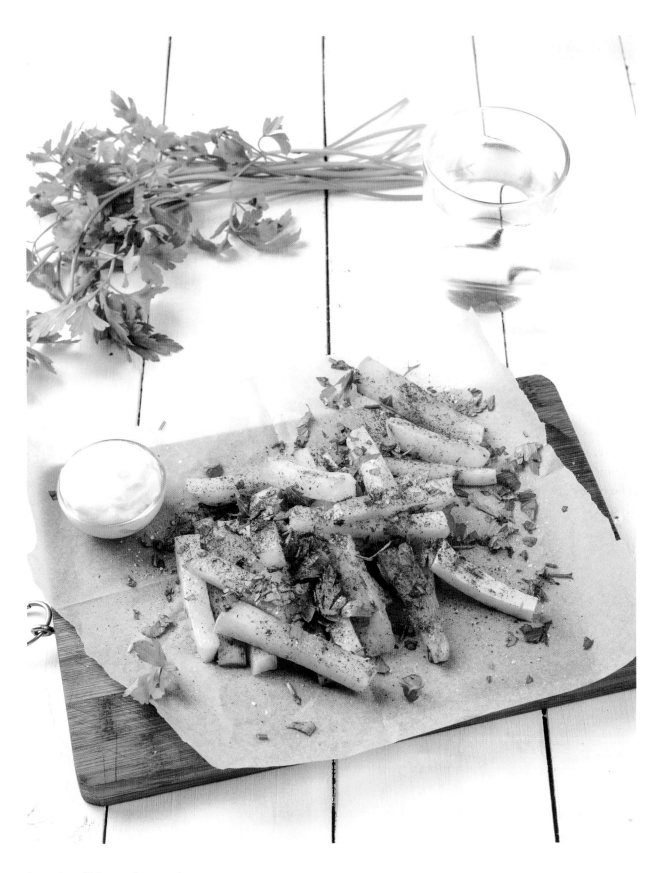

Per serving, with homemade mayonnaise:

calories: **276** | calories from fat: **213** | total fat: **23.7g** | saturated fat: **3.4g** | cholesterol: **10mg**
sodium: **245mg** | carbs: **14.7g** | dietary fiber: **8.2g** | net carbs: **6.5g** | sugars: **3g** | protein: **1.2g**

FAT:	CARBS:	PROTEIN:
77%	**21%**	**2%**

SAUTÉED ASPARAGUS WITH LEMON-TAHINI SAUCE

 COCONUT-FREE • DAIRY-FREE • EGG-FREE • NIGHTSHADE-FREE • NUT-FREE • VEGAN • VEGETARIAN

SERVES 4

PREP TIME: 5 minutes

COOK TIME: 10 minutes

This recipe is awesome as a snack or as a side to your favorite protein dish. It is also great made with broccoli instead of asparagus. The sauce is so good; don't be afraid to double or triple the recipe and use it as a dressing for the week!

16 asparagus spears, woody ends snapped off

2 tablespoons avocado oil

LEMON-TAHINI SAUCE:

2 tablespoons tahini

1 tablespoon avocado oil

2½ teaspoons lemon juice

1 small clove garlic, minced

¹⁄₁₆ teaspoon finely ground sea salt

Pinch of ground black pepper

1 to 1½ tablespoons water

1. Place the asparagus and oil in a large frying pan over medium heat. Cook, tossing the spears in the oil every once in a while, until the spears begin to brown slightly, about 10 minutes.

2. Meanwhile, make the sauce: Place the tahini, oil, lemon juice, garlic, salt, pepper, and 1 tablespoon of water in a medium-sized bowl. Whisk until incorporated. If the dressing is too thick, add the additional ½ tablespoon of water and whisk again.

3. Place the cooked asparagus on a serving plate and drizzle with the lemon tahini sauce.

| **STORE IT:** *Store in the fridge for up to 3 days. Leftovers are best enjoyed cold.*

Per serving:

| calories: **106** | calories from fat: **69** | total fat: **7.7g** | saturated fat: **1.1g** | cholesterol: **0mg** | | FAT: | CARBS: | PROTEIN: |
| sodium: **43mg** | carbs: **5.7g** | dietary fiber: **2.8g** | net carbs: **2.9g** | sugars: **2g** | protein: **3.5g** | **65%** | **22%** | **13%** |

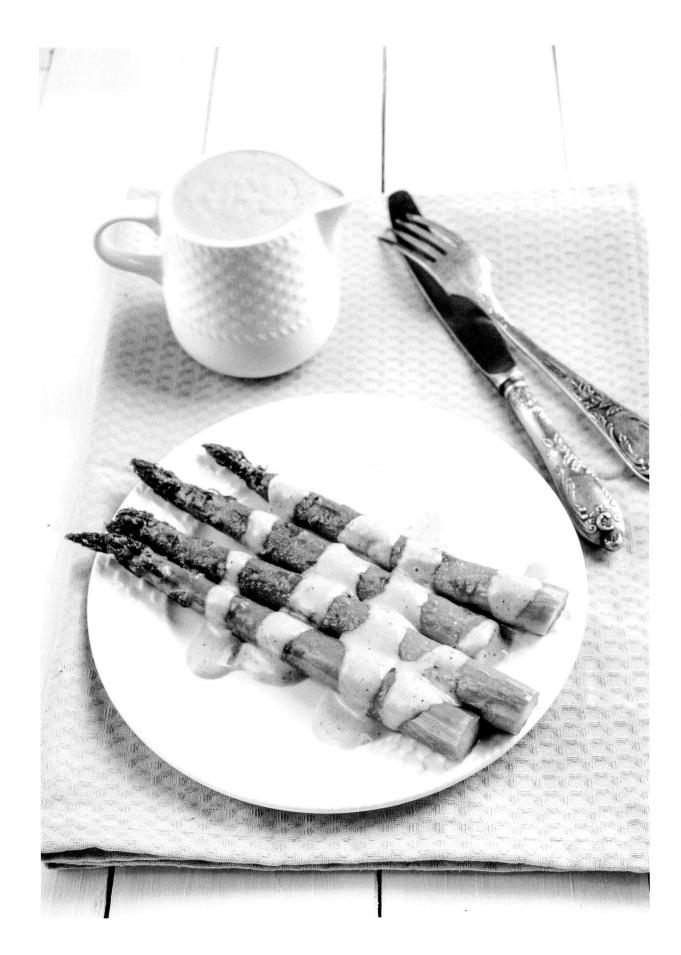

LIVER BITES

 COCONUT-FREE • DAIRY-FREE • EGG-FREE • NIGHTSHADE-FREE • NUT-FREE
OPTION: AIP

MAKES 24 bites (1 per serving)

PREP TIME: 10 minutes, plus 24 hours to soak livers

COOK TIME: 28 minutes

Another tasty way to enjoy liver! While you can enjoy these bites just as they are, serving them with some Ranch Dressing (page 76) or Green Speckled Dressing (page 80) makes for one tasty treat. Who knew we could ever say that about liver?

8 ounces (225 g) chicken livers

1 tablespoon apple cider vinegar

4 strips bacon (about 4½ oz/130 g)

1 pound (455 g) ground beef

1 cup (75 g) crushed pork rinds

12 cloves garlic, minced

1 tablespoon plus 1 teaspoon onion powder

1 teaspoon ground black pepper

1 teaspoon dried thyme leaves

½ teaspoon finely ground sea salt

1. Place the chicken livers in a medium-sized bowl and cover with water. Add the vinegar. Cover and place in the fridge for 24 to 48 hours. Rinse and drain the livers.

2. Preheat the oven to 375°F (190°C). Line a rimmed baking sheet with parchment paper or a silicone baking mat.

3. Place the livers and bacon in a high-powered blender and pulse until smooth. If using a regular blender or food processor, roughly chop the bacon beforehand.

4. Transfer the liver mixture to a medium-sized bowl and add the remaining ingredients. Mix with your hands until fully incorporated.

5. Pinch a tablespoon of the mixture, roll it into a ball between your hands, and place on the lined baking sheet. Repeat with the remaining liver mixture, making a total of 24 balls.

6. Bake the liver balls for 25 to 28 minutes, until the internal temperature reaches 165°F (74°C).

make it AIP:
Omit the black pepper.

STORE: *Keep in an airtight container in the fridge for up to 3 days or in the freezer for up to 1 month.*

REHEAT IT: *Enjoy cold, or place in a frying pan with a drop of oil, cover, and reheat on medium-low for 3 minutes.*

THAW IT: *Place in the fridge and allow to defrost completely before using the reheating instructions above.*

Per bite:

calories: **116** | calories from fat: **67** | total fat: **7.4g** | saturated fat: **2.7g** | cholesterol: **80mg**
sodium: **248mg** | carbs: **1.1g** | dietary fiber: **0.1g** | net carbs: **1g** | sugars: **0.2g** | protein: **11.4g**

FAT:	CARBS:	PROTEIN:
57%	**4%**	**39%**

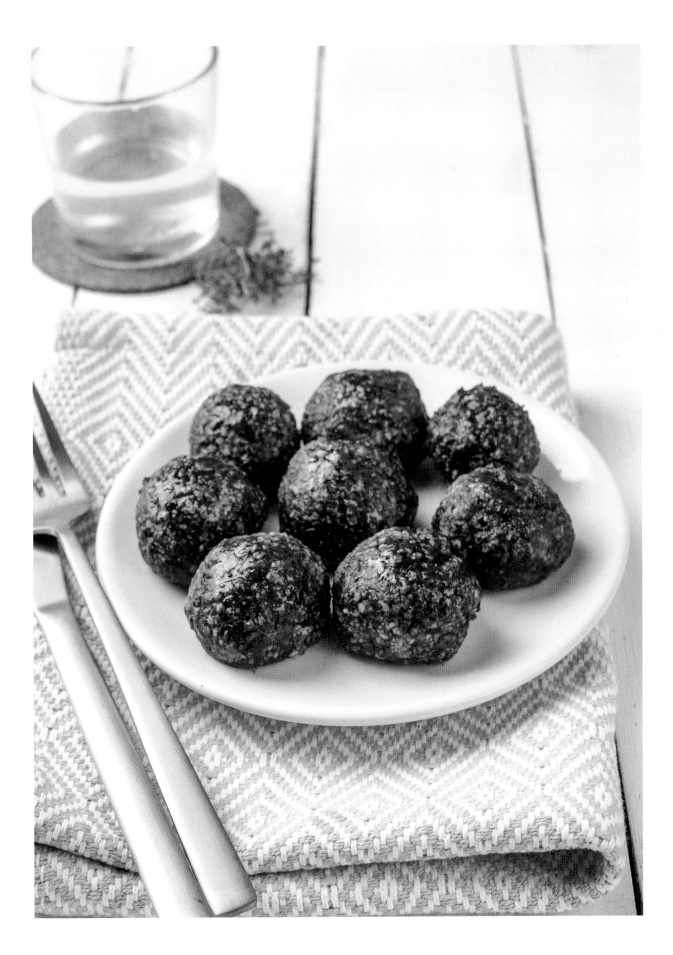

WEDGE DIPPERS

DAIRY-FREE • NIGHTSHADE-FREE • NUT-FREE • VEGETARIAN
OPTIONS: AIP • COCONUT-FREE • EGG-FREE • VEGAN

SERVES 4

PREP TIME: 5 minutes

COOK TIME: –

I know, this is such a simple idea, but I promise you'll love it and use it again and again. I love snacking on these crunchy wedges. Enjoy them on their own or as a side to your favorite protein dish. They are awesome with Teriyaki Sauce & Marinade (page 92) or Thai Dressing (page 72), too!

1 medium head iceberg lettuce (about 6 in/15 cm in diameter)

½ cup (120 ml) ranch dressing

1. Cut the head of lettuce in half, then lay the halves cut side down. Cut each half into 8 wedges, like a pie, for a total of 16 wedges.

2. Serve with the ranch dressing.

make it **AIP**:
Choose a compliant dressing.

make it **COCONUT-FREE**:
Use a store-bought ranch dressing that is coconut-free.

make it **EGG-FREE/VEGAN**:
Use an egg-free ranch dressing.

MAKE IT AT HOME
Replace store-bought ranch dressing with my homemade version.

Ranch Dressing

Per serving, with homemade ranch dressing:

calories: **132** | calories from fat: **107** | total fat: **12.3g** | saturated fat: **2.4g** | cholesterol: **0mg** | sodium: **111mg** | carbs: **4.6g** | dietary fiber: **0.9g** | net carbs: **3.7g** | sugars: **1.4g** | protein: **0.8g**

FAT:	CARBS:	PROTEIN:
84%	14%	2%

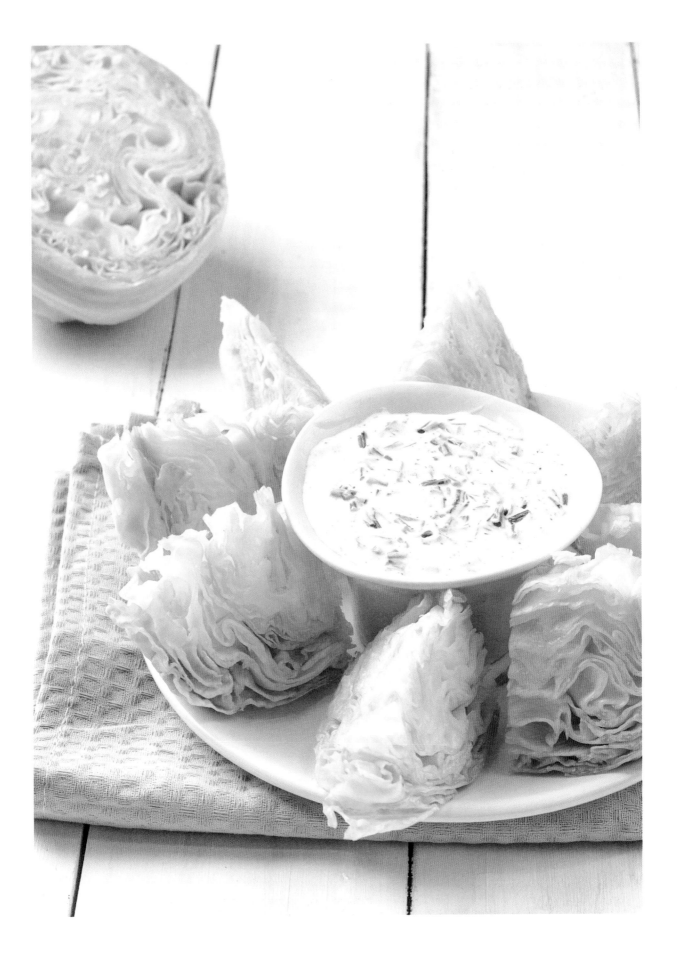

MAC FATTIES

DAIRY-FREE • EGG-FREE • VEGAN • VEGETARIAN
OPTIONS: LOW-FODMAP • NIGHTSHADE-FREE

MAKES 20 fat cups
(1 per serving)

PREP TIME: 10 minutes, plus time to freeze

COOK TIME: –

When I started keto, I thought that fat bombs could only be sweet. I loaded up on ingredients like cacao powder, stevia, erythritol, and nuts in an attempt to increase my fat intake. Those sweet fat bombs were tasty, sure, but a lot of times they spiked my desire for more sweet things, and the cycle continued. It wasn't until I swapped out the sweet (keto-friendly) treats with savory ones that I truly realized a life without a sweet tooth. If your experience has been similar, try this recipe! It can be made with any nut or seed you have. And there are four different flavors per batch, adding variety and keeping things interesting.

Thanks to Holly, one of our amazing Healthful Pursuit *readers, Mac Fatties are perfectly named. Thanks for the title idea, Holly!*

1¾ cups (280 g) roasted and salted macadamia nuts

⅓ cup (70 g) coconut oil

ROSEMARY LEMON FLAVOR:

1 teaspoon finely chopped fresh rosemary

¼ teaspoon lemon juice

SPICY CUMIN FLAVOR:

½ teaspoon ground cumin

¼ teaspoon cayenne pepper

TURMERIC FLAVOR:

½ teaspoon turmeric powder

¼ teaspoon ginger powder

GARLIC HERB FLAVOR:

1¼ teaspoons dried oregano leaves

½ teaspoon paprika

½ teaspoon garlic powder

1. Place the macadamia nuts and oil in a blender or food processor. Blend until smooth, or as close to smooth as you can get it with the equipment you're using.

2. Divide the mixture among 4 small bowls, placing ¼ cup (87 g) in each bowl.

3. To the first bowl, add the rosemary and lemon juice and stir to combine.

4. To the second bowl, add the cumin and cayenne and stir to combine.

5. To the third bowl, add the turmeric and ginger and stir to combine.

6. To the fourth bowl, add the oregano, paprika, and garlic powder and stir to combine.

7. Set a 24-well silicone or metal mini muffin pan on the counter. If using a metal pan, line 20 of the wells with mini foil liners. (Do not use paper; it would soak up all the fat.) Spoon the mixtures into the wells, using about 1 tablespoon per well.

8. Place in the freezer for 1 hour, or until firm. Enjoy directly from the freezer.

make it LOW-FODMAP/ NIGHTSHADE-FREE:
Prepare the Rosemary Lemon and Turmeric flavors only, doubling up on the ingredients. Add each flavor to half of the macadamia nut mixture instead of one-quarter.

STORE IT: *Keep in an airtight container in the freezer for up to 1 month or in the fridge for up to 3 days. They're great right out of the freezer and keep fine in the fridge, but they will soften significantly if left out at room temperature. Therefore, it's best to enjoy them directly from the freezer or fridge.*

Per fat cup:

calories: **139** | calories from fat: **127** | total fat: **14.1g** | saturated fat: **4.7g** | cholesterol: **0mg**
sodium: **37mg** | carbs: **1.9g** | dietary fiber: **1.2g** | net carbs: **0.7g** | sugars: **0.6g** | protein: **1.1g**

FAT:	CARBS:	PROTEIN:
91%	6%	3%

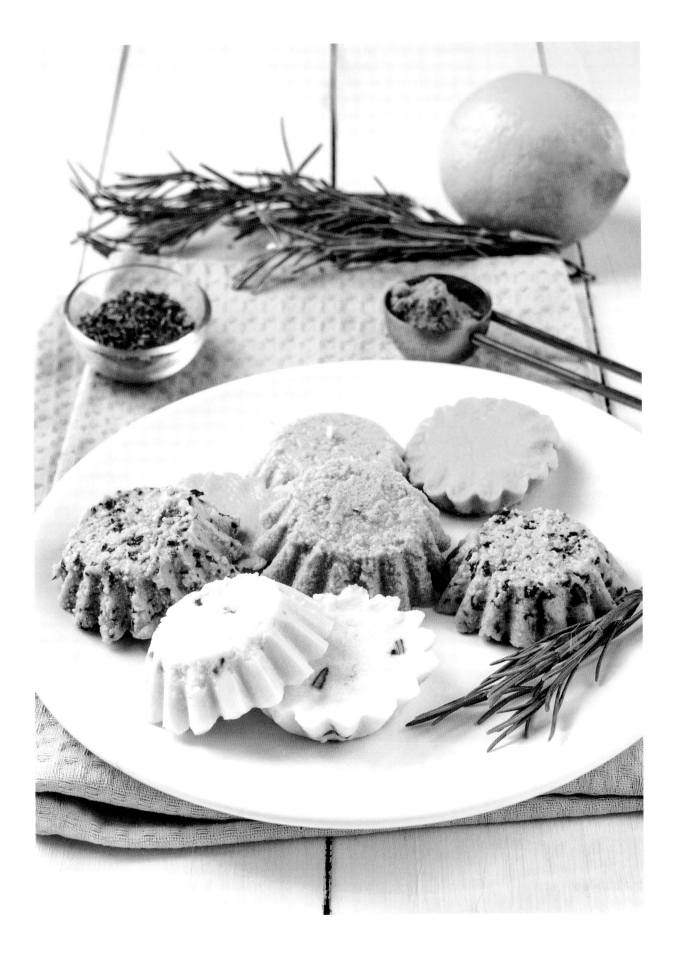

CAULIFLOWER PATTIES

NIGHTSHADE-FREE • VEGETARIAN

OPTIONS: COCONUT-FREE • DAIRY-FREE • VEGAN

MAKES 10 patties (2 per serving)

PREP TIME: 10 minutes

COOK TIME: 20 minutes

There are so many ways to enjoy cauliflower, and this is one of the best ways I know. Once you get comfortable with this recipe, you can play around with the flavors. Adding bacon is always a good idea. You can also swap out the nutritional yeast for cheese if you're okay with dairy or replace the spices with your favorite spice mix.

These patties are awesome with Bacon Dressing (page 82) or Creamy Italian Dressing (page 94).

1 medium head cauliflower (about 1½ lbs/680 g), or 3 cups (375 g) pre-riced cauliflower

2 large eggs

⅔ cup (75 g) blanched almond flour

¼ cup (17 g) nutritional yeast

1 tablespoon dried chives

1 teaspoon finely ground sea salt

1 teaspoon garlic powder

½ teaspoon turmeric powder

¼ teaspoon ground black pepper

3 tablespoons coconut oil or ghee, for the pan

make it COCONUT-FREE:
Use ghee.

make it DAIRY-FREE/VEGAN:
Use coconut oil.

1. If you're using pre-riced cauliflower, skip ahead to Step 2. Otherwise, cut the base off the head of cauliflower and remove the florets. Transfer the florets to a food processor or blender and pulse 3 or 4 times to break them up into small (¼-inch/6-mm) pieces.

2. Transfer the riced cauliflower to a medium-sized saucepan and add enough water to the pan to completely cover the cauliflower. Cover with the lid and bring to a boil over medium heat. Boil, covered, for 3½ minutes.

3. Meanwhile, place a fine-mesh strainer over a bowl.

4. Pour the hot cauliflower into the strainer, allowing the bowl to catch the boiling water. With a spoon, press down on the cauliflower to remove as much water as possible.

5. Discard the cooking water and place the cauliflower in the bowl, then add the eggs, almond flour, nutritional yeast, chives, salt, and spices. Stir until everything is incorporated.

6. Heat a large frying pan over medium-low heat. Add the oil and allow to melt completely.

7. Using a ¼-cup (60-ml) scoop, scoop up a portion of the mixture and roll between your hands to form a ball about 1¾ inches (4.5 cm) in diameter. Place in the hot oil and flatten the ball with the back of a fork until it is a patty about ½ inch (1.25 cm) thick. Repeat with the remaining cauliflower mixture, making a total of 10 patties.

8. Cook the patties for 5 minutes per side, or until golden brown. Transfer to a serving plate and enjoy!

STORE IT: *Keep in an airtight container in the fridge for up to 3 days or in the freezer for up to 1 month (no thawing needed).*

REHEAT IT: *Transfer a single serving to a microwave-safe plate, cover, and microwave for 1 minute if refrigerated or 3 minutes if frozen; or place in a frying pan with a drop of oil and fry over medium heat for about 1 minute per side if refrigerated or 4 minutes per side if frozen.*

Per serving, made with coconut oil:

| calories: **164** | calories from fat: **111** | total fat: **12.3g** | saturated fat: **7.9g** | cholesterol: **74mg** |
| sodium: **433mg** | carbs: **6.9g** | dietary fiber: **3.6g** | net carbs: **3.3g** | sugars: **2.9g** | protein: **6.6g** |

FAT:	CARBS:	PROTEIN:
68%	17%	16%

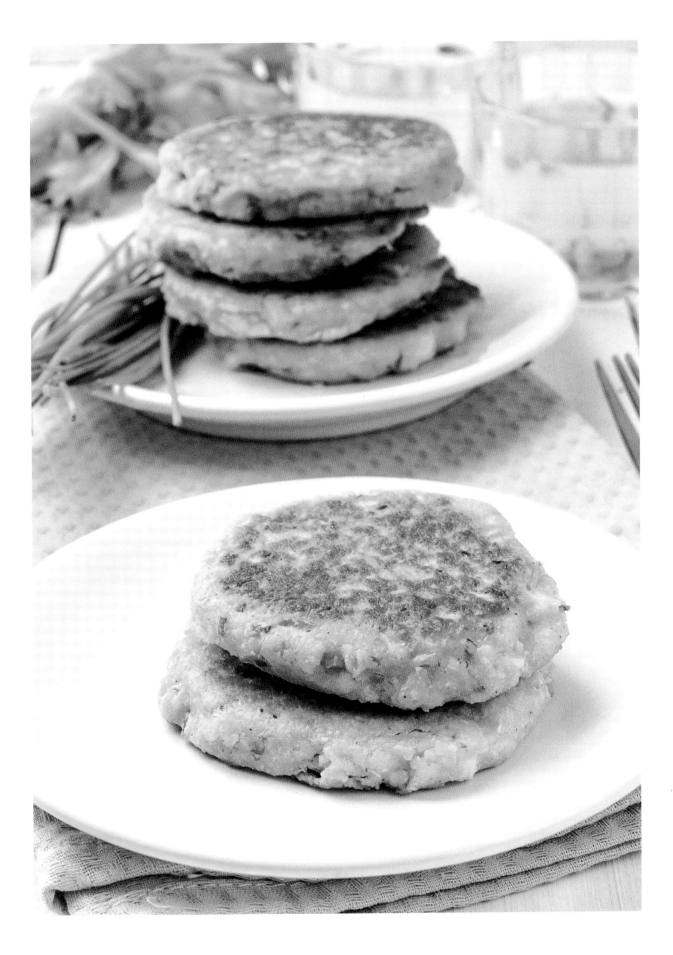

TAPENADE

COCONUT-FREE • DAIRY-FREE • EGG-FREE • NUT-FREE
OPTIONS: VEGAN • VEGETARIAN

SERVES 6
PREP TIME: 5 minutes
COOK TIME: –

I could live on tapenade. In fact, while writing this book, I nearly did! Amazing on its own or with celery sticks, pepperoni slices, or pork rinds, it makes the perfect midday snack or light meal.

This recipe calls for only one anchovy fillet. So, when you're chowing down on tapenade, you're going to be wondering, "Now, what do I do with the rest of those anchovies?" My favorite is sautéing zucchini noodles (spiral-sliced zucchini) in coconut oil with garlic, anchovies, capers, and finely chopped red bell pepper. After cooking for about 5 minutes, add fresh parsley and voilà!

1 cup (115 g) pitted black olives

1 cup (115 g) pitted green olives

¼ cup (28 g) sun-dried tomatoes in oil, drained

6 fresh basil leaves

1 tablespoon capers

1 tablespoon fresh parsley leaves

2 teaspoons fresh thyme leaves

Leaves from 1 sprig fresh oregano

1 clove garlic

1 anchovy fillet

¼ cup (60 ml) olive oil

6 medium celery stalks, cut into sticks, for serving

1. Place all the ingredients, except the olive oil and celery sticks, in a blender or food processor. Pulse until roughly chopped.

2. Add the olive oil and pulse a couple more times, just to combine.

3. Transfer to a 16-ounce (475-ml) or larger serving dish and enjoy with celery sticks.

make it VEGAN/VEGETARIAN:
Omit the anchovy.

STORE IT: *Keep in an airtight container in the fridge for up to 5 days.*

Per ¼-cup/56-g serving, tapenade only:

| calories: **167** | calories from fat: **148** | total fat: **16.4g** | saturated fat: **1.3g** | cholesterol: **3mg** | | FAT: | CARBS: | PROTEIN: |
| sodium: **716mg** | carbs: **4.1g** | dietary fiber: **0.5g** | net carbs: **3.6g** | sugars: **0g** | protein: **0.9g** | **88%** | **10%** | **2%** |

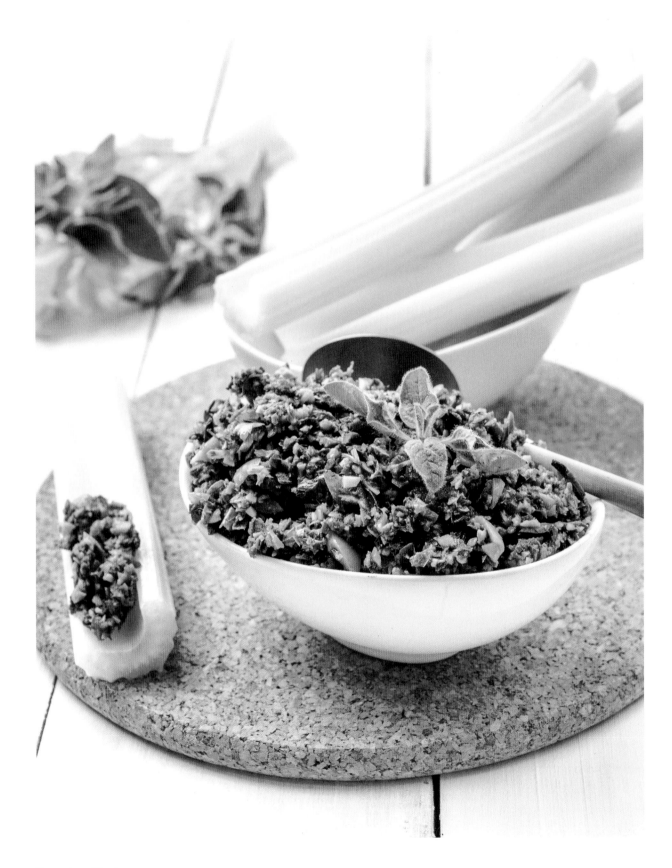

Per serving, with celery:

| calories: **171** | calories from fat: **149** | total fat: **16.5g** | saturated fat: **1.4g** | cholesterol: **3mg** |
| sodium: **748mg** | carbs: **5.5g** | dietary fiber: **1.1g** | net carbs: **4.4g** | sugars: **0.7g** | protein: **0.3g** |

| FAT: | CARBS: | PROTEIN: |
| **87%** | **12%** | **1%** |

HUMMUS CELERY BOATS

COCONUT-FREE • DAIRY-FREE • EGG-FREE • VEGAN • VEGETARIAN

OPTIONS: LOW-FODMAP • NIGHTSHADE-FREE

SERVES 10

PREP TIME: 5 minutes, plus 24 hours to soak nuts

COOK TIME: –

My favorite snack as a kid was ants on a log. Have you ever had it? You take celery sticks, fill them with nut butter, and top with raisins. How fun, eating ants for a snack! I thought it was one of the coolest things. Nowadays the nut butter has been replaced with nut-based hummus and the ants…well, who wants to eat ants? Eww. But if you do want ants on your logs, add a sprinkle of hulled sunflower seeds.

1 cup (160 g) raw macadamia nuts

3 tablespoons fresh lemon juice

2 cloves garlic

2 tablespoons olive oil

2 tablespoons tahini

Pinch of cayenne pepper

Pinch of finely ground sea salt

Pinch of ground black pepper

1 bunch celery, stalks cut crosswise into 2-inch (5-cm) pieces

1. Place the macadamia nuts in a large bowl and cover with water. Cover the bowl and place in the fridge to soak for 24 hours.

2. After 24 hours, drain and rinse the macadamia nuts. Transfer to a food processor or blender. Add the lemon juice, garlic, olive oil, tahini, cayenne, salt, and pepper and blend until smooth.

3. Spread the hummus on the celery pieces and place on a plate for serving.

make it LOW-FODMAP:
Omit the garlic. Replace the celery with 1 medium cucumber, sliced into coins.

make it NIGHTSHADE-FREE:
Omit the cayenne.

STORE IT: *Keep the assembled logs in an airtight container in the fridge for up to 2 days. If stored separately, the hummus will keep in the fridge for up to 5 days.*

Per serving of 2 tablespoons hummus spread on 5 celery pieces:

calories: **171** | calories from fat: **143** | total fat: **15.9g** | saturated fat: **2.4g** | cholesterol: **0mg**
sodium: **5mg** | carbs: **5g** | dietary fiber: **2.5g** | net carbs: **2.5g** | sugars: **1.9g** | protein: **2.1g**

FAT:	CARBS:	PROTEIN:
84%	11%	5%

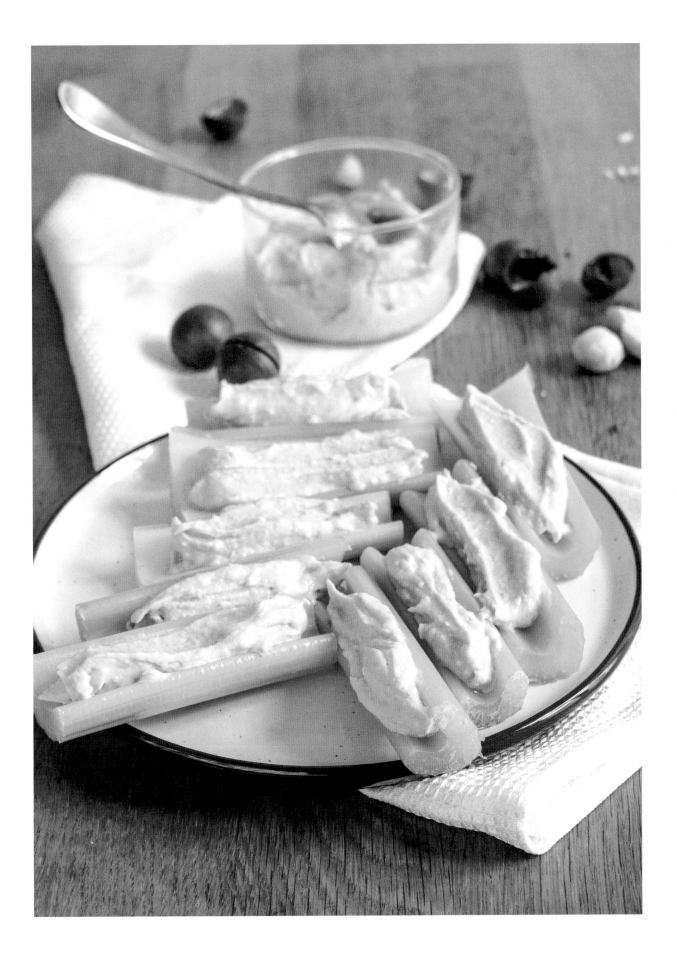

FRIED CABBAGE WEDGES

AIP • DAIRY-FREE • EGG-FREE • NIGHTSHADE-FREE • NUT-FREE • VEGETARIAN
OPTIONS: COCONUT-FREE • LOW-FODMAP • VEGAN

SERVES 6
PREP TIME: 5 minutes
COOK TIME: 15 minutes

As a keto warrior, you'll soon realize that cabbage is a wonderful keto-friendly food that goes well with just about everything. With a little creativity, you can have a lot of fun with it, too. I've seen cabbage leaves used as wraps, noodles, sandwich buns, you name it—each variation delicious! It's important to add as much variety to your eating style as you can to keep things interesting, so here's another way to enjoy cabbage outside of the traditional coleslaw.

You can easily replace the green goddess dressing with Herby Vinaigrette & Marinade (page 98) or Honey Mustard Dressing & Marinade (page 78).

1 large head green or red cabbage (about 2½ lbs/1.2 kg)

2 tablespoons coconut oil or avocado oil

2 teaspoons garlic powder

½ teaspoon finely ground sea salt

¾ cup (180 ml) green goddess dressing

SPECIAL EQUIPMENT:
12 (4-in/10-cm) bamboo skewers

1. Cut the cabbage in half through the core, from top to bottom. Working with each half separately, remove the core by cutting a triangle around it and pulling it out. Then lay the half cut side down and cut into 6 wedges. Press a bamboo skewer into each wedge to secure the leaves. Repeat with the other half.

2. Heat the oil in a large frying pan over medium-low heat.

3. Place the cabbage wedges in the frying pan and sprinkle with the garlic powder and salt. Cook for 10 minutes on one side, or until lightly browned, then cook for 5 minutes on the other side. Serve with the dressing on the side.

STORE IT: *Store in an airtight container in the fridge for up to 3 days.*

make it COCONUT-FREE:
Use avocado oil.

make it LOW-FODMAP:
Omit the garlic powder.

make it VEGAN:
Use an egg-free dressing.

MAKE IT AT HOME

Replace store-bought green goddess dressing with my homemade version.

Green Speckled Dressing

Per serving, made with coconut oil, with Green Speckled Dressing:

							FAT:	CARBS:	PROTEIN:
calories: **252**	calories from fat: **189**	total fat: **20.9g**	saturated fat: **3.7g**	cholesterol: **8mg**			**75%**	**20%**	**5%**
sodium: **284mg**	carbs: **13.1g**	dietary fiber: **5.3g**	net carbs: **7.8g**	sugars: **6.9g**	protein: **3g**				

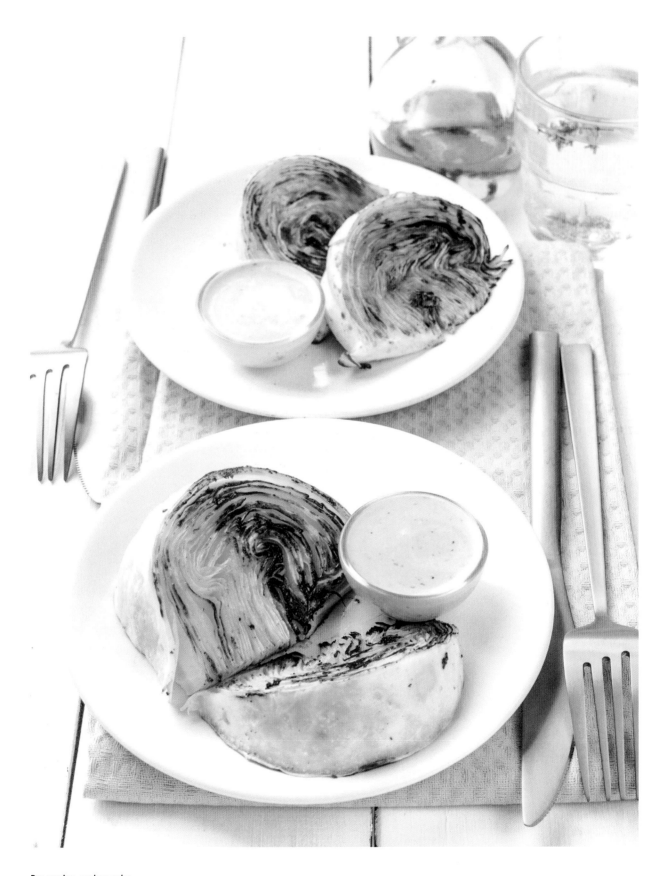

Per serving, wedges only:

calories: **102** | calories from fat: **41** | total fat: **4.5g** | saturated fat: **1.7g** | cholesterol: **4mg**

sodium: **194mg** | carbs: **12.7g** | dietary fiber: **5.3g** | net carbs: **7.4g** | sugars: **6.9g** | protein: **2.8g**

FAT:	CARBS:	PROTEIN:
40%	**50%**	**10%**

SALAMI CHIPS WITH BUFFALO CHICKEN DIP

 DAIRY-FREE • EGG-FREE • NUT-FREE

OPTIONS: AIP • LOW-FODMAP • NIGHTSHADE-FREE

SERVES 6

PREP TIME: 10 minutes (not including time to cook chicken)

COOK TIME: 10 minutes

Whether you make the dip or not, this recipe is worth it for the chips alone! Baking sliced salami (pepperoni works as well) makes it ultra-crisp and great for snacking.

8 ounces (225 g) salami, cut crosswise into 24 slices

BUFFALO CHICKEN DIP:

1 cup (240 ml) full-fat coconut milk

¾ cup (140 g) shredded cooked chicken

⅓ cup (22 g) nutritional yeast

1 tablespoon coconut aminos

1 tablespoon hot sauce

2 teaspoons onion powder

1½ teaspoons garlic powder

1 teaspoon turmeric powder

½ teaspoon finely ground sea salt

¼ teaspoon ground black pepper

¼ cup (17 g) roughly chopped fresh parsley

1. Preheat the oven to 400°F (205°C). Line 2 rimmed baking sheets with parchment paper or silicone baking mats.

2. Set the salami slices on the lined baking sheets. Bake for 8 to 10 minutes, until the centers look crisp and the edges are just slightly turned up.

3. Meanwhile, make the dip: Place the dip ingredients in a small saucepan. Bring to a simmer over medium-high heat, then reduce the heat to medium-low and cook, uncovered, for 6 minutes, or until thickened, stirring often.

4. Transfer the salami chips to a serving plate and the dip to a serving bowl. Stir the parsley into the dip and dig in!

make it AIP/NIGHTSHADE-FREE: Look for salami that uses compliant ingredients. Omit the hot sauce in the dip. For AIP, also omit the black pepper.

make it LOW-FODMAP: Omit the onion powder and garlic powder. Replace 1 tablespoon of the coconut milk with garlic-infused oil.

STORE IT: *Keep the chips and dip in separate airtight containers in the fridge. The dip will keep for up to 3 days; the chips, up to 5 days.*

REHEAT IT: *The dip can be enjoyed warm or cold. To reheat it, place it in a microwave-safe dish, cover, and microwave on high for 3 minutes, stirring halfway through.*

Per serving:

calories: **294** | calories from fat: **191** | total fat: **21.2g** | saturated fat: **12.8g** | cholesterol: **54mg** | sodium: **830mg** | carbs: **6.5g** | dietary fiber: **2.1g** | net carbs: **4.4g** | sugars: **1.9g** | protein: **19.5g**

FAT:	CARBS:	PROTEIN:
65%	**9%**	**26%**

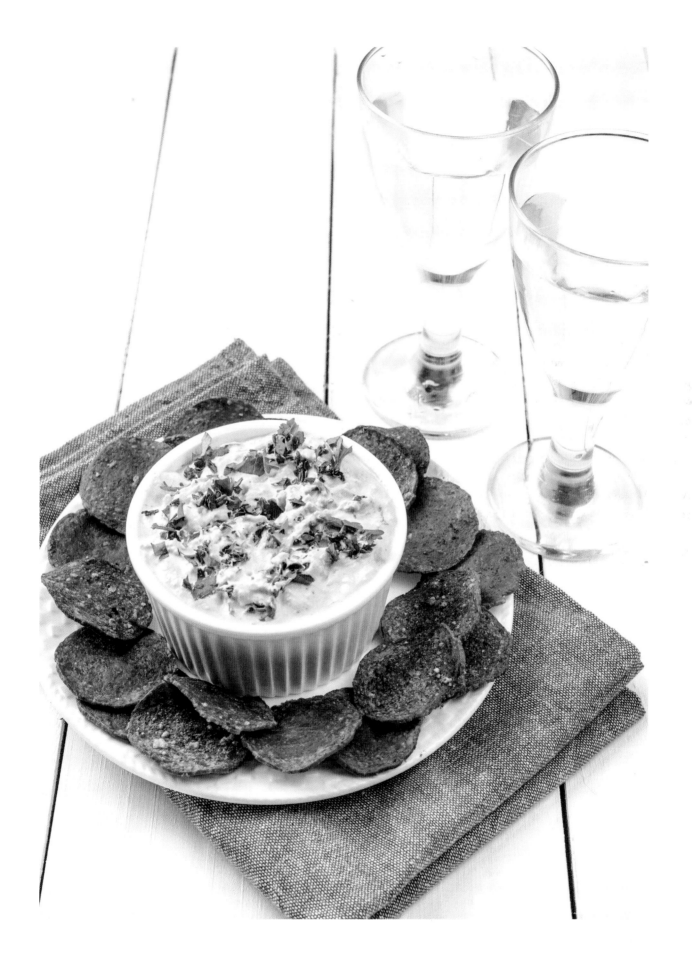

DAIRY-FREE
(BUT JUST AS GOOD) QUESO

DAIRY-FREE • EGG-FREE

OPTIONS: COCONUT-FREE • VEGAN • VEGETARIAN

SERVES 5

PREP TIME: 10 minutes, plus 12 hours to soak cashews

COOK TIME: 10 minutes

Kids and adults alike go crazy for this recipe, whether they're keto or not! If you have taco seasoning kicking around, replace all the spices, including the salt, with 2 tablespoons of taco seasoning. My all-time favorite way to enjoy this queso is with pork rinds. But don't limit yourself to using it as a dip; it doubles as a super delicious sauce when dolloped onto your favorite savory dishes.

1 cup (130 g) raw cashews

½ cup (120 ml) nondairy milk

¼ cup (17 g) nutritional yeast

½ teaspoon finely ground sea salt

¼ cup (60 ml) avocado oil

1 medium yellow onion, sliced

2 cloves garlic, roughly chopped

1 tablespoon chili powder

1 teaspoon ground cumin

¾ teaspoon garlic powder

¼ teaspoon onion powder

½ teaspoon dried oregano leaves

⅛ teaspoon paprika

⅛ teaspoon cayenne pepper

3½ ounces (100 g) pork rinds, or 2 medium zucchinis, cut into sticks, for serving (optional)

1. Place the cashews in a 12-ounce (350-ml) or larger sealable container. Cover with water. Seal and place in the fridge to soak for 12 hours.

2. After 12 hours, drain and rinse the cashews, then place them in a food processor or blender along with the milk, nutritional yeast, and salt. Set aside.

3. Heat the oil in a medium-sized frying pan over medium-low heat until shimmering. Add the onion, garlic, and spices and toss to coat the onion with the seasonings. Stir the mixture every couple of minutes until the onion begins to soften, about 10 minutes.

4. Transfer the onion mixture to the food processor or blender. Cover and blend until smooth.

5. Enjoy the queso with pork rinds or zucchini sticks, if desired.

make it COCONUT-FREE:
Opt for a nondairy milk not made from coconut, like almond or hazelnut milk.

make it VEGAN/VEGETARIAN:
Serve with zucchini sticks.

STORE IT: *Keep in an airtight container in the fridge for up to 3 days.*

Per ¼-cup/76-g serving, made with almond milk, queso only:

calories: **300**	calories from fat: **218**	total fat: **24.2g**	saturated fat: **4.1g**	cholesterol: **0mg**
sodium: **228mg**	carbs: **14.2g**	dietary fiber: **2.9g**	net carbs: **11.3g**	sugars: **2.5g**	protein: **6.5g**

FAT:	CARBS:	PROTEIN:
73%	**18%**	**9%**

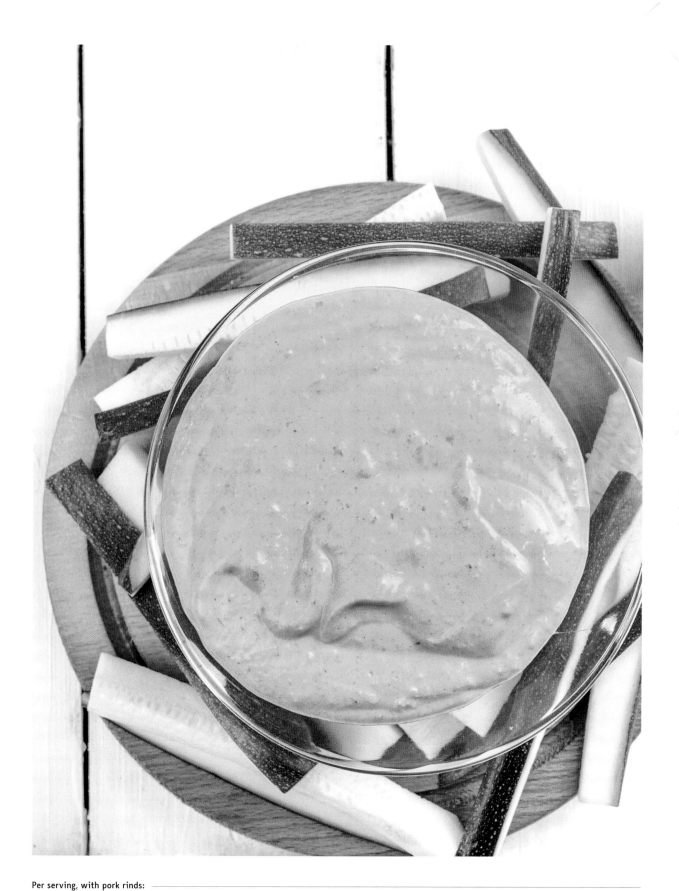

Per serving, with pork rinds:

					FAT:	CARBS:	PROTEIN:
calories: **416**	calories from fat: **300**	total fat: **31.4g**	saturated fat: **6.9g**	cholesterol: **29mg**	**68%**	**13%**	**19%**
sodium: **613mg**	carbs: **14.2g**	dietary fiber: **2.9g**	net carbs: **11.3g**	sugars: **2.5g**	protein: **19.3g**		

TOASTED ROSEMARY NUTS

EGG-FREE • LOW-FODMAP • VEGETARIAN
OPTIONS: COCONUT-FREE • DAIRY-FREE • NIGHTSHADE-FREE • VEGAN

SERVES 5
PREP TIME: 5 minutes
COOK TIME: 10 minutes

I used almonds for this recipe because it's what I had on hand, but you can use any nuts you'd like. The slight differences will be seen in the cook time and measurement for each type of nut: for pecans, use 1½ cups (210 g) and cook on low for 2 to 3 minutes; for cashews, use 1¼ cups (200 g) and cook on low for 6 minutes; for walnuts, use 1½ cups (180 g) and cook on low for 3 minutes.

2 tablespoons coconut oil or ghee

2 teaspoons finely chopped fresh rosemary leaves

1¼ teaspoons finely ground sea salt

1 teaspoon erythritol

½ teaspoon ground cumin

⅛ teaspoon ground black pepper

Pinch of cayenne pepper

1¼ cups (200 g) raw almonds

1. Melt the oil in a large frying pan over low heat. Once melted, add the rosemary, salt, erythritol, cumin, black pepper, and cayenne. Stir, then add the almonds.

2. Cook, stirring the almonds every 30 seconds, for a total of 5 to 8 minutes, until the nuts begin to brown slightly. Remove from the heat and allow to cool completely before enjoying.

make it **COCONUT-FREE:**
Use ghee.

make it **DAIRY-FREE/VEGAN:**
Use coconut oil.

make it **NIGHTSHADE-FREE:**
Omit the cayenne.

STORE IT: *Store in an airtight container in the fridge for up to 1 week or in the freezer for up to 1 month. The nuts can be enjoyed straight from the freezer, no thawing needed.*

Per ¼-cup/40-g serving, made with coconut oil:

calories: **300**	calories from fat: **230**	total fat: **25.6g**	saturated fat: **6.3g**	cholesterol: **0mg**
sodium: **469mg**	carbs: **9g**	dietary fiber: **5.2g**	net carbs: **3.8g**	sugars: **1.7g**	protein: **8.5g**

FAT:	CARBS:	PROTEIN:
77%	**12%**	**11%**

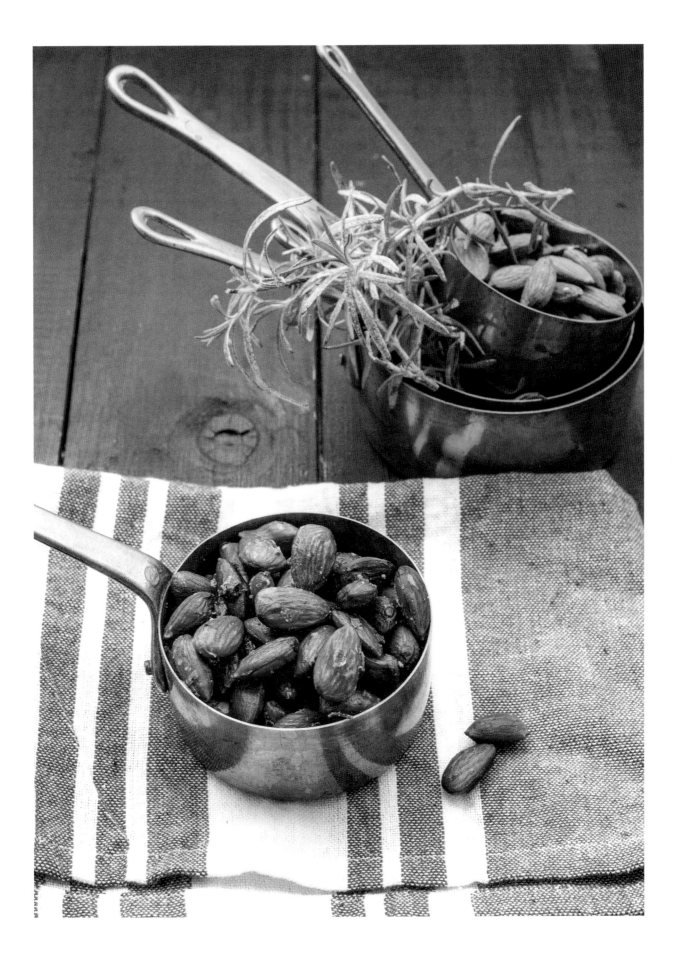

CHIMICHURRI

COCONUT-FREE · DAIRY-FREE · EGG-FREE · NUT-FREE
OPTIONS: AIP · LOW-FODMAP · VEGAN · VEGETARIAN

MAKES 1½ cups (320 g) (6 servings)

PREP TIME: 5 minutes, plus 20 minutes to rest

COOK TIME: –

My first experience with chimichurri was back in 2009. I'd ordered a vegan (gasp!) sandwich with chimichurri on the side for dipping. It was extravagant, but I never thought to make it at home. Fast-forward to 2018: My husband and I booked a sailing trip in Mexico and enjoyed chimichurri at every meal. Come the end of that seven-day trip, I told Kevin, "Babe, chimichurri has to be a recipe in my next book." And here we are! If you haven't had chimichurri before, you are missing out. And if you have, now you know how to make it yourself!

Generally, chimichurri is served with bread. If you have a favorite keto bread recipe, use it! Otherwise, it goes fabulously with pork rinds, mixed into zucchini noodles, or on steak.

I added a healthy dose of oregano oil to this recipe because oregano oil is a potent antibiotic that has the potential to heal many ailments, and it is a great addition to any no-cook recipe that calls for oregano. In addition to its antibiotic properties, it is anti-inflammatory; aids in gut health; assists with yeast infections; balances cholesterol; helps with acne, dandruff, warts, psoriasis, muscle pain, and varicose veins; and so many other things. You can find oregano oil in many health food stores or pharmacies. It comes as a liquid or gel capsule. I like to buy the gel caps because they're more versatile. To use them in a recipe, I just cut one open and add a few drops to what I'm making.

If you don't want to use oregano oil, simply double the amount of fresh oregano.

Additionally, I use flat-leaf parsley here because I prefer the texture of it over curly parsley for chimichurri. You'll know it's flat-leaf because it looks a little like cilantro.

⅔ packed cup (40 g) fresh flat-leaf parsley (leaves and stems)

¼ cup plus 2 tablespoons (90 ml) red wine vinegar

3 cloves garlic

2 tablespoons fresh oregano leaves

8 drops oregano oil, or 2 tablespoons additional fresh oregano leaves

1 teaspoon red pepper flakes

½ teaspoon finely ground sea salt

¼ teaspoon ground black pepper

1 cup (240 ml) olive oil

4¼ ounces (120 g) pork rinds, for serving (optional)

1. Place all the ingredients, except the oil and pork rinds, in a blender or food processor. Pulse until the parsley is broken up into ⅛-inch (3-mm) pieces.

2. If serving right away, transfer the mixture to a serving bowl. Add the oil and stir to combine; allow the chimichurri to sit for at least 20 minutes before serving with the pork rinds.

If serving later, transfer the mixture to a 16-ounce (475-ml) or larger airtight container. Add the oil, cover, and shake until incorporated, then place in the fridge. Set the container on the counter for 20 minutes before serving with the pork rinds.

STORE IT: *Keep in an airtight container in the fridge for up to 5 days.*

Per ¼-cup/52-g serving, chimichurri only:

calories: **317**	calories from fat: **296**	total fat: **34g**	saturated fat: **4.8g**	cholesterol: **0mg**
sodium: **160mg**	carbs: **2.4g**	dietary fiber: **1.2g**	net carbs: **1.2g**	sugars: **0.4g**	protein: **0.4g**

FAT:	CARBS:	PROTEIN:
97%	**3%**	**0%**

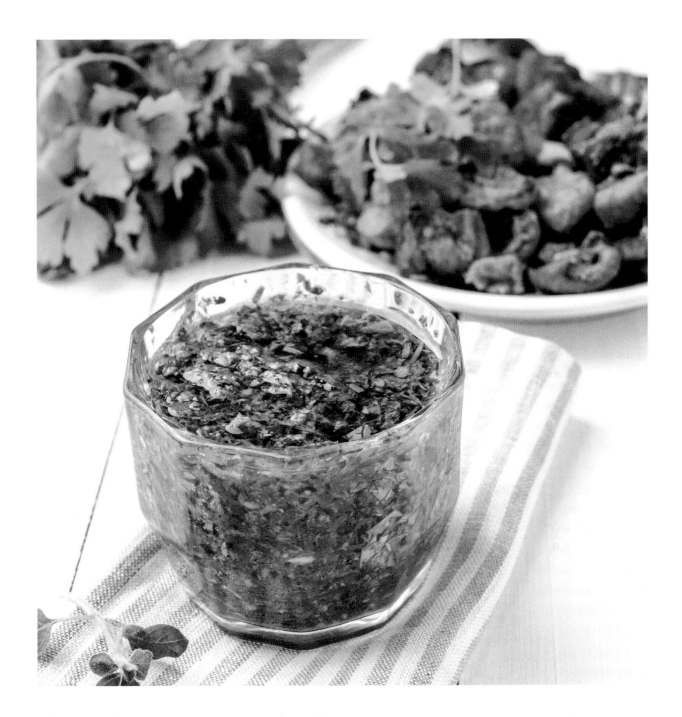

USE IN THESE RECIPES

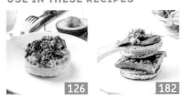

126
Full Meal Deal

182
Chimichurri Steak Bunwiches

make it **AIP:**
Omit the red pepper flakes and black pepper.

make it **LOW-FODMAP:**
Omit the garlic and replace ½ cup (120 ml) of the olive oil with garlic-infused oil.

make it **VEGAN/VEGETARIAN:**
Skip the pork rinds and serve with a handful of celery sticks per person.

Per serving, with pork rinds:

| calories: **419** | calories from fat: **356** | total fat: **40g** | saturated fat: **6.8g** | cholesterol: **0mg** |
| sodium: **455mg** | carbs: **2.4g** | dietary fiber: **1.2g** | net carbs: **1.2g** | sugars: **0.4g** | protein: **12.4g** |

FAT:	CARBS:	PROTEIN:
86%	**2%**	**12%**

BREADED MUSHROOM NUGGETS

COCONUT-FREE • DAIRY-FREE • VEGETARIAN
OPTION: NIGHTSHADE-FREE

SERVES 4

PREP TIME: 15 minutes

COOK TIME: 50 minutes

Oh, tasty! This is a great recipe for when you have guests over or you want to fancy up your snacking game. Because mushrooms are naturally wet, this recipe doesn't keep well, meaning that the mushrooms won't have a crunchy coating forever. If you know you'll have leftovers and you're not one for soggy mushrooms, it's better to halve the recipe. They still taste great soggy, and they're awesome on a salad, but I felt I should let you know so that you can decide.

24 cremini mushrooms (about 1 lb/455 g)

2 large eggs

½ cup (55 g) blanched almond flour

1 teaspoon garlic powder

1 teaspoon paprika

½ teaspoon finely ground sea salt

2 tablespoons avocado oil

½ cup (120 ml) honey mustard dressing, for serving (optional)

SPECIAL EQUIPMENT (optional):

Toothpicks

1. Preheat the oven to 350°F (177°C). Line a rimmed baking sheet with parchment paper or a silicone baking mat.

2. Break the stems off the mushrooms or cut them short so that the stems are level with the caps.

3. Crack the eggs into a small bowl and whisk.

4. Place the almond flour, garlic powder, paprika, and salt in a medium-sized bowl and whisk to combine.

5. Dip one mushroom at a time into the eggs, then use the same hand to drop it into the flour mixture, being careful not to get the flour mixture on that hand. Rotate the mushroom in the flour mixture with a fork to coat on all sides, then transfer it to the lined baking sheet. Repeat with the remaining mushrooms.

6. Drizzle the coated mushrooms with the oil. Bake for 50 minutes, or until the tops begin to turn golden.

7. Remove from the oven and serve with the dressing, if using. If serving to friends and family, provide toothpicks.

make it NIGHTSHADE-FREE:
Omit the paprika.

MAKE IT AT HOME

Replace store-bought honey mustard dressing with my homemade version.

78

Honey Mustard Dressing & Marinade

Per serving, with Honey Mustard Dressing & Marinade:

| calories: **332** | calories from fat: **263** | total fat: **29.3g** | saturated fat: **3.7g** | cholesterol: **93mg** |
| sodium: **398mg** | carbs: **9.3g** | dietary fiber: **2g** | net carbs: **7.3g** | sugars: **4.5g** | protein: **8g** |

FAT:	CARBS:	PROTEIN:
79%	**11%**	**10%**

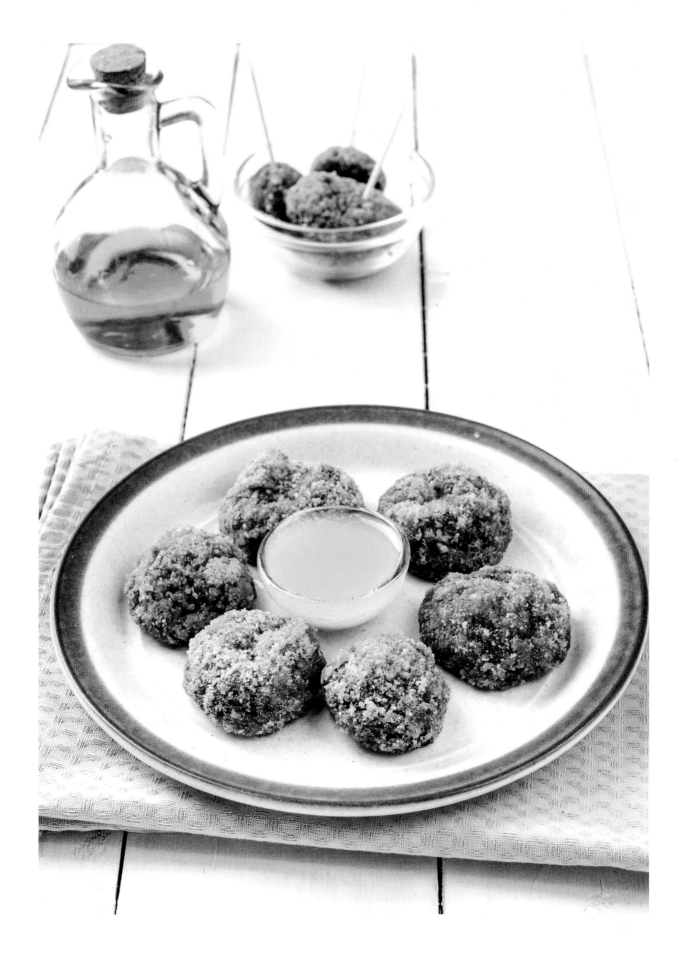

CUCUMBER SALMON COINS

COCONUT-FREE • DAIRY-FREE • NIGHTSHADE-FREE • NUT-FREE
OPTIONS: EGG-FREE • LOW-FODMAP

SERVES 2

PREP TIME: 5 minutes

COOK TIME: –

After a long day of flying to Guelph, Ontario, for a book tour, Kevin and I decided to grab lunch at a cute little café before getting ready for the event. Each of us ordered a plate of salmon coins and asked the server to swap out the crackers for cucumber slices. The dish was so good that I knew I'd have to re-create it for this book.

If you don't have a garlic press, you can mince the garlic using the smallest holes of a box grater. It works like a charm!

¼ cup (52 g) mayonnaise

Grated zest of ½ lemon

1 tablespoon plus 1 teaspoon lemon juice

1 teaspoon Dijon mustard

1 clove garlic, minced

¼ teaspoon finely ground sea salt

⅛ teaspoon ground black pepper

1 English cucumber (about 12 in/ 30.5 cm long), sliced crosswise into coins

8 ounces (225 g) smoked salmon, separated into small pieces

2 fresh chives, sliced

1. Place the mayonnaise, lemon zest, lemon juice, mustard, garlic, salt, and pepper in a small bowl and whisk to combine.

2. Divide the cucumber coins between 2 plates. Top each coin with a piece of smoked salmon, then drizzle with the mayonnaise mixture and sprinkle with sliced chives.

3. Serve right away or store in the fridge for up to 1 day.

make it EGG-FREE:
Use egg-free mayonnaise (see recipe on page 102).

make it LOW-FODMAP:
Omit the garlic.

MAKE IT AT HOME

Replace store-bought mayonnaise with my homemade version.

Mayonnaise

Per serving, made with homemade mayonnaise:

| calories: **337** | calories from fat: **226** | total fat: **25.1g** | saturated fat: **4.1g** | cholesterol: **36mg** | | FAT: | CARBS: | PROTEIN: |
| sodium: **2200mg** | carbs: **5.4g** | dietary fiber: **1.7g** | net carbs: **3.7g** | sugars: **3.3g** | protein: **22.4g** | **67%** | **6%** | **27%** |

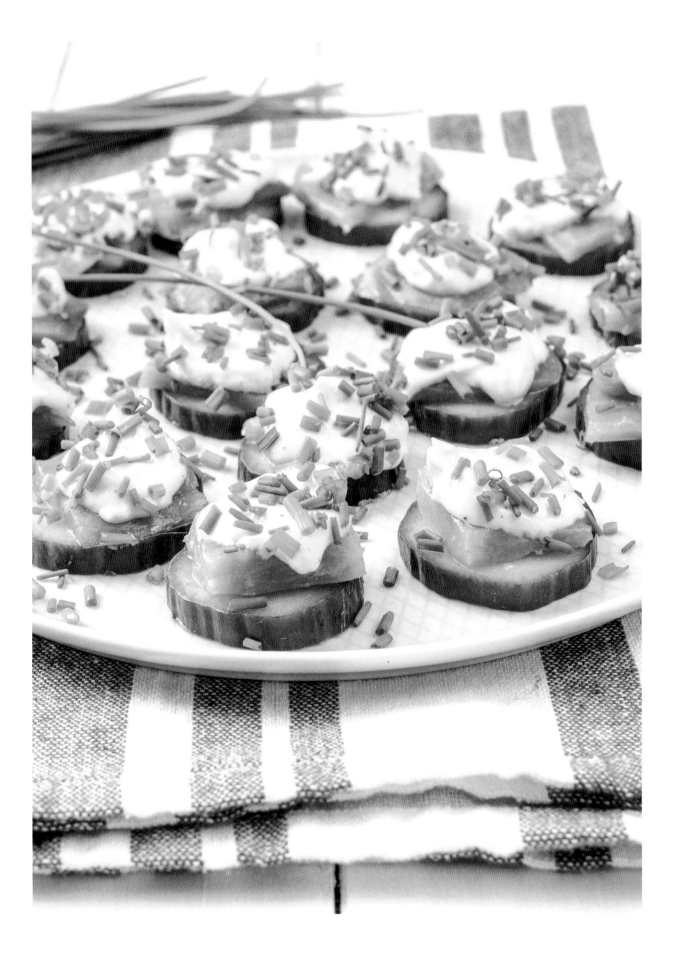

RADISH CHIPS & PESTO

 COCONUT-FREE • DAIRY-FREE • EGG-FREE • NIGHTSHADE-FREE • VEGAN • VEGETARIAN

SERVES 2

PREP TIME: 10 minutes (not including time to soak almonds)

COOK TIME: –

Radishes! They're crunchy, delicious, and perfect for dipping.

PESTO:

1 cup (60 g) fresh basil leaves

⅓ heaping cup (60 g) raw almonds, soaked in water for 12 hours, drained, and rinsed

⅓ cup (25 g) fresh parsley leaves and stems

1 small clove garlic

2 tablespoons olive oil

1 tablespoon apple cider vinegar

1½ teaspoons lemon juice

⅛ teaspoon finely ground sea salt

20 medium radishes (about 3¼ oz/ 90 g), thinly sliced, for serving

1. Place all the ingredients for the pesto in a food processor or high-powered blender. Blend on high until smooth.

2. Transfer the pesto to a serving bowl. Place the sliced radishes on a plate and serve.

Per serving:

calories: **337** | calories from fat: **265** | total fat: **29.4g** | saturated fat: **3.2g** | cholesterol: **0mg**

sodium: **144mg** | carbs: **10.2g** | dietary fiber: **5.4g** | net carbs: **4.8g** | sugars: **2.4g** | protein: **8.1g**

FAT:	CARBS:	PROTEIN:
79%	11%	10%

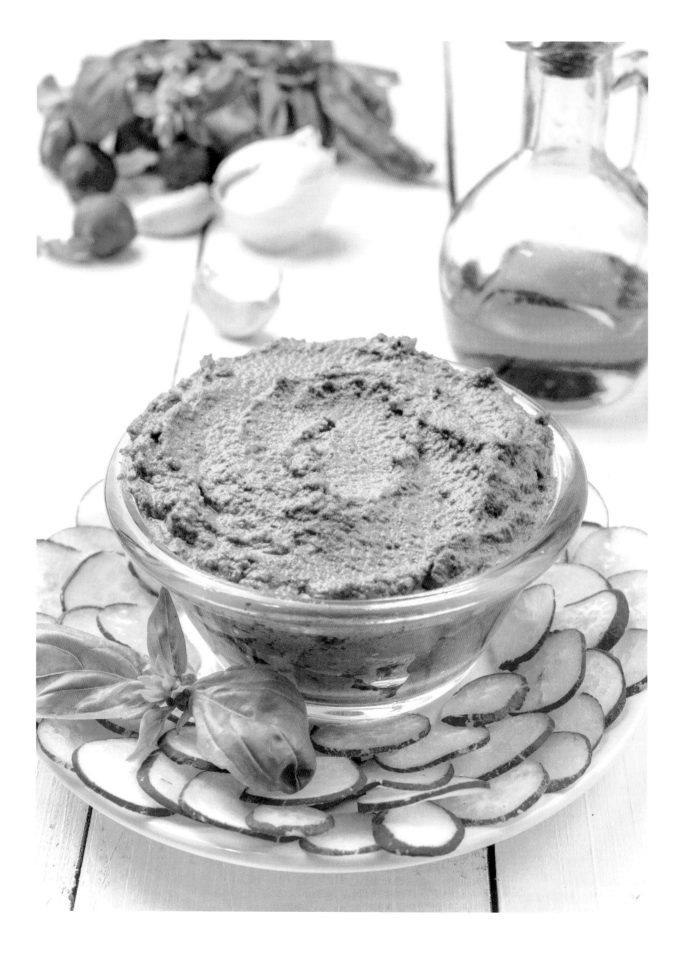

BLT DIP

COCONUT-FREE • DAIRY-FREE
OPTION: EGG-FREE

SERVES 10

PREP TIME: 10 minutes
(not including time to
soak cashews)

COOK TIME: 15 minutes

Dig into this party favorite game-friendly snack, made keto and dairy-free! Smooth "cream cheese" is topped with chunky bacon bits, tomatoes, lettuce, and green onions. Keep it low-carb by serving it with sliced cucumber, zucchini, or jicama.

8 strips bacon (about 8 oz/225 g)

BLT DIP:

Warm bacon grease, reserved from cooking bacon (above)

1½ cups (240 g) raw cashews, soaked in water for 12 hours, drained, and rinsed

⅓ cup (70 g) mayonnaise

¼ cup (40 g) collagen peptides or protein powder (optional)

2 tablespoons apple cider vinegar

2 tablespoons lemon juice

2 teaspoons paprika or smoked paprika

2 tablespoons diced yellow onions

1 clove garlic

½ teaspoon finely ground sea salt

¼ teaspoon ground black pepper

TOPPINGS:

1 cup (115 g) sliced iceberg lettuce

1 small tomato, diced

Crumbled bacon (from above)

2 green onions, sliced

1 English cucumber (about 12 in/ 30.5 cm long), sliced crosswise into coins, for serving

1. Cook the bacon in a large frying pan over medium heat until crispy, about 15 minutes, then remove from the pan. When the bacon has cooled, crumble it.

2. Make the dip: Pour the warm bacon grease into a food processor or high-powered blender. Add the soaked cashews, mayonnaise, collagen (if using), vinegar, lemon juice, paprika, onions, garlic, salt, and pepper. Pulse until smooth, about 2 minutes.

3. Transfer the mixture to a 9-inch (23-cm) pie plate. Top with the lettuce, tomato, bacon, and green onions. Serve with the cucumber coins.

MAKE IT AT HOME

Replace store-bought mayonnaise with my homemade version.

Mayonnaise

make it EGG-FREE:
Use egg-free mayonnaise (see recipe on page 102).

Per serving, made with homemade mayonnaise and collagen, with 2 cucumber coins:

| calories: **378** | calories from fat: **248** | total fat: **27.5g** | saturated fat: **7.1g** | cholesterol: **38mg** | FAT: | CARBS: | PROTEIN: |
| sodium: **931mg** | carbs: **12.7g** | dietary fiber: **1.4g** | net carbs: **11.3g** | sugars: **2.8g** | protein: **20g** | **65%** | **13%** | **21%** |

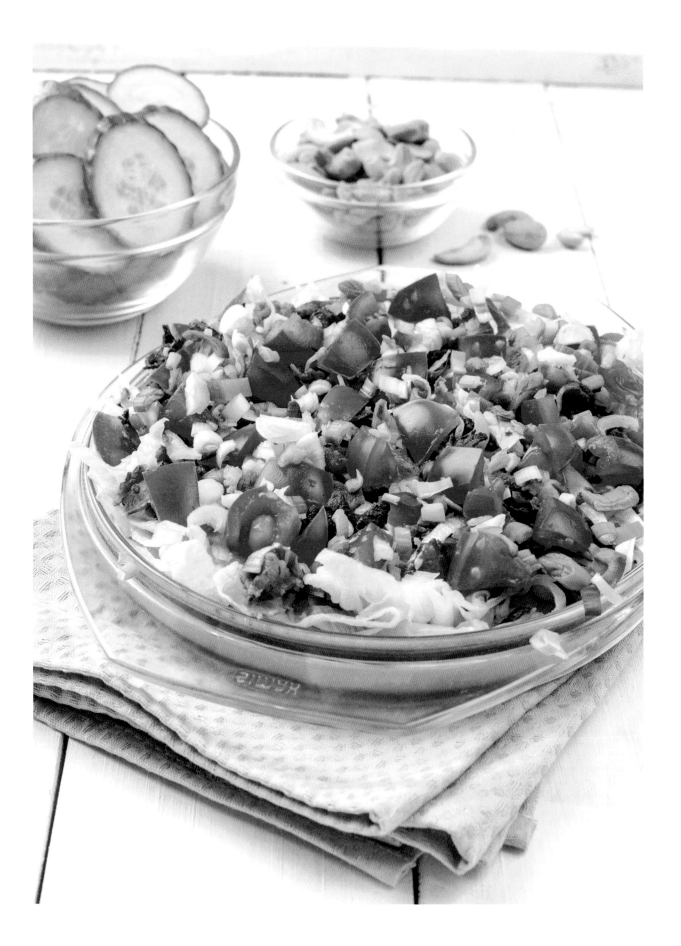

TUNA CUCUMBER BOATS

COCONUT-FREE • DAIRY-FREE • NIGHTSHADE-FREE • NUT-FREE
OPTIONS: EGG-FREE • LOW-FODMAP

SERVES 1

PREP TIME: 5 minutes

COOK TIME: –

I'm a fan of boat things, so much so that my little family lives on a boat! But really, shaping your vegetables into boats—like I did with the Creamy Spinach Zucchini Boats (page 214) and the Hummus Celery Boats (page 274)—is an easy way to make a quick meal with balanced macros and to get your veggies in at the same time. You can turn just about any vegetable into a boat—bell pepper, cucumber, zucchini, celery, eggplant, butternut squash, lettuce. Heck, there's a whole cookbook dedicated to the art of the edible vegetable boat.

If you don't want to use mayonnaise in this recipe, replace it with an equal amount of Herby Vinaigrette & Marinade (page 98).

1 English cucumber (about 12 in/ 30.5 cm long)

1 (5-oz/142-g) can flaked tuna packed in water, drained

1 dill pickle, finely diced

3 tablespoons mayonnaise

2 tablespoons finely diced red onions

2 teaspoons finely chopped fresh parsley

1 teaspoon lemon juice

1 clove garlic, minced

½ teaspoon Dijon mustard

1. Cut the cucumber in half lengthwise, scoop out the seeds, and then cut each piece in half crosswise. Set aside.

2. Place the remaining ingredients in a medium-sized bowl and mix until incorporated.

3. Spoon the tuna mixture into the hollowed-out cucumber pieces, piling it high. Set on a plate and enjoy!

make it EGG-FREE:
Use egg-free mayonnaise (see recipe on page 102) or Herby Vinaigrette & Marinade (page 98).

make it LOW-FODMAP:
Replace the red onions with 1 green onion, sliced, and omit the garlic.

MAKE IT AT HOME

Replace store-bought mayonnaise with my homemade version.

104

Mayonnaise

Per serving, made with homemade mayonnaise:
calories: **527** | calories from fat: **310** | total fat: **34.4g** | saturated fat: **4.5g** | cholesterol: **83mg** | sodium: **1054mg** | carbs: **12.7g** | dietary fiber: **4.2g** | net carbs: **8.5g** | sugars: **7.7g** | protein: **41.7g**

FAT:	CARBS:	PROTEIN:
59%	10%	31%

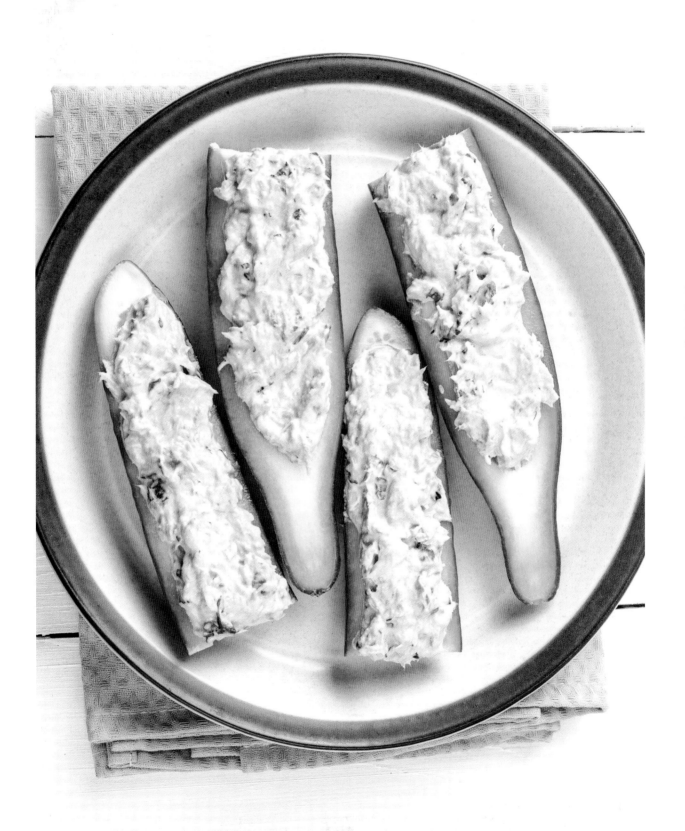

ZUCCHINI CAKES WITH LEMON AIOLI

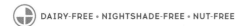 **DAIRY-FREE • NIGHTSHADE-FREE • NUT-FREE**

MAKES 8 small cakes
(4 per serving)

PREP TIME: 20 minutes

COOK TIME: 22 minutes

These cakes are ridiculously good. They are creamy on the inside and crisp on the outside. You'll think there is cheese inside…but there isn't! The full-on bacon flavor pairs so well with the zucchini; you'll be mega impressed. If you don't want to pair the cakes with the Lemon Aioli, they also go great with Chimichurri (page 284), Creamy Italian Dressing (page 94), or Honey Mustard Dressing & Marinade (page 78).

CAKES:

3 lightly packed cups (450 g) shredded zucchini (about 3 medium zucchinis)

4 strips bacon (about 4 oz/110 g)

1 teaspoon finely ground sea salt

1 large egg

1 tablespoon coconut flour

1 tablespoon arrowroot starch or tapioca starch

¾ teaspoon garlic powder

¾ teaspoon onion powder

½ teaspoon dried oregano leaves

¼ teaspoon ground black pepper

LEMON AIOLI:

¼ cup (52 g) mayonnaise

Grated zest of ½ lemon

1 tablespoon plus 1 teaspoon lemon juice

1 teaspoon Dijon mustard

1 clove garlic, minced

¼ teaspoon finely ground sea salt

⅛ teaspoon ground black pepper

1. Place the shredded zucchini in a strainer set over the sink. Sprinkle with the salt and allow to sit for 15 minutes.

2. Meanwhile, cook the bacon in a large frying pan over medium heat until crispy, about 10 minutes. Remove the bacon from the pan, leaving the grease in the pan. When the bacon has cooled, crumble it.

3. While the bacon is cooking, make the aioli: Put the mayonnaise, lemon zest, lemon juice, mustard, garlic, salt, and pepper in a small bowl and whisk to incorporate. Set aside.

4. When the zucchini is ready, squeeze it over and over again to get out as much of the water as you can.

5. Transfer the zucchini to a large mixing bowl and add the remaining ingredients for the cakes. Stir until fully incorporated.

6. Set the frying pan with the bacon grease over medium-low heat. Scoop up 2 tablespoons of the zucchini mixture, roll it into a ball between your hands, and place in the hot pan. Repeat with the remaining mixture, making a total of 8 balls. Press each ball with the back of a fork until the cakes are about ½ inch (1.25 cm) thick.

7. Cook the cakes for 4 to 6 minutes per side, until golden. Serve with the aioli.

MAKE IT AT HOME

Replace store-bought mayonnaise with my homemade version.

Mayonnaise

STORE IT: *Keep the cakes and aioli in separate airtight containers in the fridge for up to 3 days.*

REHEAT IT: *Transfer a single serving of the cakes to a microwave-safe plate, cover, and microwave for 2 minutes; or place in a frying pan with a drop of oil and fry over medium heat for about 1 minute per side.*

Per serving, made with homemade mayonnaise:

| calories: **636** | calories from fat: **474** | total fat: **52.7g** | saturated fat: **12.5g** | cholesterol: **155mg** |
| sodium: **2300mg** | carbs: **12.2g** | dietary fiber: **3.3g** | net carbs: **8.9g** | sugars: **5g** | protein: **27.5g** |

FAT:	CARBS:	PROTEIN:
75%	**8%**	**17%**

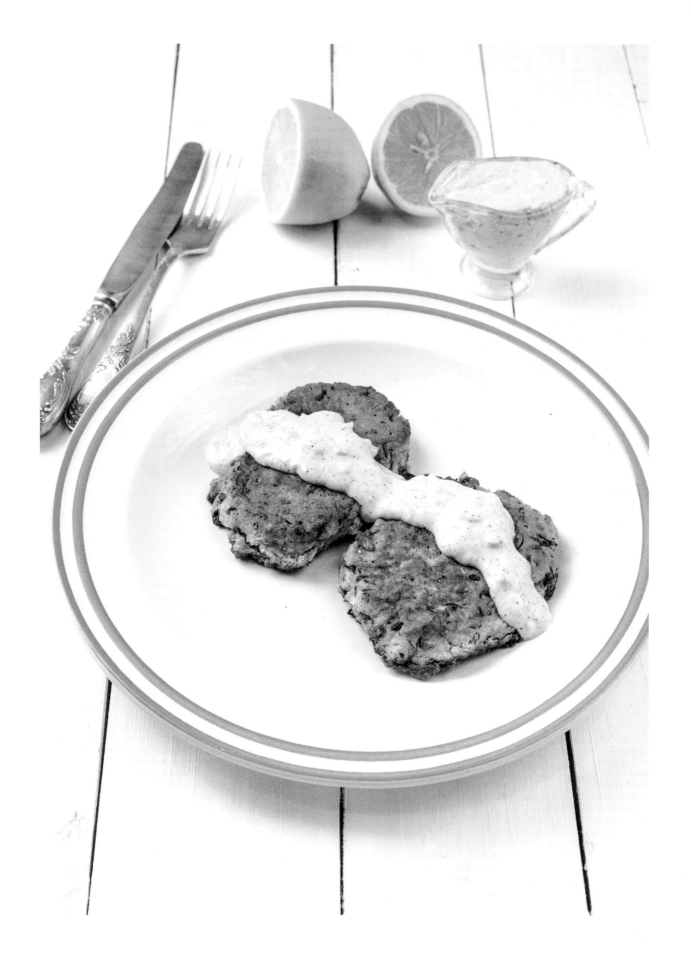

KETO DIET SNACK PLATE

SERVES 1

PREP TIME: 5 minutes
(not including time to
hard-boil egg)

COOK TIME: –

Let's not overthink keto meals, okay? A lot of keto folks swear against snacking, and that's fair. We shouldn't have to snack too often while burning fat. But snacking is a perfectly safe activity, and if you're hungry but not too hungry, snack-y but not too interested in making something elaborate, this plate will do the trick!

If you don't want to use mayonnaise for dipping, Chimichurri (page 284), Avocado Lime Dressing (page 84), and Herby Vinaigrette & Marinade (page 98) are also great options.

3 ounces (85 g) sliced salami

6 jalapeño-stuffed olives

¼ cup (28 g) sauerkraut

1 medium Hass avocado, peeled, pitted, and sliced (about 4 oz/110 g of flesh)

1 large egg, hard-boiled, peeled, and cut in half

1 tablespoon mayonnaise

1 (0.35-oz/10-g) package roasted seaweed sheets

Place all the items on a plate and dig in!

MAKE IT AT HOME

Replace store-bought mayonnaise with my homemade version.

104

Mayonnaise

Per serving, made with homemade mayonnaise:

calories: **657**	calories from fat: **519**	total fat: **57.7g**	saturated fat: **16.3g**	cholesterol: **229mg**
sodium: **1561mg**	carbs: **14.9g**	dietary fiber: **9.4g**	net carbs: **5.5g**	sugars: **2.8g**	protein: **19.7g**

FAT:	CARBS:	PROTEIN:
79%	**9%**	**12%**

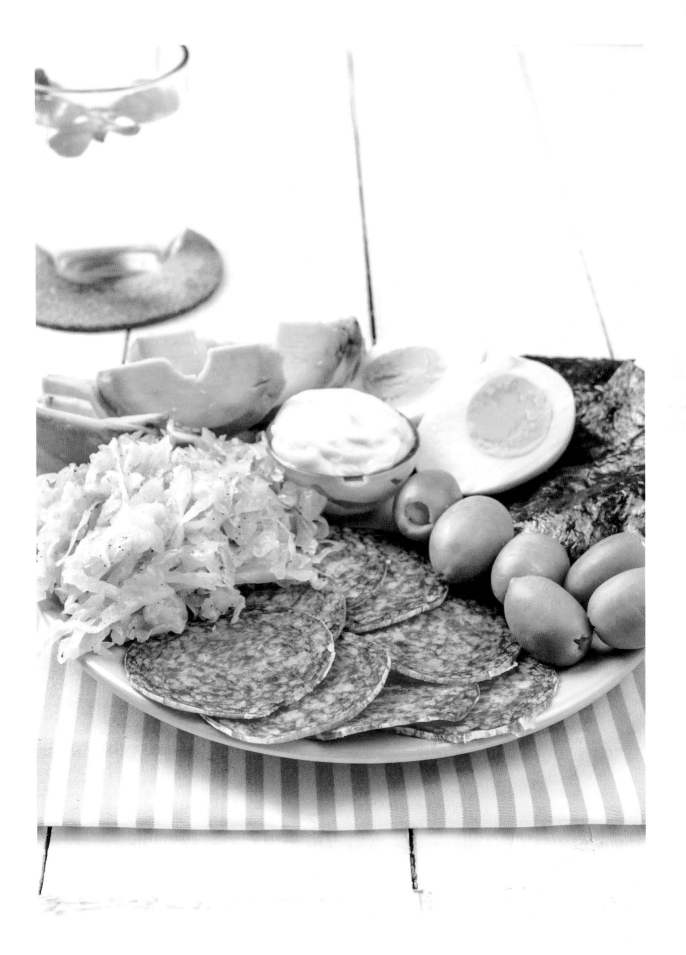

BACON-WRAPPED AVOCADO FRIES

AIP • COCONUT-FREE • DAIRY-FREE • EGG-FREE • NIGHTSHADE-FREE • NUT-FREE

SERVES 4
PREP TIME: 10 minutes
COOK TIME: 18 minutes

Sometimes avocado gets a little boring—gasp, did I just write that? Let's do something about that, shall we?

These fries are awesome dipped in Ranch Dressing (page 76) or Green Speckled Dressing (page 80).

2 medium Hass avocados, peeled and pitted (about 8 oz/220 g of flesh)

16 strips bacon (about 1 lb/455 g), cut in half lengthwise

1. Cut each avocado into 8 fry-shaped pieces, making a total of 16 fries.

2. Wrap each avocado fry in 2 half-strips of bacon. Once complete, place in a large frying pan.

3. Set the pan over medium heat and cover with a splash guard. Fry for 6 minutes on each side and on the bottom, or until crispy, for a total of 18 minutes.

4. Remove from the heat and enjoy immediately!

Per serving:

calories: **723**	calories from fat: **525**	total fat: **58.3g**	saturated fat: **17.9g**	cholesterol: **125mg**
sodium: **2631mg**	carbs: **6.4g**	dietary fiber: **3.7g**	net carbs: **2.7g**	sugars: **0.3g**	protein: **43.2g**

FAT:	CARBS:	PROTEIN:
73%	**3%**	**24%**

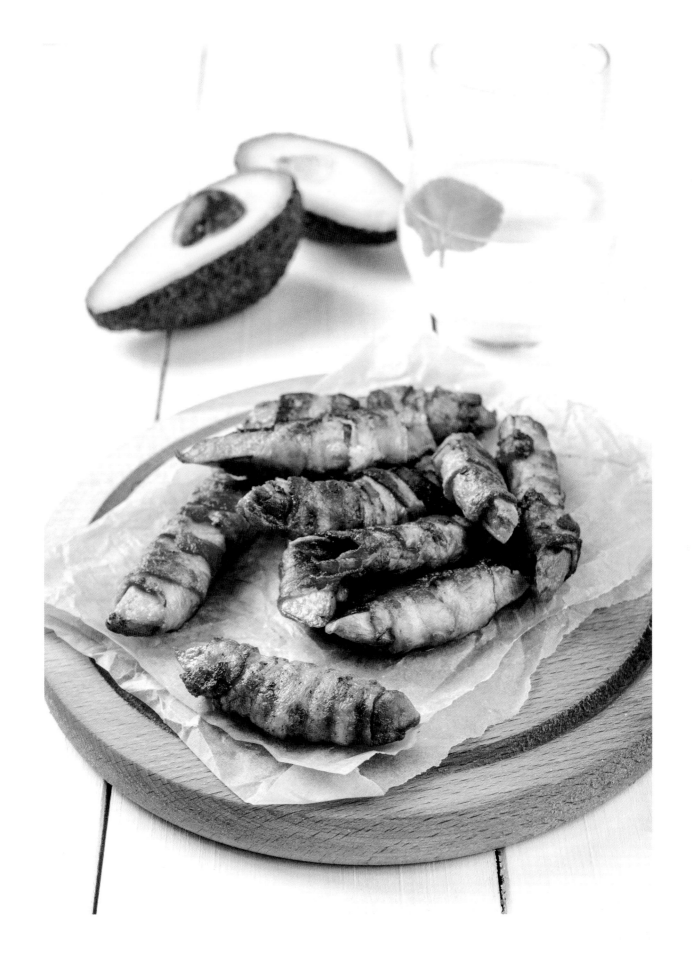

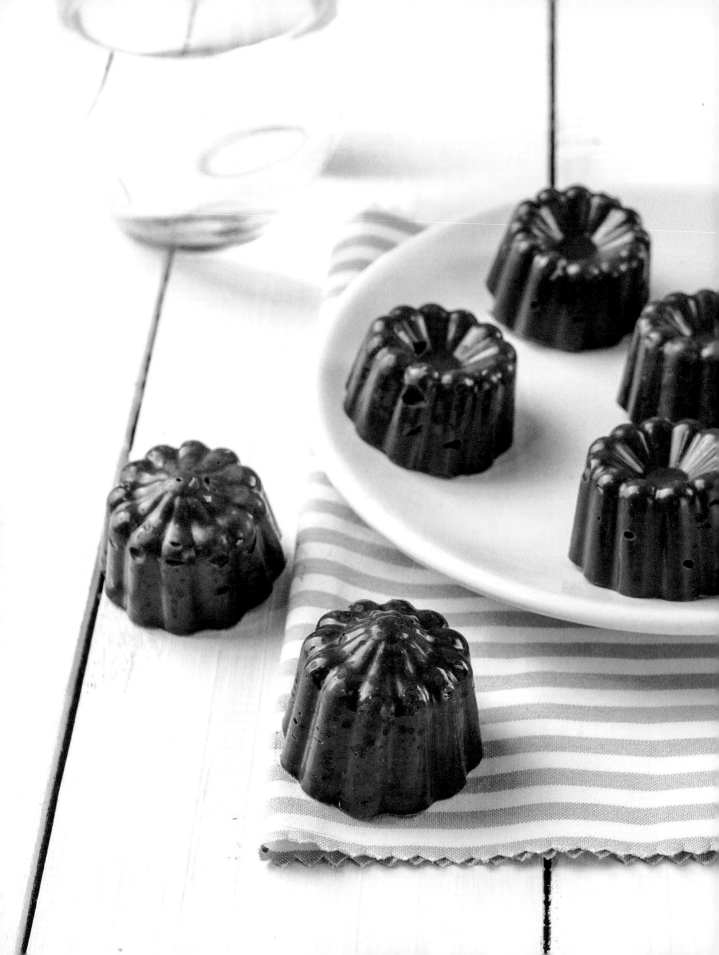

9.

SWEET SNACKS

KETONE GUMMIES

AIP • COCONUT-FREE • DAIRY-FREE • EGG-FREE • LOW-FODMAP • NIGHTSHADE-FREE • NUT-FREE

MAKES 8 gummies (1 per serving)

PREP TIME: 10 minutes, plus 30 minutes to set

COOK TIME: 5 minutes

If you don't have a pack of exogenous ketones on hand, don't worry about it! This recipe can be made without them, and it'll still taste great. There's no need to buy extra things you don't require, and exogenous ketones are one of those items that are nice to have, but not a requirement. If you like exogenous ketones and find that you thrive on them, great. But don't break the budget because you think they're essential to your success. I use them sporadically, when I find I need them, but I don't go hog wild because they're a little pricey. If you don't use exogenous ketones in this recipe, simply add 2 drops of liquid stevia or 2 teaspoons of confectioners'-style erythritol in their place. Easy as that!

½ cup (120 ml) lemon juice

8 hulled strawberries (fresh or frozen and defrosted)

2 tablespoons unflavored gelatin

2 teaspoons exogenous ketones

SPECIAL EQUIPMENT (optional):

Silicone mold with eight 2-tablespoon or larger cavities

1. Have on hand your favorite silicone mold. I like to use a large silicone ice cube tray and spoon 2 tablespoons of the mixture into each cavity, which makes 8 gummies total. If you do not have a silicone mold, you can use an 8-inch (20-cm) square silicone or metal baking pan; if using a metal pan, line it with parchment paper, draping some over the sides for easy removal.

2. Place the lemon juice, strawberries, and gelatin in a blender or food processor and pulse until smooth. Transfer the mixture to a small saucepan and set over low heat for 5 minutes, or until it becomes very liquid-y and begins to simmer.

3. Remove from the heat and stir in the exogenous ketones.

4. Divide the mixture evenly among 8 cavities of the mold or pour into the baking pan. Transfer to the fridge and allow to set for 30 minutes. If using a baking pan, cut into 8 squares.

STORE IT: *Keep in an airtight container in the fridge for up to 5 days.*

Per gummy:

calories: **19** | calories from fat: **1.8** | total fat: **0.2g** | saturated fat: **0.1g** | cholesterol: **0mg** | sodium: **10mg** | carbs: **1.2g** | dietary fiber: **0.3g** | net carbs: **0.9g** | sugars: **0.9g** | protein: **3.2g**

FAT:	CARBS:	PROTEIN:
9%	25%	66%

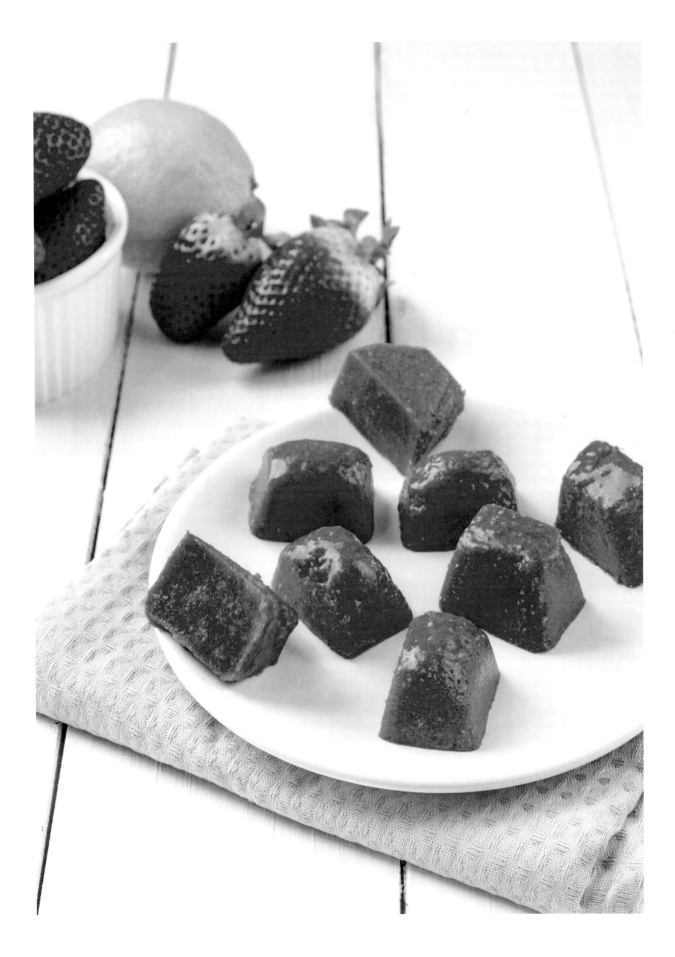

STRAWBERRY SHORTCAKE COCONUT ICE

DAIRY-FREE • EGG-FREE • LOW-FODMAP • NIGHTSHADE-FREE • NUT-FREE • VEGAN • VEGETARIAN
OPTIONS: AIP • COCONUT-FREE

SERVES 4

PREP TIME: 5 minutes

COOK TIME: –

If you don't like coconut and you can do dairy, this recipe is amazing made with heavy cream. You know, the real stuff. Or so I've been told. I've made it for friends a bunch of times, and they go crazy over the cream version! It's still great with coconut cream, but it's nice to have options.

9 hulled strawberries (fresh or frozen and defrosted)

⅓ cup (85 g) coconut cream

1 tablespoon apple cider vinegar

2 drops liquid stevia, or 2 teaspoons erythritol

3 cups (420 g) ice cubes

1. Place the strawberries, coconut cream, vinegar, and sweetener in a blender or food processor. Blend until smooth.

2. Add the ice and pulse until crushed.

3. Divide among four ¾-cup (180-ml) or larger bowls and serve immediately.

make it **AIP**:
Use stevia.

make it **COCONUT-FREE**:
Swap out the coconut cream for cashew milk, macadamia nut milk, or, if you can handle dairy, heavy cream. (Note that using cashew milk would make it higher in FODMAPs, if that is a concern for you.)

Per serving:

calories: **61** | calories from fat: **45** | total fat: **5g** | saturated fat: **4.4g** | cholesterol: **0mg** | sodium: **4mg** | carbs: **3.3g** | dietary fiber: **1g** | net carbs: **2.3g** | sugars: **2g** | protein: **0.7g**

FAT:	CARBS:	PROTEIN:
74%	21%	5%

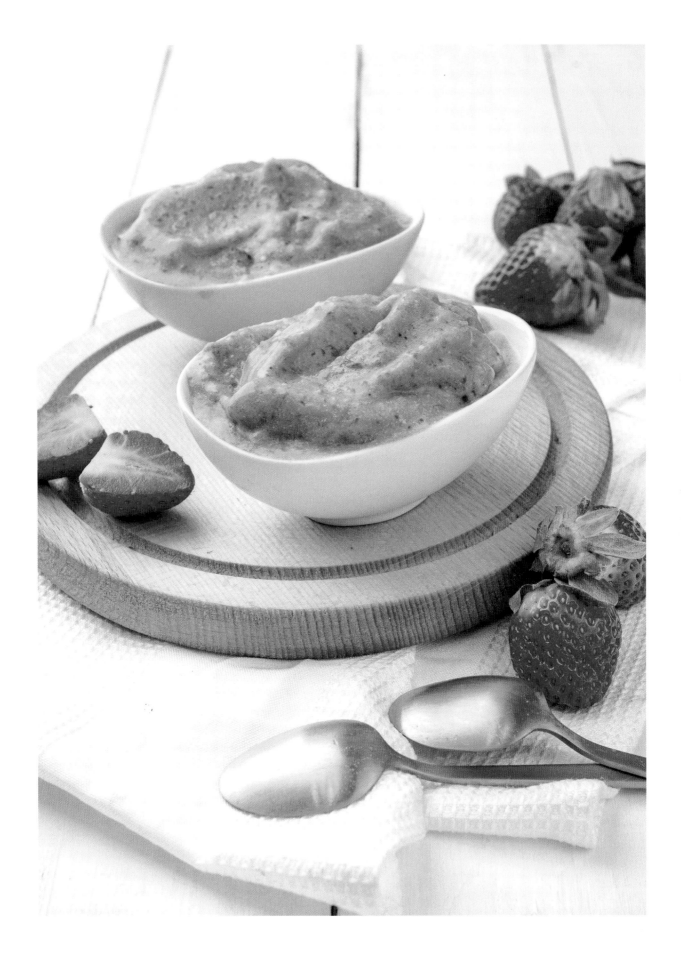

GRANDMA'S MERINGUES

DAIRY-FREE • LOW-FODMAP • NIGHTSHADE-FREE • NUT-FREE • VEGETARIAN
OPTION: COCONUT-FREE

**MAKES 12 meringues
(2 per serving)**

**PREP TIME: 10 minutes,
plus 1 hour to cool in oven**

COOK TIME: 1 hour

My grandma, maybe like yours, was a fabulous baker. Each time my sister and I would go to her house, she'd have something special in the freezer. Christina's favorites: chocolate chip cookies and sherbet. My favorites: butter tarts and meringues. Grandma would cut up fresh berries and scatter them on top of her meringues...they were so tasty, but not at all keto. So, here's Grandma's recipe made keto!

Be sure not to get any egg yolk in your meringue batter. That'll make the meringues flatten before you even start. This is why it's best to crack your eggs over a separate bowl. Save those yolks for a batch of Edana's Macadamia Crack Bars (page 326).

2 large egg whites, room temperature

¼ teaspoon cream of tartar

Pinch of finely ground sea salt

½ cup (80 g) confectioners'-style erythritol

½ teaspoon vanilla extract

FOR SERVING:

24 fresh strawberries, sliced

¾ cup (190 g) coconut cream

12 fresh mint leaves

1. Preheat the oven to 225°F (108°C). Line a rimmed baking sheet with parchment paper or a silicone baking mat.

2. Place the egg whites, cream of tartar, and salt in a very clean large bowl. Make sure that the bowl does not have any oil residue in it. Using a handheld electric mixer or stand mixer, mix on low speed until the mixture becomes foamy.

3. Once foamy, increase the speed to high. Slowly add the erythritol, 1 tablespoon at a time, mixing all the while. Add a tablespoon about every 20 seconds.

4. Keep beating until the mixture is shiny and thick and peaks have formed; it should be nearly doubled in volume. (The peaks won't be as stiff as in a traditional meringue.) Fold in the vanilla.

5. Using a large spoon, dollop the meringue mixture onto the lined baking sheet, making a total of 12 meringues.

6. Bake for 1 hour without opening the oven door. After 1 hour, turn off the oven and keep the meringues in the cooling oven for another hour, then remove.

7. To serve, place 2 meringues on each plate. Top each serving with 4 sliced strawberries, 2 tablespoons of coconut cream, and 2 mint leaves.

make it COCONUT-FREE:
Replace the coconut cream with heavy cream if you can tolerate dairy.

STORE IT: *Store the meringues in an airtight container on the counter for up to 3 days; store the strawberries, cream, and mint in the refrigerator for up to 3 days. If the meringues become a bit chewy, you can set them in a 225°F (108°C) oven for a couple of minutes to crisp them up again before serving.*

Per serving:

calories: **100**	calories from fat: **68**	total fat: **7.6g**	saturated fat: **6.6g**	cholesterol: **0mg**
sodium: **56mg**	carbs: **5.8g**	dietary fiber: **1.8g**	net carbs: **4g**	sugars: **3.5g**	protein: **2.3g**

FAT:	CARBS:	PROTEIN:
68%	23%	9%

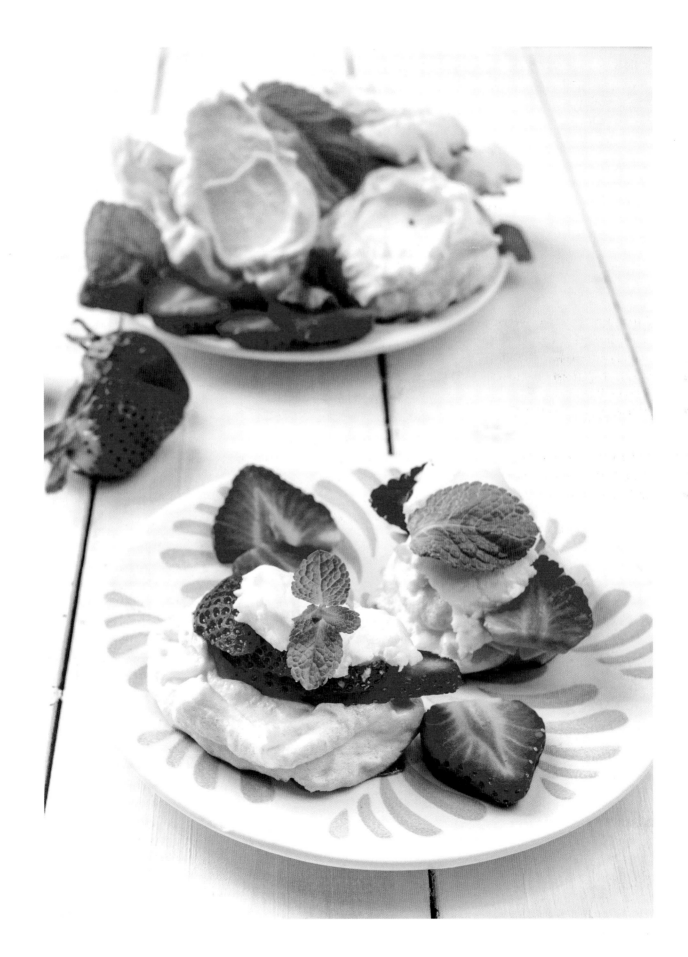

HAYSTACK COOKIES

EGG-FREE • LOW-FODMAP • NIGHTSHADE-FREE • NUT-FREE • VEGETARIAN

OPTIONS: DAIRY-FREE • VEGAN

MAKES 20 cookies (2 per serving)

PREP TIME: 10 minutes, plus 45 minutes to chill

COOK TIME: 5 minutes

Around the time my husband and I were getting ready to move into our motor home full-time and travel about, we were gifted a ginormous box of monk fruit–sweetened chocolate. Like, actually ginormous—144 bars, to be exact. It was so much chocolate that I had to start getting creative on how to use it. After all, there was only so much room in the motor home for chocolate bars!

That's when I started playing around with haystack recipes and discovered that coconut milk is an essential addition to a good haystack. (If you don't like coconut milk and can eat dairy, heavy cream would be amazing in this recipe.)

The MCT oil powder does nothing to the consistency or flavor of the end product. Instead, it increases the amount of fat in the recipe, which may be a goal for you! If you decide to go for it, use an unsweetened, unflavored MCT oil powder. My favorite brand is Perfect Keto.

½ cup (95 g) erythritol

¼ cup (60 ml) full-fat coconut milk

3 tablespoons coconut oil, ghee, or cacao butter

¼ cup (20 g) cocoa powder

⅓ cup (30 g) unflavored MCT oil powder (optional)

2 cups (200 g) unsweetened shredded coconut

1. Line a rimmed baking sheet or large plate with parchment paper or a silicone baking mat.

2. Place the erythritol, coconut milk, and oil in a large frying pan. Slowly bring to a simmer over medium-low heat, whisking periodically to prevent burning; this should take about 5 minutes.

3. When the mixture reaches a simmer, remove from the heat and stir in the cocoa powder. Once fully combined, stir in the MCT oil powder, if using, and then the shredded coconut.

4. Using a 1-tablespoon measuring spoon, carefully scoop out a portion of the mixture and press it into the spoon. Place the haystack on the lined baking sheet and repeat, making a total of 20 cookies.

5. Refrigerate for 30 to 45 minutes before enjoying.

make it DAIRY-FREE/VEGAN: Do not use ghee.

STORE IT: *Keep in an airtight container in the fridge for up to 5 days or in the freezer for up to 1 month.*

THAW IT: *Let the haystacks sit out on the counter for 1 minute before enjoying.*

Per serving, made with coconut oil, without MCT oil powder:

					FAT:	CARBS:	PROTEIN:
calories: **122**	calories from fat: **107**	total fat: **11.9g**	saturated fat: **9.6g**	cholesterol: **0mg**	83%	13%	4%
sodium: **4mg**	carbs: **4.2g**	dietary fiber: **2.5g**	net carbs: **1.7g**	sugars: **1.2g**	protein: **1.3g**		

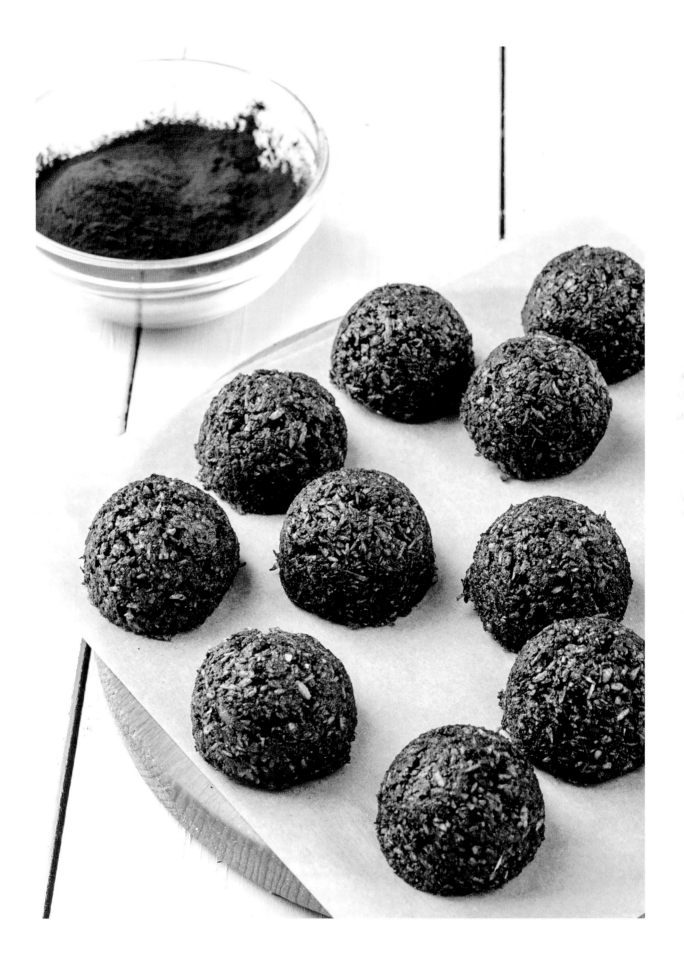

CHEESECAKE BALLS

EGG-FREE • LOW-FODMAP • NIGHTSHADE-FREE • VEGETARIAN
OPTIONS: COCONUT-FREE • DAIRY-FREE • VEGAN

MAKES 12 balls (1 per serving)

PREP TIME: 15 minutes, plus 1 hour 20 minutes to chill

COOK TIME: –

With so many dairy-free options out there, fat bombs made with cream cheese are available to all. If you can do dairy, make this recipe with actual cream cheese. If you can't, head to your local health food store and ask where the dairy-free cream cheese is hidden.

Why the different types of erythritol in this recipe? Since it's no-bake, using confectioners'-style erythritol makes sense so you don't have little granules of sugar in each bite. But, for the cinnamon sugar topping, having granules isn't a bad thing. If you have only granulated erythritol on hand, you can make it confectioners'-style by pulsing it in your blender or food processor until it's powdered.

ALMOND FLOUR CENTER:

½ cup (55 g) blanched almond flour

2 tablespoons coconut oil or ghee

1 tablespoon confectioners'-style erythritol

CREAM CHEESE LAYER:

1 (8-oz/225-g) package cream cheese (dairy-free or regular)

3 tablespoons coconut oil or ghee

¼ cup plus 2 tablespoons (60 g) confectioners'-style erythritol

2 teaspoons ground cinnamon

CINNAMON SUGAR TOPPING:

¼ cup (48 g) granulated erythritol

2 teaspoons ground cinnamon

make it COCONUT-FREE: Use ghee.

make it DAIRY-FREE/VEGAN: Use coconut oil and dairy-free cream cheese.

STORE IT: *Keep in an airtight container in the fridge for up to 1 week or in the freezer for up to 1 month.*

THAW IT: *Let the balls sit out on the counter for 15 to 20 minutes before serving.*

1. Line a rimmed baking sheet or tray that will fit into your freezer with parchment paper.

2. Make the almond flour center: Place the almond flour, oil, and erythritol in a small bowl. Knead with your hands until incorporated. Separate the mixture into 12 pieces and roll into balls. Place the balls on the lined baking sheet and place in the freezer.

3. Make the cream cheese layer: Place the cream cheese, oil, and erythritol in a small bowl and combine with a fork or handheld mixer. Divide the mixture evenly between 2 bowls. To one bowl, add the cinnamon and mix until incorporated. Place both bowls in the freezer until the cream cheese has hardened but is still workable and not completely frozen through, about 1 hour.

4. Place the ingredients for the cinnamon sugar topping in a small bowl and whisk with a fork to combine. Set aside.

5. Once the cream cheese mixtures have chilled sufficiently, scoop a teaspoon each of the cinnamon cream cheese mixture and the plain cream cheese mixture and place them side by side on the lined baking sheet. Take the almond flour balls out of the freezer and place one ball between a pair of cream cheese pieces. Pick up the pile and roll between your palms until the almond flour ball is in the middle and the cream cheese surrounds it. Roll the ball in the cinnamon sugar mixture until coated. Place the coated ball back on the lined baking sheet and place in the freezer.

6. Repeat with the remaining almond flour balls, cream cheese mixtures, and cinnamon sugar topping, placing the coated balls on the baking sheet in the freezer as you complete them.

7. Place the coated balls in the freezer to chill for 20 minutes before enjoying.

Per ball, made with coconut oil and dairy-free cream cheese:

| calories: **126** | calories from fat: **113** | total fat: **12.5g** | saturated fat: **7.4g** | cholesterol: **0mg** | | FAT: | CARBS: | PROTEIN: |
| sodium: **75mg** | carbs: **2g** | dietary fiber: **0.8g** | net carbs: **1.2g** | sugars: **0g** | protein: **1.4g** | **89%** | **6%** | **5%** |

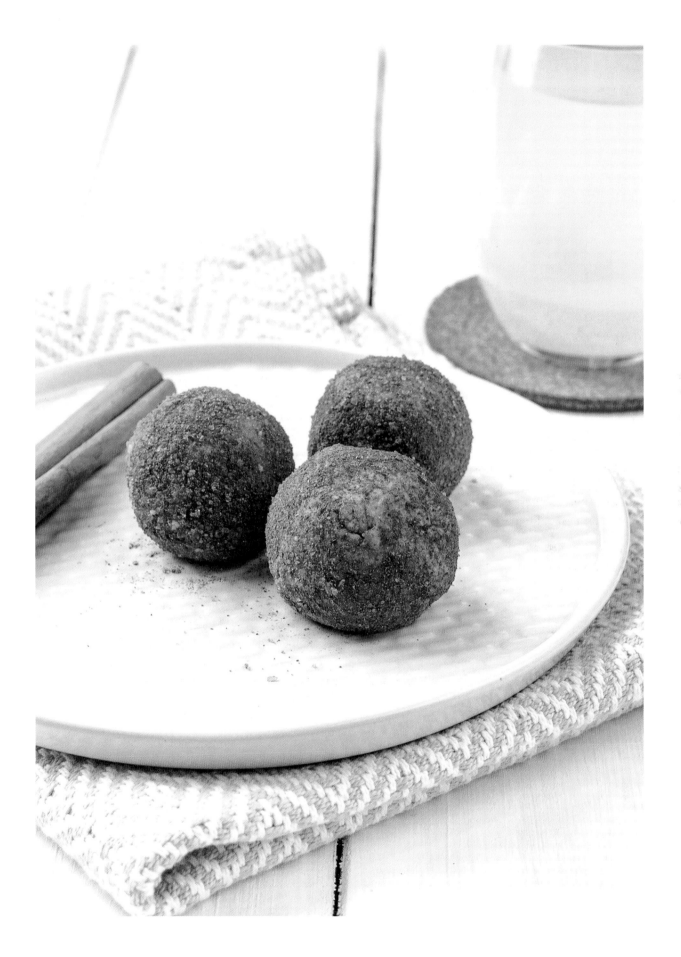

CINNAMON BOMBS

 EGG-FREE • LOW-FODMAP • NIGHTSHADE-FREE • VEGETARIAN

OPTIONS: AIP • COCONUT-FREE • DAIRY-FREE • NUT-FREE • VEGAN

MAKES 8 bombs (1 per serving)

PREP TIME: 5 minutes, plus 15 or 30 minutes to chill

COOK TIME: –

When I'm in a hurry and need something fatty, this is my go-to fat bomb. It's easy, the ingredients are commonplace, and (most importantly) it's fat-tastic!

Personalize this recipe based on your needs by adding ¼ cup (25 g) of unflavored MCT oil powder, 1 teaspoon of exogenous ketones, or 2 teaspoons of mushroom elixirs, such as chaga, cordyceps, or reishi.

⅓ cup (85 g) smooth unsweetened nut or seed butter or coconut butter

3 tablespoons melted coconut oil, cacao butter, or ghee

¾ teaspoon ground cinnamon

2 drops liquid stevia, or 2 teaspoons confectioners'-style erythritol

SPECIAL EQUIPMENT (optional):

Silicone mold with eight 1-tablespoon or larger cavities

1. Have on hand your favorite silicone mold. I like to use a large silicone ice cube tray and spoon 1 tablespoon of the mixture into each cavity, which makes 8 cubes total. If you do not have a silicone mold, making this into a bark works well, too. Simply use an 8-inch (20-cm) square silicone or metal baking pan; if using a metal pan, line it with parchment paper, draping some over the sides for easy removal.

2. Place all the ingredients in a medium-sized bowl and stir until well mixed and smooth.

3. Divide the mixture evenly among 8 cavities of the silicone mold or pour into the baking pan. Transfer to the fridge and allow to set for 15 minutes if using cacao butter or 30 minutes if using ghee or coconut oil. If using a baking pan, break the bark into 8 pieces for serving.

> **STORE IT:** *Keep in an airtight container in the fridge for up to 10 days or in the freezer for up to 2 months. Enjoy straight from the freezer, no thawing needed.*

make it AIP:
Use coconut butter. Do not use ghee. Use stevia or enjoy unsweetened.

make it COCONUT-FREE:
Use a nut or seed butter. Do not use coconut oil.

make it DAIRY-FREE/VEGAN:
Do not use ghee.

make it NUT-FREE:
Use sunflower seed butter or coconut butter.

Per serving, made with almond butter and coconut oil:

calories: **134** | calories from fat: **113** | total fat: **12.5g** | saturated fat: **5.2g** | cholesterol: **0mg**
sodium: **0mg** | carbs: **2.6g** | dietary fiber: **1.8g** | net carbs: **0.8g** | sugars: **0.4g** | protein: **2.9g**

FAT:	CARBS:	PROTEIN:
84%	7%	9%

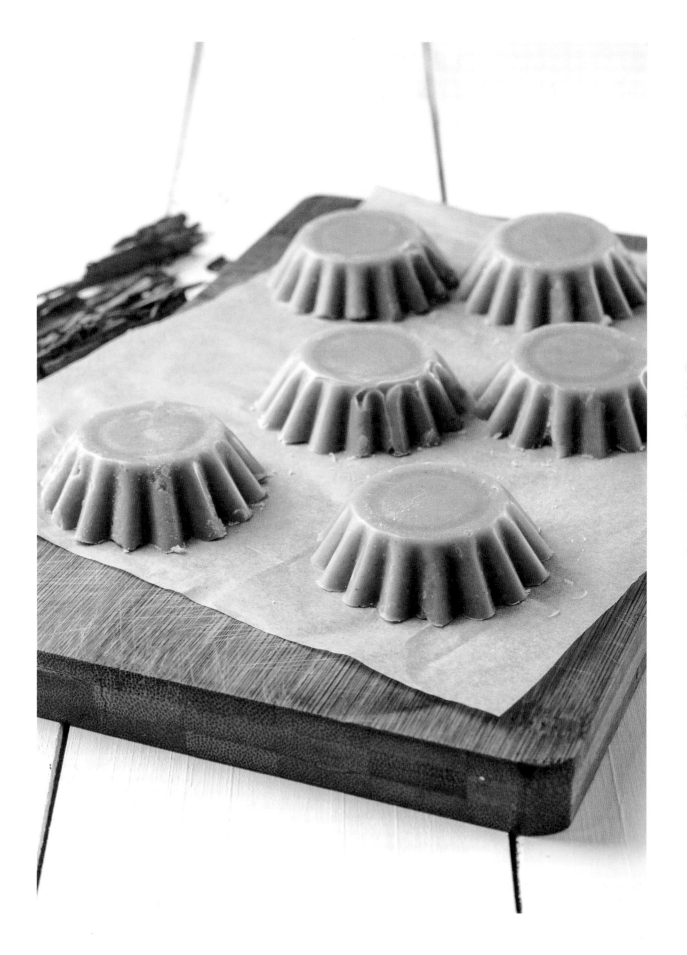

SUPERPOWER FAT BOMBS

EGG-FREE • LOW-FODMAP • NIGHTSHADE-FREE • NUT-FREE

OPTIONS: COCONUT-FREE • DAIRY-FREE • VEGAN • VEGETARIAN

MAKES 8 bombs (1 per serving)

PREP TIME: 10 minutes, plus 15 or 30 minutes to chill

COOK TIME: –

This is a great recipe if you're a superfood junkie and love collecting new ingredients to try but don't really know how to use them. Literally anything will work here, so don't feel limited to the superfoods listed below. Here are some ideas for making this recipe your own: Add 1 teaspoon of exogenous ketones, 1 teaspoon of maca powder, 1 teaspoon of turmeric powder, or 2 teaspoons of mushroom elixirs, such as chaga, cordyceps, or reishi. Or try different protein powders or swap out the coffee granules for matcha powder.

What are cacao nibs, you ask? They're little bits of raw cacao, completely unsweetened and in their natural state.

⅔ cup (145 g) coconut oil, cacao butter, or ghee, melted

¼ cup (40 g) collagen peptides or protein powder

¼ cup (25 g) unflavored MCT oil powder

2 tablespoons cocoa powder

2 tablespoons roughly ground flax seeds

1 tablespoon cacao nibs

1 teaspoon instant coffee granules

4 drops liquid stevia, or 1 tablespoon plus 1 teaspoon confectioners'-style erythritol

Pinch of finely ground sea salt

SPECIAL EQUIPMENT (optional):

Silicone mold with eight 2-tablespoon or larger cavities

1. Have on hand your favorite silicone mold. I like to use a large silicone ice cube tray and spoon 2 tablespoons of the mixture into each well, which makes 8 cubes total. If you do not have a silicone mold, making this into a bark works well, too. Simply use an 8-inch (20-cm) square silicone or metal baking pan; if using a metal pan, line it with parchment paper, draping some over the sides for easy removal.

2. Place all the ingredients in a medium-sized bowl and stir until well mixed and smooth.

3. Divide the mixture evenly among 8 cavities in the silicone mold or pour into the baking pan. Transfer to the fridge and allow to set for 15 minutes if using cacao butter or 30 minutes if using ghee or coconut oil. If using a baking pan, break the bark into 8 pieces for serving.

make it COCONUT-FREE:
Use cacao butter or ghee.

make it DAIRY-FREE:
Do not use ghee.

make it VEGAN:
Do not use ghee or collagen. Opt for a plant-based protein powder.

make it VEGETARIAN:
Do not use collagen. Opt for a plant- or egg-based protein powder.

STORE IT: *Keep in an airtight container in the fridge for up to 10 days or in the freezer for up to 2 months. Enjoy straight from the freezer, no thawing needed.*

Per serving, made with coconut oil and collagen:

calories: **136** | calories from fat: **110** | total fat: **12.3g** | saturated fat: **6.8g** | cholesterol: **0mg** | sodium: **84mg** | carbs: **3g** | dietary fiber: **2.4g** | net carbs: **0.6g** | sugars: **0g** | protein: **5.8g**

FAT:	CARBS:	PROTEIN:
76%	8%	16%

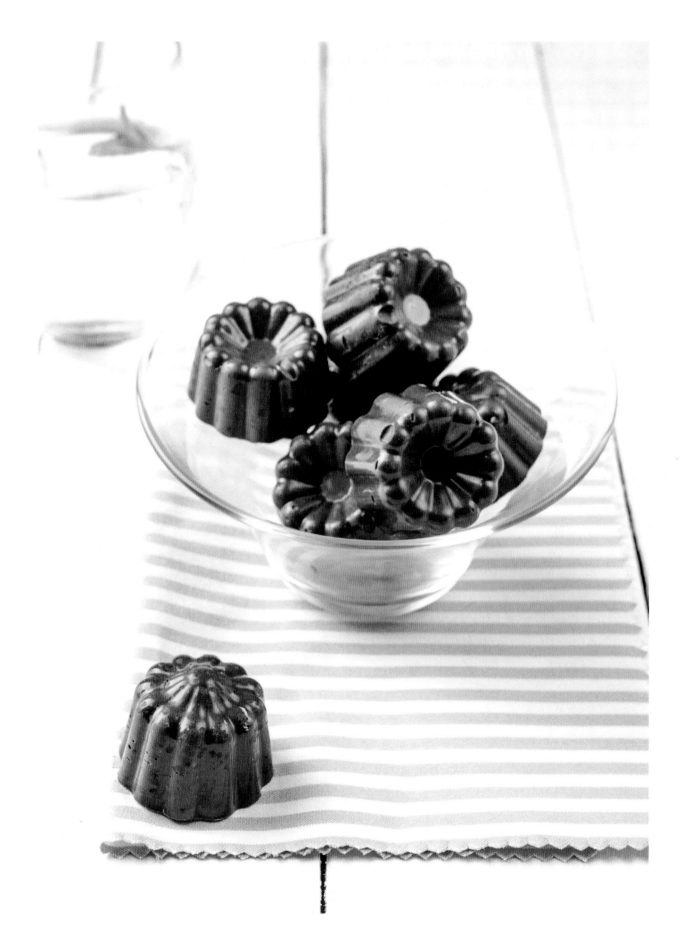

JELLY CUPS

EGG-FREE • LOW-FODMAP • NIGHTSHADE-FREE

OPTIONS: AIP • COCONUT-FREE • DAIRY-FREE • NUT-FREE

MAKES 16 jelly cups (1 per serving)

PREP TIME: 10 minutes, plus 30 minutes to chill

COOK TIME: 5 minutes

Like collagen peptides, gelatin is packed with health benefits, but unlike collagen, it has gelling properties. It's a bit cumbersome to use, so I wouldn't be surprised if you're not cooking with gelatin as often as you thought you might. If you have a tub of gelatin in your pantry collecting dust, you can give it a purpose by making these simple jelly cups! (Looking for another recipe to use up the gelatin in your pantry? Try the Ketone Gummies on page 304.)

You can have loads of fun with this recipe. Try swapping out the butter base for melted chocolate, using 7½ ounces (200 g) of chopped stevia-sweetened baking chocolate or 1 cup (225 g) of stevia-sweetened chocolate chips, or replacing the raspberries in the jelly filling with any fresh berry of your choice.

BUTTER BASE:

⅔ cup (170 g) coconut butter or smooth unsweetened nut or seed butter

⅔ cup (145 g) coconut oil, ghee, or cacao butter, melted

2 teaspoons vanilla extract

7 drops liquid stevia, or 2 teaspoons confectioners'-style erythritol

JELLY FILLING:

½ cup (70 g) fresh raspberries

¼ cup (60 ml) water

3 drops liquid stevia, or 1 teaspoon confectioners'-style erythritol

1½ teaspoons unflavored gelatin

SPECIAL EQUIPMENT:

16 mini muffin cup liners, or 1 silicone mini muffin pan

make it AIP:
Use coconut butter. Do not use ghee.

make it COCONUT-FREE:
Use a nut or seed butter. Almond butter is great here! Opt for ghee or cacao butter.

make it DAIRY-FREE:
Do not use ghee.

make it NUT-FREE:
Use coconut butter or a seed butter. Sunflower seed butter is great!

1. Set 16 mini muffin cup liners on a tray or have on hand a silicone mini muffin pan.

2. Make the base: Place the coconut butter, melted oil, vanilla, and sweetener in a medium-sized bowl and stir to combine.

3. Take half of the base mixture and divide it equally among the 16 mini muffin cup liners or 16 wells of the mini muffin pan, filling each about one-quarter full. Place the muffin cup liners (or muffin pan) in the fridge. Set the remaining half of the base mixture aside.

4. Make the jelly filling: Place the raspberries, water, and sweetener in a small saucepan and bring to a simmer over medium heat. Simmer for 5 minutes, then sprinkle with the gelatin and mash with a fork. Transfer to the fridge to set for 15 minutes.

5. Pull the muffin cup liners and jelly filling out of the fridge. Using a ½-teaspoon measuring spoon, scoop out a portion of the jelly and roll it into a ball between your palms, then flatten it into a disc about 1 inch (2.5 cm) in diameter (or in a diameter to fit the size of the liners you're using). Press into a chilled butter base cup. Repeat with the remaining jelly filling and cups. Then spoon the remaining butter base mixture over the tops.

6. Place in the fridge for another 15 minutes before serving.

STORE IT: *Keep in the fridge for up to 5 days.*

Per serving, made with coconut butter and coconut oil:

calories: **151** | calories from fat: **136** | total fat: **15.1g** | saturated fat: **13.2g** | cholesterol: **0mg**
sodium: **4mg** | carbs: **2.9g** | dietary fiber: **1.9g** | net carbs: **1g** | sugars: **0.9g** | protein: **0.9g**

FAT:	CARBS:	PROTEIN:
90%	8%	2%

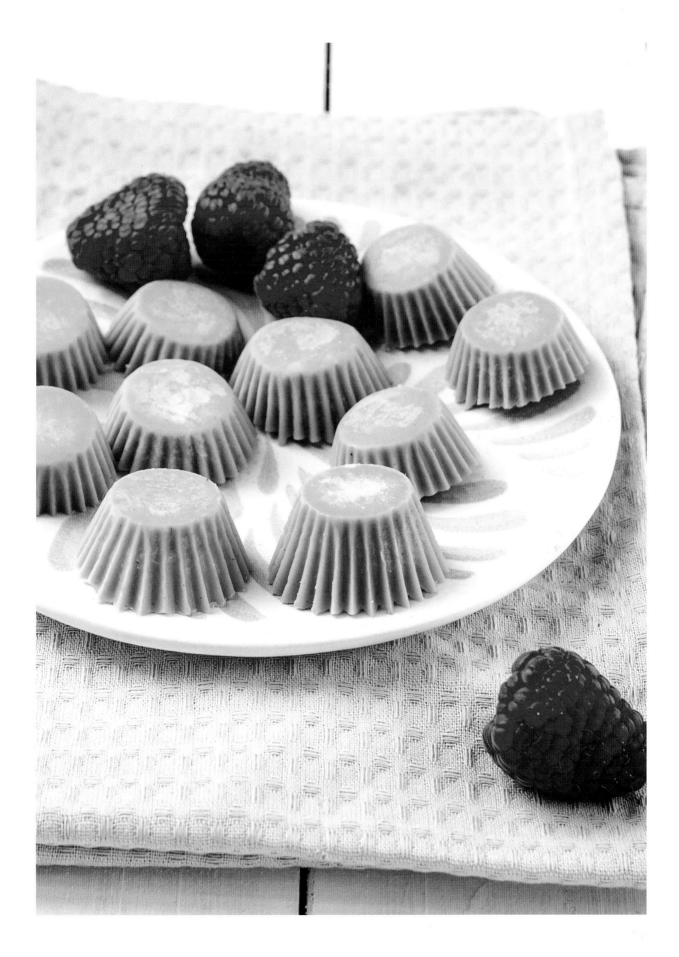

FUDGE BOMBS

EGG-FREE • LOW-FODMAP • NIGHTSHADE-FREE • VEGETARIAN
OPTIONS: COCONUT-FREE • DAIRY-FREE • NUT-FREE • VEGAN

MAKES 8 bombs (1 per serving)

PREP TIME: 5 minutes, plus 15 to 30 minutes to chill

COOK TIME: –

This recipe is another of my whip-it-up-quick fat bomb snacks, like the Cinnamon Bombs on page 314. If you want to get crazy, try topping each piece with a fresh raspberry. It's delicious!

½ cup (125 g) smooth unsweetened nut or seed butter

⅓ cup (75 g) melted coconut oil, cacao butter, or ghee

3 tablespoons cocoa powder

3 drops liquid stevia, or 3 teaspoons erythritol

SPECIAL EQUIPMENT (optional):

Silicone mold with eight 2-tablespoon or larger cavities

1. Have on hand your favorite silicone mold. I like to use a large silicone ice cube tray and spoon 2 tablespoons of the mixture into each cavity, which makes 8 cubes total. If you do not have a silicone mold, making this into a bark works well, too. Simply use an 8-inch (20-cm) square silicone or metal baking pan; if using a metal pan, line it with parchment paper, draping some over the sides for easy removal.

2. Place all the ingredients in a medium-sized bowl and stir until well mixed and smooth.

3. Divide the mixture evenly among 8 cavities of the mold or pour into the baking pan. Transfer to the fridge and allow to set for 15 minutes if using cacao butter or 30 minutes if using coconut oil or ghee. If using a baking pan, break the bark into 8 pieces for serving.

> **STORE IT:** *Keep in an airtight container in the fridge for up to 10 days or in the freezer for up to 2 months. Enjoy straight from the freezer, no thawing needed.*

make it COCONUT-FREE:
Use cacao butter or ghee.

make it DAIRY-FREE/VEGAN:
Do not use ghee.

make it NUT-FREE:
Use a seed butter.

Per serving, made with almond butter and coconut oil:

	FAT:	CARBS:	PROTEIN:
calories: **168**	calories from fat: **145**	total fat: **16.1g**	saturated fat: **4.1g**	cholesterol: **0mg**	**80%**	**10%**	**10%**
sodium: **0mg**	carbs: **4.8g**	dietary fiber: **3.1g**	net carbs: **1.7g**	sugars: **0.7g**	protein: **4.7g**			

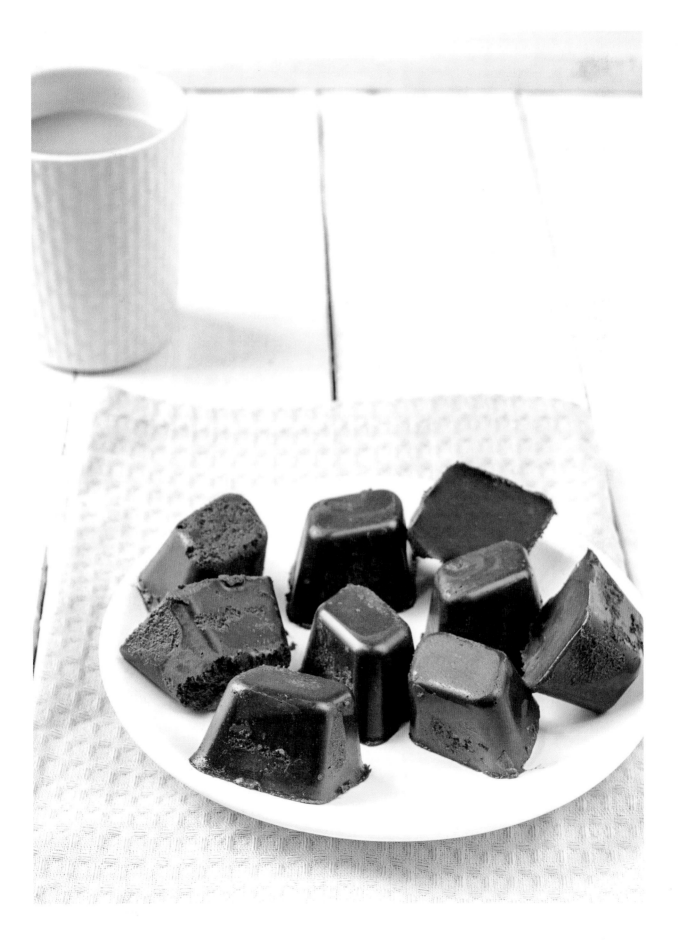

BROWNIE CAKE

NIGHTSHADE-FREE • VEGETARIAN
OPTIONS: COCONUT-FREE • DAIRY-FREE

SERVES 8

PREP TIME: 10 minutes, plus 30 minutes to cool

COOK TIME: 25 minutes

This is a perfect recipe for wowing your friends with keto, impressing family members when they come over for dinner, or just making for your little family on a Saturday movie night.

¾ cup (120 g) confectioners'-style erythritol, divided

½ cup plus 3 tablespoons (143 g) coconut oil, ghee, or cacao butter, melted, divided

2 large eggs

2 teaspoons vanilla extract

¾ cup (85 g) blanched almond flour

¼ cup plus 2 tablespoons (30 g) cocoa powder, divided

1 teaspoon baking powder

1. Preheat the oven to 350°F (177°C). Line an 8-inch (20-cm) round cake pan or square baking pan with parchment paper.

2. Combine ½ cup (95 g) of the erythritol, ½ cup (120 ml) of the melted oil, the eggs, and vanilla in a large mixing bowl.

3. In a separate bowl, place the almond flour, ¼ cup (20 g) of the cocoa powder, and the baking powder and whisk with a fork.

4. Add the dry mixture to the wet mixture and mix until smooth.

5. Transfer the batter to the lined pan and smooth with the back of a spoon. Bake for 23 to 25 minutes, until a toothpick inserted in the middle comes out clean. Allow to cool for 30 minutes.

6. Meanwhile, prepare the frosting: Place the remaining ¼ cup (25 g) of erythritol, 3 tablespoons of melted oil, and 2 tablespoons of cocoa powder in a small bowl. Whisk to combine.

7. If you're serving the cake right away, as soon as it's cool, cut into 8 equal pieces, place on plates, and drizzle with the frosting. If you're serving it later, cover the entire cake with the frosting while it's still in the pan and set in the fridge for at least 20 minutes before serving.

make it **COCONUT-FREE:**
Use ghee or cacao butter.

make it **DAIRY-FREE:**
Do not use ghee.

STORE IT: *Keep in an airtight container in the fridge for up to 5 days or in the freezer for up to 1 month.*

THAW IT: *Set on the counter for 20 to 30 minutes before serving.*

Per serving, made with coconut oil:

calories: **207**	calories from fat: **196**	total fat: **21.8g**	saturated fat: **17g**	cholesterol: **47mg**
sodium: **19mg**	carbs: **3.3g**	dietary fiber: **1.5g**	net carbs: **1.8g**	sugars: **0.4g**	protein: **2.9g**

FAT:	CARBS:	PROTEIN:
89%	**6%**	**5%**

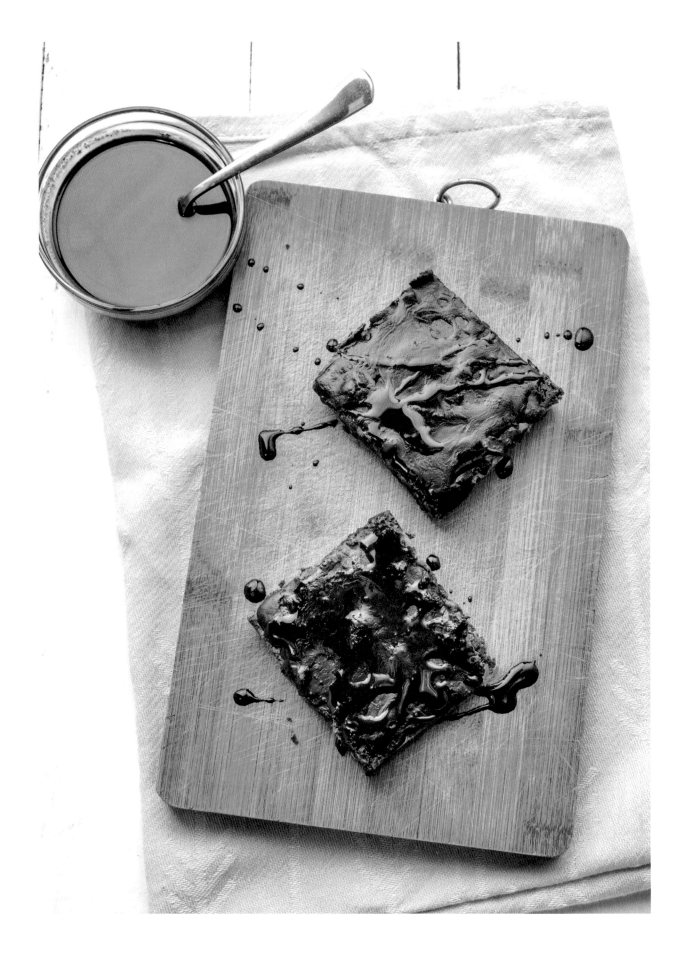

CINNAMON SUGAR MUFFINS

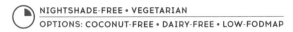
NIGHTSHADE-FREE • VEGETARIAN
OPTIONS: COCONUT-FREE • DAIRY-FREE • LOW-FODMAP

MAKES 12 muffins (1 per serving)

PREP TIME: 15 minutes

COOK TIME: 18 minutes

I use hulled hemp seeds in this recipe to boost the protein, but if you don't have hemp seeds around and don't feel like buying them, simply omit them, or replace them with ½ cup (80 g) of collagen peptides. Please note that this recipe is low-FODMAP because almond flour is safe in amounts of less than ¼ cup (55 g) per serving. Just be sure not to eat more than one muffin per day.

2 cups (220 g) blanched almond flour

⅔ cup (130 g) erythritol

1 tablespoon plus 1 teaspoon baking powder

1 tablespoon plus 1 teaspoon ground cinnamon

½ teaspoon finely ground sea salt

4 large eggs

½ cup (120 ml) milk (nondairy or regular)

½ cup (120 ml) melted coconut oil or ghee

2 teaspoons vanilla extract

⅔ cup (100 g) hulled hemp seeds

CINNAMON SUGAR TOPPING:

2 tablespoons melted coconut oil or ghee

¼ cup (45 g) granulated erythritol

2 teaspoons ground cinnamon

make it COCONUT-FREE:
Use ghee.

make it DAIRY-FREE:
Use a nondairy milk. Do not use ghee.

make it LOW-FODMAP:
Use almond, macadamia nut, or hemp milk.

1. Preheat the oven to 350°F (177°C). Line a standard-size 12-well muffin pan with muffin liners, or use a silicone muffin pan, which won't require liners.

2. Place the almond flour, erythritol, baking powder, cinnamon, and salt in a large bowl. Mix until combined.

3. In a small bowl, whisk the eggs, milk, melted oil, and vanilla. Add the egg mixture to the flour mixture and stir until fully combined. Fold in the hemp seeds.

4. Divide the batter evenly among the muffin wells, filling each about three-quarters full. Bake for 15 to 18 minutes, until the tops are golden. Remove from the oven and let cool in the pan.

5. Meanwhile, prepare the cinnamon sugar topping: Place the melted oil in a small dish, then place the erythritol and cinnamon in another small bowl and stir to combine.

6. Once the muffins are cool enough to handle, brush the top of a muffin with melted oil and then, holding it above the cinnamon sugar bowl, sprinkle with the cinnamon sugar. Gently shake off the excess and repeat with the remaining muffins.

STORE IT: *Store in an airtight container in the fridge for up to 1 week or in the freezer for up to 1 month.*

THAW IT: *Set on the counter to defrost completely before enjoying.*

Per muffin, made with almond milk and coconut oil:

| calories: **281** | calories from fat: **233** | total fat: **25.9g** | saturated fat: **12g** | cholesterol: **62mg** |
| sodium: **110mg** | carbs: **7g** | dietary fiber: **3.2g** | net carbs: **3.8g** | sugars: **0g** | protein: **5g** |

FAT:	CARBS:	PROTEIN:
83%	10%	7%

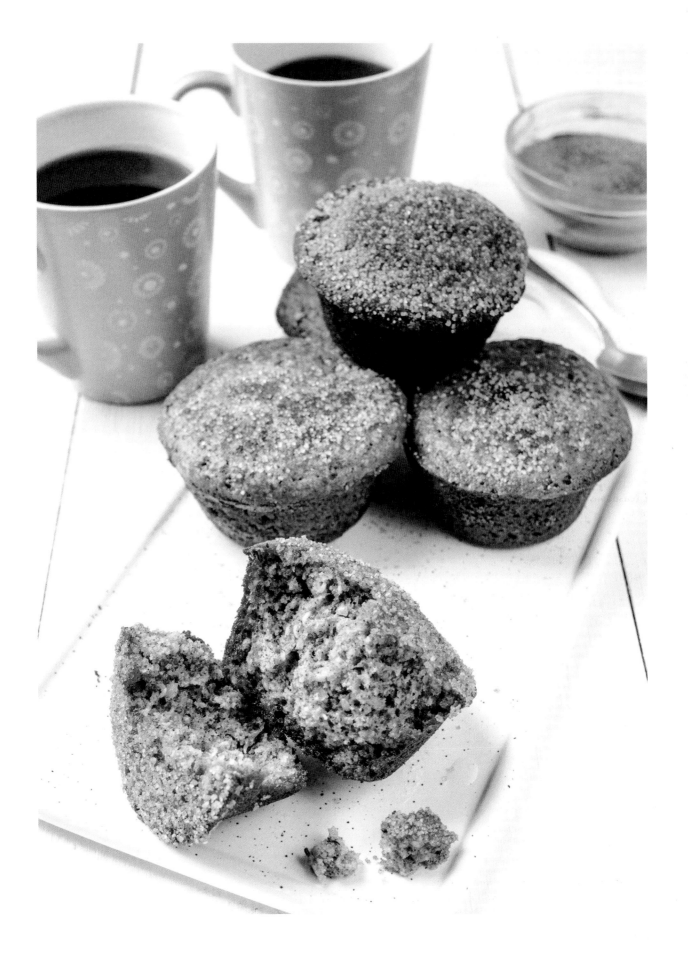

EDANA'S MACADAMIA CRACK BARS

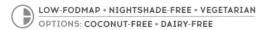
LOW-FODMAP • NIGHTSHADE-FREE • VEGETARIAN
OPTIONS: COCONUT-FREE • DAIRY-FREE

MAKES 12 bars (1 per serving)

PREP TIME: 15 minutes, plus 2 hours to cool/chill

COOK TIME: 35 minutes

We decided to sail the Gulf Stream at night before a gnarly weather system made it most uncomfortable to cross. It was our first Gulf Stream crossing at night, so snacks were essential in order to stay awake. Our training captain, Edana, was sitting at the helm when I asked if she wanted a piece of my macadamia bar. She broke off a piece, and her reaction was priceless. Her face lit up with joy, and she said quite loudly, "WHOA! This is SO good. What? Oh my, yes. Whoa, so good. What is this? How? How did you make this?"

This one's for you, Edana!

BASE:

1¼ cups (140 g) blanched almond flour

⅓ cup (65 g) erythritol

⅓ cup (70 g) coconut oil, ghee, or cacao butter, melted

1 teaspoon vanilla extract

¼ teaspoon finely ground sea salt

COCONUT CREAM LAYER:

½ cup (95 g) erythritol

½ cup (125 g) coconut cream

¼ cup (55 g) coconut oil, ghee, or cacao butter, melted

2 large egg yolks

1 teaspoon vanilla extract

TOPPINGS:

1 cup (160 g) raw macadamia nuts, roughly chopped

1 cup (100 g) unsweetened shredded coconut

1. Preheat the oven to 350°F (177°C). Line an 8-inch (20-cm) square baking pan with parchment paper, draping it over two opposite sides of the pan for easy lifting.

2. Place the base ingredients in a large mixing bowl and stir to combine. Press into the prepared pan and par-bake for 10 to 12 minutes, until the top is only lightly browned. Remove from the oven and lower the oven temperature to 300°F (150°C).

3. Meanwhile, make the coconut cream layer: Place the erythritol, coconut cream, melted oil, egg yolks, and vanilla in a large mixing bowl. Whisk until smooth.

4. Pour the coconut cream mixture over the par-baked base. Top with the macadamia nuts, then the shredded coconut.

5. Return the pan to the oven and bake for 25 minutes, or until the edges are lightly browned.

6. Let cool in the pan on the counter for 1 hour before transferring to the fridge to chill for another hour. Once chilled, cut into 2-inch (5-cm) squares.

make it COCONUT-FREE:
Do not use coconut oil. Use heavy cream instead of coconut cream (if you can tolerate dairy). Omit the shredded coconut topping.

make it DAIRY-FREE:
Do not use ghee.

STORE IT: *Keep in an airtight container in the fridge for up to 5 days or in the freezer for up to 1 month. Can be eaten directly from the freezer.*

Per bar, made with coconut oil:

calories: **303**	calories from fat: **276**	total fat: **30.7g**	saturated fat: **14.8g**	cholesterol: **35mg**
sodium: **44mg**	carbs: **5.6g**	dietary fiber: **3.2g**	net carbs: **2.4g**	sugars: **1.9g**	protein: **2g**

FAT:	CARBS:	PROTEIN:
90%	**7%**	**3%**

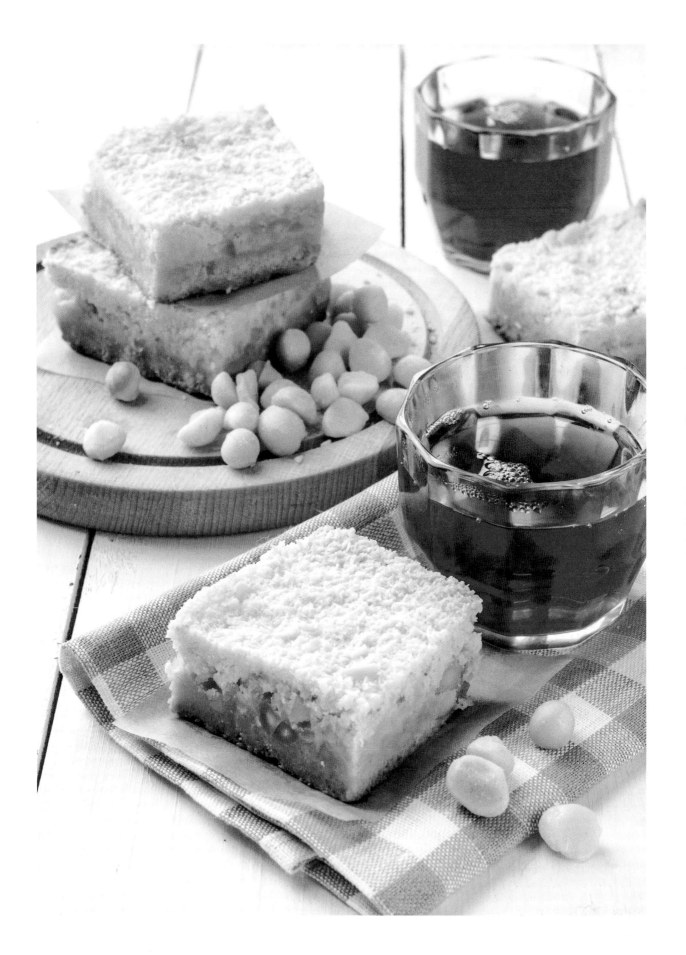

N'OATMEAL BARS

DAIRY-FREE • EGG-FREE • LOW-FODMAP • NIGHTSHADE-FREE • NUT-FREE • VEGAN • VEGETARIAN

MAKES 16 bars (1 per serving)

PREP TIME: 25 minutes, plus 3 hours to chill

COOK TIME: –

Gone are the days when you mourned the loss of oats on your ketogenic diet. After making this recipe, you'll realize just how versatile hulled hemp seeds (aka hemp hearts) are, and you'll swap out oats for hemp seeds in all your favorite recipes! Hemp seeds have gained in popularity over the years; however, not all shops or countries will carry them. If you're in one of those places, you can easily replace them with coarsely ground hulled sunflower seeds. The key is, when you grind the sunflower seeds, to pulse them only once or twice. They need to be broken up just a little, not a lot.

These bars are so good that I sometimes cut them larger, as shown, for a heartier snack.

1 cup (180 g) coconut oil

½ cup (95 g) erythritol, divided

2 cups (300 g) hulled hemp seeds

½ cup (50 g) unsweetened shredded coconut

⅓ cup (33 g) coconut flour

½ teaspoon vanilla extract

10 ounces (285 g) unsweetened baking chocolate, roughly chopped

½ cup (120 ml) full-fat coconut milk

1. Line a 9-inch (23-cm) square baking pan with parchment paper, draping it over all sides of the pan for easy lifting.

2. Place the coconut oil and half of the erythritol in a medium-sized saucepan and melt over medium heat, about 2 minutes. Continue to Step 3 if using confectioners'-style erythritol; if using granulated erythritol, continue to cook until the granules can no longer be felt on the back of the spoon.

3. Add the hulled hemp seeds, shredded coconut, coconut flour, and vanilla, stirring until coated. Set aside half of the mixture for the topping. Press the remaining half of the mixture into the prepared pan.

4. Transfer the pan with the base layer to the refrigerator for at least 10 minutes, until set.

5. Meanwhile, prepare the chocolate layer: Place the remaining erythritol, the baking chocolate, and coconut milk in a small saucepan over low heat. Stir frequently until melted and smooth.

6. Take the base out of the fridge and spoon the chocolate mixture over the base layer, spreading it evenly with a knife or the back of a spoon. If the base hasn't totally set, a couple of hulled hemp seeds will lift up and mix in with the chocolate, so don't rush it.

7. Crumble the reserved hemp seed mixture over the chocolate layer, pressing in gently. Cover and refrigerate for 2 to 3 hours or overnight.

8. Cut into 16 bars and enjoy!

STORE IT: *Store in an airtight container in the fridge for up to 5 days or in the freezer for up to 1 month.*

THAW IT: *Set the bars on the counter for 10 to 15 minutes before enjoying.*

Per bar:

calories: **311** | calories from fat: **267** | total fat: **29.7g** | saturated fat: **18.5g** | cholesterol: **0mg** | sodium: **16mg** | carbs: **9.5g** | dietary fiber: **5.2g** | net carbs: **4.3g** | sugars: **1.3g** | protein: **7.9g**

FAT:	CARBS:	PROTEIN:
80%	**11%**	**9%**

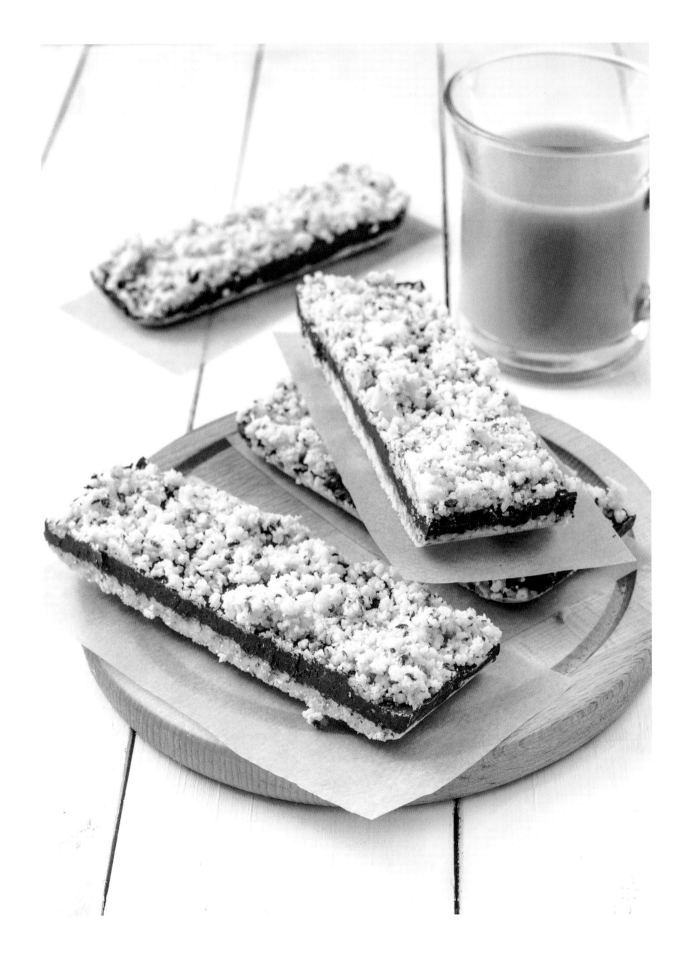

BLUEBERRY CRUMBLE WITH CREAM TOPPING

EGG-FREE · NIGHTSHADE-FREE · VEGETARIAN
OPTIONS: DAIRY-FREE · VEGAN

SERVES 6

PREP TIME: 5 minutes

COOK TIME: 25 minutes

As summer transitions into fall, blueberries go on sale, and we just can't eat them fast enough! That was until I realized I could freeze them right in the clamshell and then vacuum-seal pounds and pounds of frozen blueberries for use during the winter months. I'm still carting around blueberries from last fall! If you practice this tactic (and you will, now that you know), you'll make good use of this recipe.

18 ounces (510 g) fresh or frozen blueberries

1 cup (110 g) blanched almond flour

⅓ cup (70 g) coconut oil or ghee, room temperature

⅓ cup (65 g) erythritol

2 tablespoons coconut flour

1 teaspoon ground cinnamon

1 cup (250 g) coconut cream, or 1 cup (240 ml) full-fat coconut milk, for serving

make it **DAIRY-FREE/VEGAN:**
Do not use ghee.

1. Preheat the oven to 350°F (177°C).

2. Place the blueberries in an 8-inch (20-cm) square baking pan.

3. Place the almond flour, oil, erythritol, coconut flour, and cinnamon in a medium-sized bowl and mix with a fork until crumbly. Crumble over the top of the blueberries.

4. Bake for 22 to 25 minutes, until the top is golden.

5. Remove from the oven and let sit for 10 minutes before dividing among 6 serving bowls. Top each bowl with 2 to 3 tablespoons of coconut cream.

STORE IT: *Keep in an airtight container in the fridge for up to 3 days or in the freezer for up to 1 month. If freezing, freeze the blueberry crumble without the coconut cream topping.*

REHEAT IT: *Transfer a single serving to a microwave-safe bowl, cover, and microwave for 1 minute.*

THAW IT: *Set on the counter for 30 minutes before following the reheating instructions above.*

Per serving, made with coconut oil and topped with coconut cream:

calories: **388** | calories from fat: **300** | total fat: **33.4g** | saturated fat: **16.5g** | cholesterol: **0mg**
sodium: **1mg** | carbs: **17g** | dietary fiber: **4.3g** | net carbs: **12.7g** | sugars: **9.1g** | protein: **4.9g**

FAT:	CARBS:	PROTEIN:
77%	18%	5%

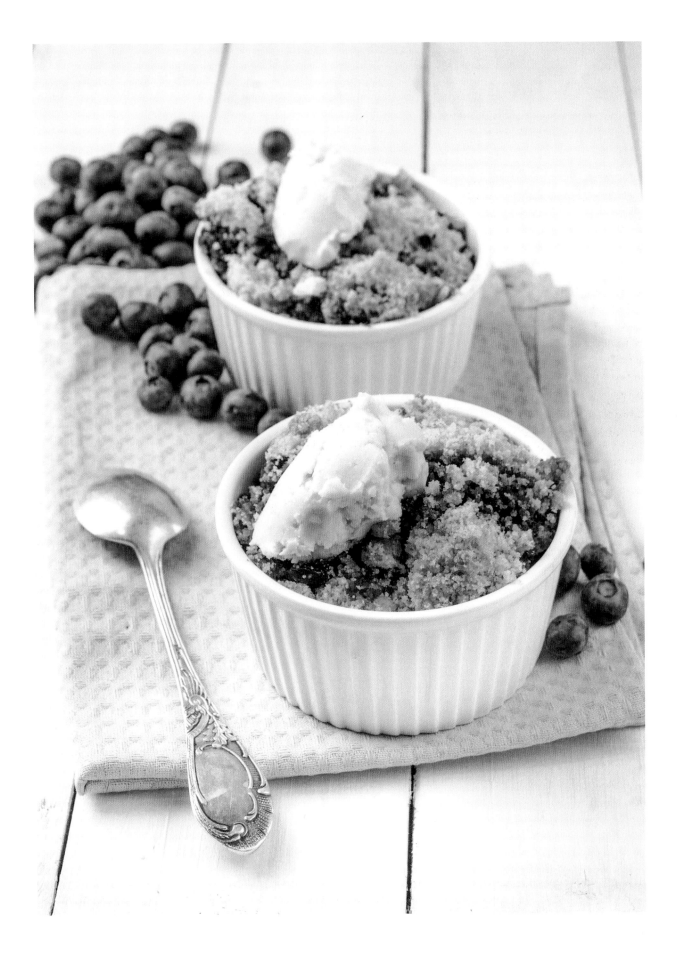

CHOCOLATE SOFT-SERVE ICE CREAM

DAIRY-FREE • EGG-FREE • NIGHTSHADE-FREE
OPTIONS: **AIP • NUT-FREE • VEGAN • VEGETARIAN**

SERVES 4

PREP TIME: 10 minutes, plus 30 to 45 minutes to freeze

COOK TIME: —

I love ice cream, and I really enjoy making it, but with such a small kitchen, I decided to donate my ice cream maker. Gasp! If you don't have an ice cream maker, either, this is the best way to make ice cream. The most crucial part of the process is separating the ice cream mixture into small serving bowls, setting them in the freezer, and checking on them often to mash up the mixture with a fork. The resulting ice cream will have the consistency of soft-serve, close to that of Wendy's famous Frosty. DO NOT let the mixture get too frozen. You're not making ice cubes here! Just keep mashing and returning the bowls to the freezer; two rounds is usually enough. You'll think it's not soft-serve consistency when you first take it out of the freezer, but as you start mashing, it'll take form.

The only downside to this recipe is that it can't be stored, as it would freeze solid and be impossible to get back to the correct consistency. As soon as you make it, you have to eat it. Shoot, I'm telling you to eat all the ice cream in one go. Whatever will you do?!

If you want to pump up the fat in your bowl of ice cream, make a batch of Chocolate Sauce (page 96) and drizzle it over the top.

1 (13½-oz/400-ml) can full-fat coconut milk

¼ cup (40 g) collagen peptides or protein powder (optional)

¼ cup (25 g) unflavored MCT oil powder (optional)

2 tablespoons smooth unsweetened almond butter

2 tablespoons cocoa powder

3 drops liquid stevia, or 1 tablespoon erythritol

1 teaspoon vanilla extract

1. Place all the ingredients in a blender or food processor. Blend until smooth and fully incorporated.

2. Divide the mixture among 4 freezer-safe serving bowls and place in the freezer for 30 minutes. At the 30-minute mark, remove from the freezer and mash with a fork until the ice cream is smooth. If it's still too runny and doesn't develop the consistency of soft-serve as you mash it, freeze for another 15 minutes, then mash with a fork again.

3. Enjoy immediately.

make it AIP:
Replace the cocoa powder with carob powder. Use stevia or enjoy unsweetened.

make it NUT-FREE:
Replace the almond butter with sunflower seed butter.

make it VEGAN/VEGETARIAN:
Omit the collagen.

Per serving, without collagen/protein powder or MCT oil powder:

						FAT:	CARBS:	PROTEIN:
calories: **478**	calories from fat: **419**	total fat: **46.6g**	saturated fat: **33.8g**	cholesterol: **0mg**		**88%**	**7%**	**5%**
sodium: **13mg**	carbs: **9g**	dietary fiber: **4.6g**	net carbs: **4.4g**	sugars: **3.4g**	protein: **5.8g**			

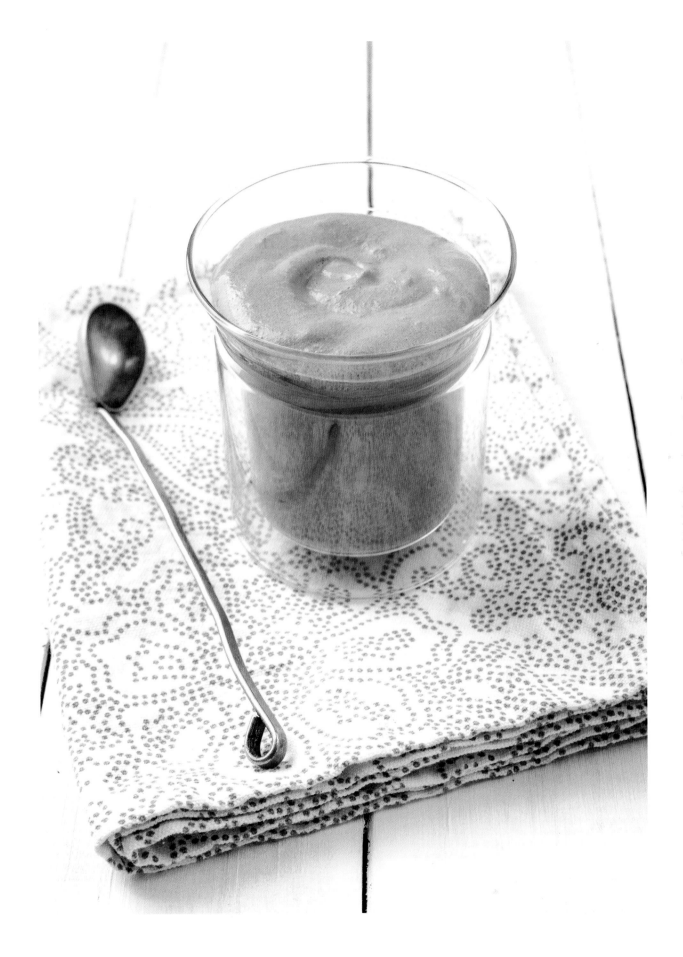

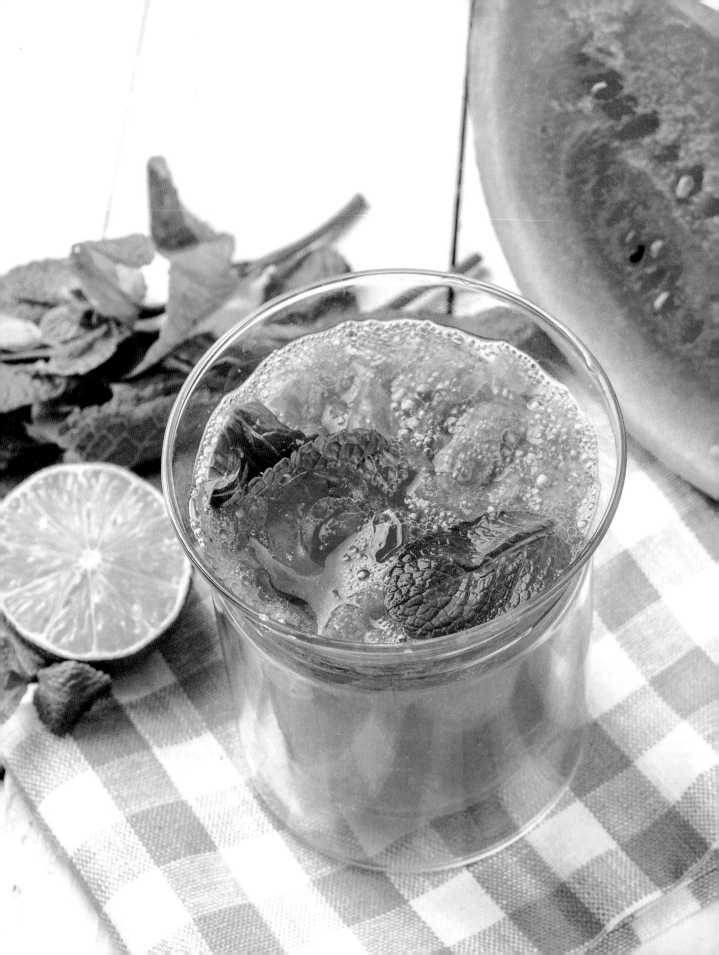

10.

EXTRA SIPS

KETO ARNOLD PALMER

COCONUT-FREE • DAIRY-FREE • EGG-FREE • LOW-FODMAP • NIGHTSHADE-FREE • NUT-FREE • VEGAN • VEGETARIAN
OPTION: AIP

MAKES two 17-ounce (500-ml) servings

PREP TIME: 10 minutes (not including time to brew tea)

COOK TIME: –

I could drink this by the gallon, and I have on multiple occasions. A common way to boost your electrolytes on keto is to drink keto lemonade, which is a mixture of water, fresh lemon juice, Himalayan salt, and a keto-friendly sweetener. But, after years on keto, the daily grind of lemonade gets a little old. Let's spice things up and swap out the plain water for tea! You can use any sort of tea here. I chose a decaffeinated black tea, but you could use rooibos, green, white, or whatever you like.

If you're in need of digestive healing, add 4 teaspoons of aloe vera; it works nicely in this recipe.

4 cups (950 ml) brewed black tea (decaf or regular), chilled

¼ cup (60 ml) lemon juice

2 teaspoons erythritol, or 6 drops liquid stevia

½ teaspoon finely ground Himalayan salt

Place all the ingredients in a large jug or pitcher that holds at least 34 ounces (1 L). Mix with a large spoon.

make it AIP:
Use stevia or enjoy unsweetened.

STORE IT: *Store covered in the fridge for up to 5 days.*

Per serving:

calories: **6** | calories from fat: **1.8** | total fat: **0.2g** | saturated fat: **0.2g** | cholesterol: **0mg**
sodium: **376mg** | carbs: **0.7g** | dietary fiber: **0.1g** | net carbs: **0.6g** | sugars: **0.6g** | protein: **0.2g**

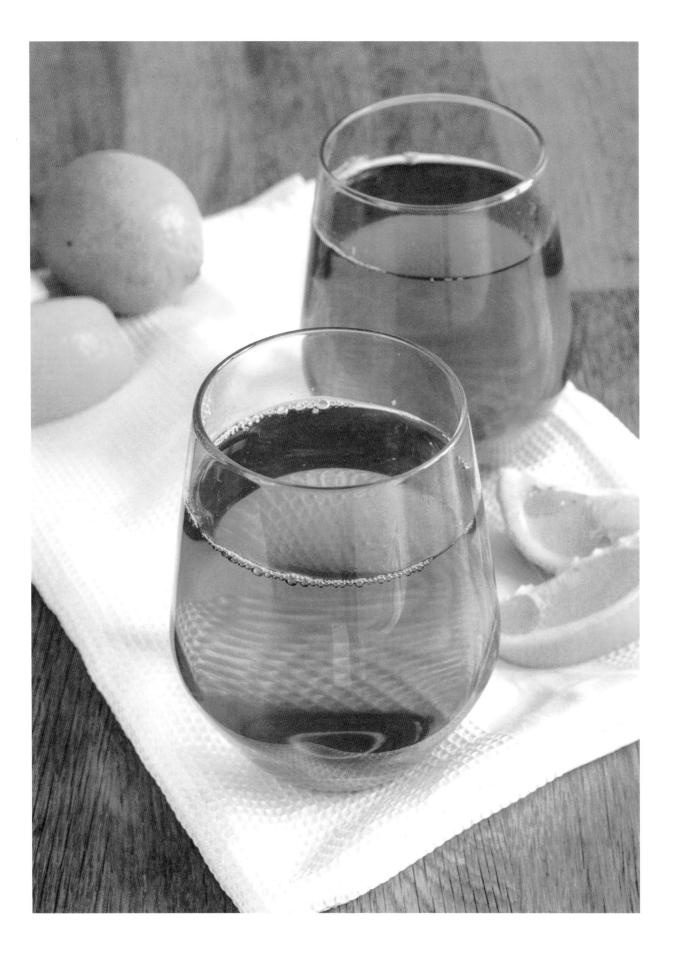

TURMERIC KETO LEMONADE

COCONUT-FREE • DAIRY-FREE • EGG-FREE • LOW-FODMAP • NIGHTSHADE-FREE • NUT-FREE • VEGAN • VEGETARIAN
OPTION: AIP

MAKES two 12-ounce (350-ml) servings

PREP TIME: 5 minutes, plus time to cool and chill

COOK TIME: 5 minutes

Electrolytes! Ensuring that you have enough electrolytes in your keto diet is a key to success. Also, your body odor won't stink, your legs won't twitch, and you won't get headaches—all great things to avoid. Not only is this lemonade packed with electrolytes, but it also includes healing roots like ginger and turmeric. I've used the powdered versions here, but if you have access to fresh ginger and turmeric, replace the powders with 2 teaspoons each of the fresh stuff—minced or grated.

Boiling helps activate the compounds in the ginger and turmeric; however, if you want to skip the boiling step, simply put all the ingredients in a 1-quart (950-ml) jar, shake, refrigerate until chilled, and enjoy! I like to keep batches of this lemonade in the fridge for when I get thirsty.

2½ cups (590 ml) water

1 teaspoon ginger powder

1 teaspoon turmeric powder

¼ cup (60 ml) lemon juice

2 teaspoons aloe vera (optional)

2 teaspoons erythritol, or 2 drops liquid stevia (optional)

¼ teaspoon finely ground Himalayan salt

Pinch of ground black pepper

6 fresh mint leaves

1 small lemon, cut into wedges

1. Place the water, ginger, and turmeric in a medium-sized saucepan and bring to a boil. Once boiling, remove from the heat, then add the lemon juice, aloe vera (if using), sweetener (if using), salt, and pepper. Stir with a spoon and allow to cool completely, about 1 hour.

2. Transfer the mixture to a 24-ounce (710-ml) or larger airtight container. Add the mint leaves, then squeeze in the lemon juice and drop the wedges into the lemonade. Refrigerate until cold. If you don't care for the grittiness of the herbs in this drink, you can strain them out with a fine-mesh strainer or cheesecloth before serving.

3. When ready to enjoy, divide between two 12-ounce (350-ml) or larger glasses.

make it AIP:
Use stevia or enjoy unsweetened. Omit the black pepper.

STORE IT: *Store in an airtight container in the fridge; it will keep for up to 2 days if stored with the mint leaves or up to 4 days without the mint leaves.*

Per serving, without aloe vera:

calories: **13** | calories from fat: **4** | total fat: **0.4g** | saturated fat: **0.3g** | cholesterol: **0mg**
sodium: **204mg** | carbs: **2g** | dietary fiber: **0.5g** | net carbs: **1.5g** | sugars: **0.7g** | protein: **0.4g**

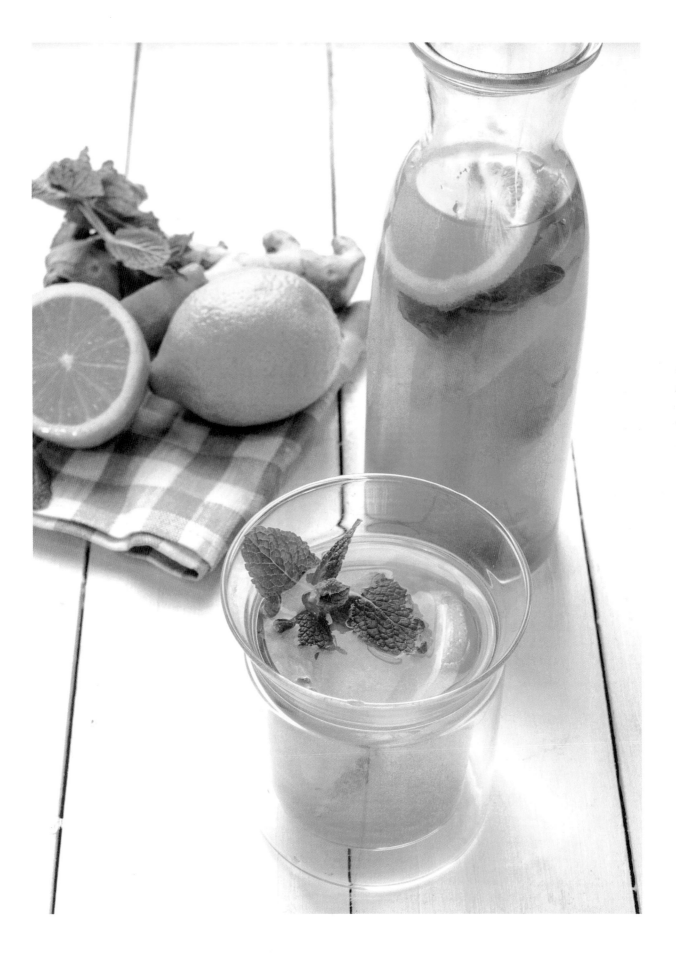

EGG CREAM

EGG-FREE • LOW-FODMAP • NIGHTSHADE-FREE • VEGETARIAN
OPTIONS: COCONUT-FREE • DAIRY-FREE • NUT-FREE • VEGAN

MAKES one 14-ounce (415-ml) serving

PREP TIME: 1 minute

COOK TIME: –

During a TV binge session of Billions, *I heard one of the main characters, Chuck Rhoades, mention an egg cream drink that has no egg and no cream, and it enticed me. So, I did a quick search and found a recipe laden with sugar. Here's my take on a low-carb egg cream…maybe Chuck would approve?*

3 tablespoons milk (nondairy or regular)

2 teaspoons cocoa powder

½ teaspoon erythritol, or 2 drops liquid stevia

12 ounces (355 ml) sparkling water, chilled

1. Place the milk, cocoa powder, and sweetener in a 16-ounce (475-ml) or larger glass. Whisk the ingredients with a fork until fully incorporated.

2. Slowly pour in the sparkling water. If you fill the glass too fast, everything will bubble over, so take your time. Best enjoyed immediately.

make it **COCONUT-FREE:**
Use a nut milk.

make it **DAIRY-FREE/VEGAN:**
Use a nondairy milk.

make it **NUT-FREE:**
Use coconut milk or dairy milk.

Per serving, made with lite coconut milk:

calories: **22** | calories from fat: **10** | total fat: **1.1g** | saturated fat: **0.9g** | cholesterol: **0mg**
sodium: **1mg** | carbs: **2.1g** | dietary fiber: **1.2g** | net carbs: **0.9g** | sugars: **0g** | protein: **0.9g**

FAT:	CARBS:	PROTEIN:
45%	**38%**	**17%**

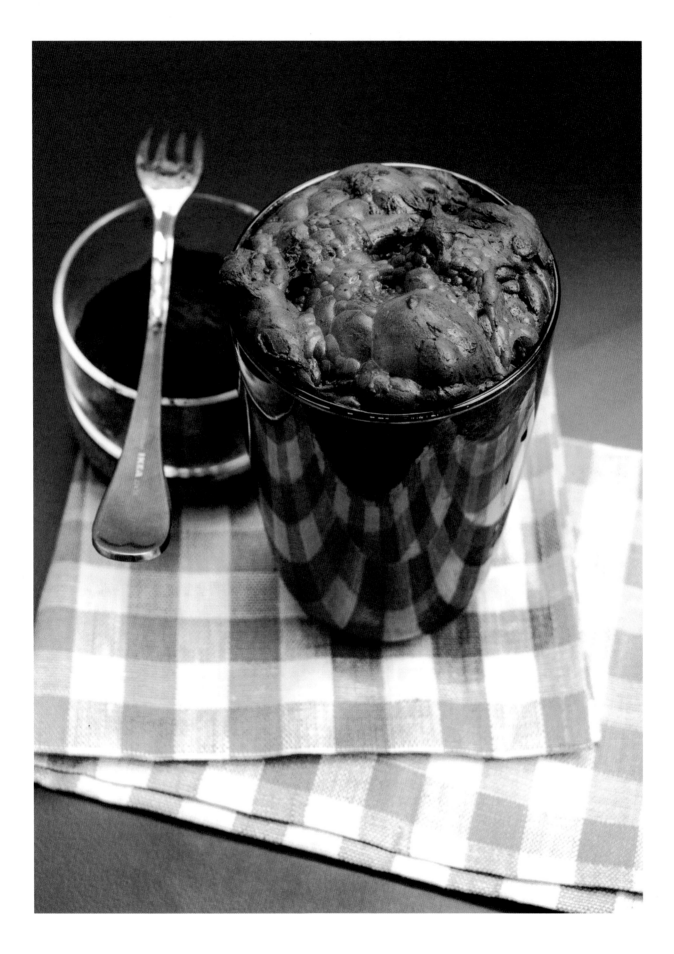

CASHEW MILK

COCONUT-FREE • DAIRY-FREE • EGG-FREE • NIGHTSHADE-FREE • VEGAN • VEGETARIAN

MAKES 1 quart (950 ml) (4 servings)

PREP TIME: 5 minutes, plus 12 hours to soak cashews

COOK TIME: –

You don't have to make your own nondairy milk, but if you're trying to be economical with your approach to a ketogenic diet and you're looking to be a touch more plant-based, preparing your own cashew milk is a fabulous idea. Cashew milk is ultra-creamy, perfect for coffees, smoothies, shakes, and curries. It'll keep in the fridge for up to four days but can be frozen if you find that you just can't get through a whole batch in that time.

About the optional add-ins: If you are only going to drink this milk, add the MCT oil powder and vanilla; it tastes great with both! If you will be using the milk for cooking, omit the MCT oil powder and vanilla to make a neutral-flavored milk that can handle high heat. (Adding MCT oil powder to milk limits its cooking applications; MCT oil, from which the powder is derived, has a moderate smoke point.)

1 cup (130 g) raw cashews

4 cups (950 ml) water

⅛ teaspoon finely ground Himalayan salt

¼ cup (25 g) unflavored MCT oil powder (optional)

1½ teaspoons vanilla extract (optional)

1. Place the cashews in a 12-ounce (350-ml) or larger sealable container. Cover with water. Seal and place in the fridge for 12 hours.

2. After 12 hours, strain and rinse the nuts, then place in a blender or food processor along with the 4 cups (950 ml) of fresh water and the salt. Blend or pulse on high for 1 to 2 minutes, until the cashews are completely pulverized. If you used a high-powered blender, skip to Step 4.

3. To strain the milk, set a fine-mesh strainer in or drape a piece of cheesecloth over a bowl that holds at least 48 ounces (1.4 L). Slowly pour the cashew mixture through the strainer or cheesecloth, allowing the milk to drip into the bowl. If you're using a strainer, press on the pulverized nuts with a spoon to release the excess liquid. If using cheesecloth, pick up the sides of the cloth and wring out the excess liquid.

4. If you do not wish to include the optional add-ins, skip to Step 5. If using the optional add-ins, pour the strained milk back into the blender or food processor, then add the MCT oil powder and/ or vanilla and blend or pulse on low for 10 seconds, just until incorporated.

5. Transfer the milk to a 1-quart (950-ml) or larger airtight container.

> **STORE IT:** *Keep in the fridge for up to 4 days or in the freezer for up to 1 month.*
>
> **THAW IT:** *Remove from the freezer and allow to thaw on the counter until at least 50% defrosted, then place in the fridge until ready to use.*

Per 1-cup/240-ml serving, without MCT oil powder:

calories: **23** | calories from fat: **16** | total fat: **1.7g** | saturated fat: **0g** | cholesterol: **0mg**
sodium: **160mg** | carbs: **1.3g** | dietary fiber: **0g** | net carbs: **1.3g** | sugars: **1g** | protein: **0.7g**

FAT:	CARBS:	PROTEIN:
66%	**22%**	**12%**

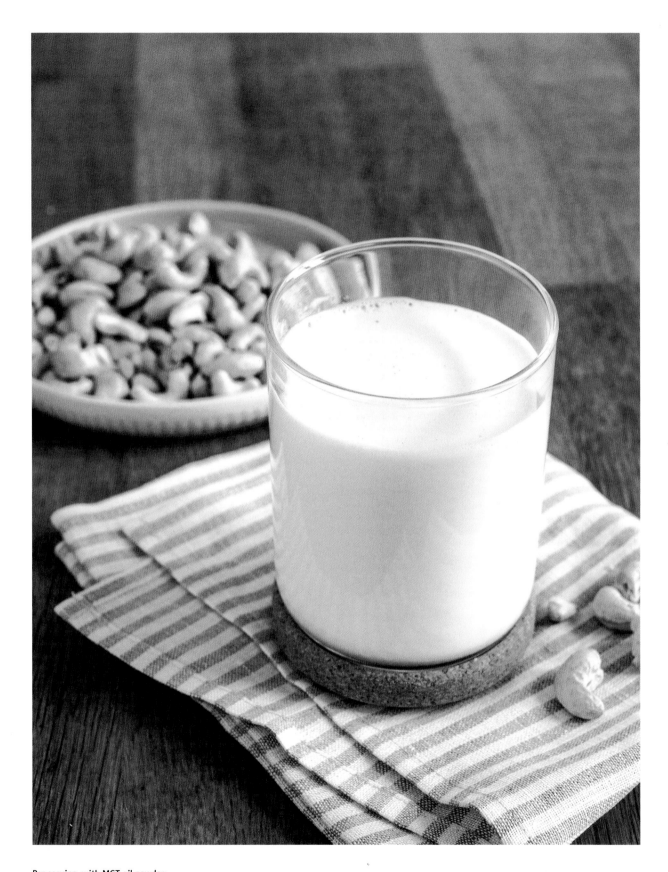

Per serving, with MCT oil powder:

| calories: **42** | calories from fat: **31** | total fat: **3.5g** | saturated fat: **1.8g** | cholesterol: **0mg** |
| sodium: **160mg** | carbs: **1.8g** | dietary fiber: **0.5g** | net carbs: **1.3g** | sugars: **1g** | protein: **0.9g** |

| FAT: | CARBS: | PROTEIN: |
| **75%** | **17%** | **8%** |

COCONUT MILK

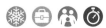

 AIP • DAIRY-FREE • EGG-FREE • NIGHTSHADE-FREE • NUT-FREE • VEGAN • VEGETARIAN

**MAKES 1 quart (950 ml)
(4 servings)**

PREP TIME: 5 minutes

COOK TIME: –

Sometimes a grocery store has a sale on fresh coconuts where you can purchase four coconuts for the price of 1 quart (950 ml) of store-bought coconut milk. Watch for that type of deal and buy as many fresh coconuts as you can! What do you do with all those coconuts? I remove the meat and freeze it for later use, or I make a couple of batches of milk and freeze the milk. Reserve the coconut water for smoothies or replace some of the plain water in the recipes in this chapter with coconut water.

If purchasing a fresh coconut has you concerned about how to open it, many grocery stores offer fresh coconut flesh already cut up and ready to go. Or just follow the directions in the how-to sidebar, opposite.

See "About the optional add-ins" in the Cashew Milk recipe on page 342 for milk-making strategies regarding the optional add-ins.

10 ounces (285 g) fresh coconut flesh (from 1 whole coconut, about 1¾ pounds/800 g)

4 cups (950 ml) water

¼ cup (25 g) unflavored MCT oil powder (optional)

1½ teaspoons vanilla extract (optional)

1. Place the coconut and water in a blender or food processor. Blend or pulse on high for 1 to 2 minutes, until the coconut pieces are completely pulverized.

2. To strain the milk, set a fine-mesh strainer in or drape a piece of cheesecloth over a bowl that holds at least 48 ounces (1.4 L). Slowly pour the coconut mixture through the strainer or cheesecloth, allowing the milk to drip into the bowl. If you're using a strainer, press on the pulverized coconut flesh with a spoon to release the excess liquid. If you're using cheesecloth, pick up the sides of the cloth and wring out the excess liquid.

3. If you do not wish to include the optional add-ins, skip to Step 4. If using the optional add-ins, pour the strained coconut milk back into the blender or food processor, then add the MCT oil powder and/or vanilla and blend or pulse on low for 10 seconds, just until incorporated.

4. Transfer the milk to a 1-quart (950-ml) airtight container.

> **STORE IT:** *Keep in the fridge for up to 4 days or in the freezer for up to 1 month.*
>
> **THAW IT:** *Remove from the freezer and allow to thaw on the counter until at least 50% defrosted, then place in the fridge until ready to use.*

Per 1-cup/240-ml serving, without MCT oil powder:

calories: **46**	calories from fat: **40**	total fat: **4.5g**	saturated fat: **4g**	cholesterol: **0mg**
sodium: **23mg**	carbs: **1.2g**	dietary fiber: **0g**	net carbs: **1.2g**	sugars: **0.4g**	protein: **0.2g**

FAT:	CARBS:	PROTEIN:
88%	**10%**	**2%**

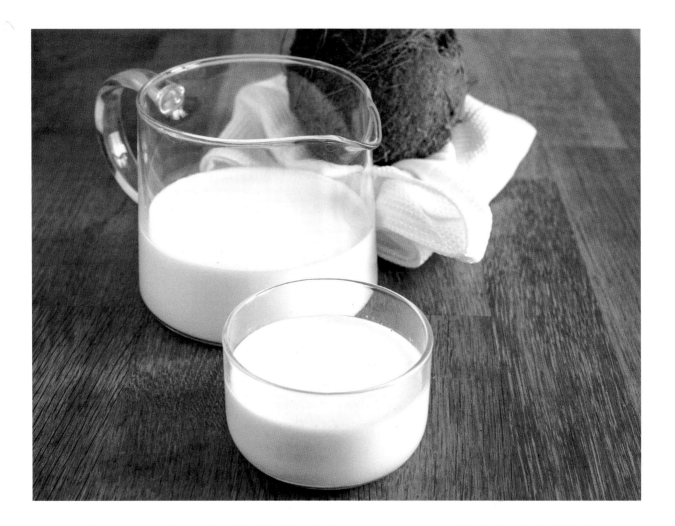

HOW TO REMOVE THE FLESH FROM A COCONUT

There are three holes at the top of a coconut, and one hole will be weaker than the other two. Poke each one with the tip of a sharp knife. When the knife slides easily into a hole, you've found the weakest link! Pierce the coconut hole with your knife.

Flip the coconut over onto a cup or bowl and allow it to drain. Reserve the coconut water for later use. (I recommend that you whip up a batch of electrolyte-filled lemonade using 1 cup (240 ml) coconut water, 1 cup (240 ml) filtered water, ¼ cup (60 ml) lemon juice, ¼ teaspoon finely ground Himalayan salt, and a drop of liquid stevia.)

Preheat the oven to 375°F (190°C). Place the drained coconut on a baking sheet. Bake for 10 minutes, or until you see a crack develop either from the hole or on the side. Remove the coconut from the oven and allow it to cool for a couple of minutes. Then wrap it in a tea towel and throw it into a clean, sturdy garbage bag. (The black ones meant for yard work are perfect.)

Now it's time to smash the life out of your coconut: Go outside to your front steps or a concrete area. Lift the coconut over your head and bash it into the concrete. Do this a couple of times until you feel the pieces break, or until you feel your stress wash away. It's a therapeutic experience. If there are observers, open the bag to reveal the coconut pieces before you go back inside. This will prevent awkward conversations with the neighbors later.

Separate the shell from your dear coconut: Wedge a knife in between the flesh and the hard shell to separate the shell from the meat. You'll be left with white meat covered in a light brown fiber. Peel away the fiber with a vegetable peeler, as you would the skin of a potato. You've now successfully opened your coconut.

Per serving, with MCT oil powder:

| calories: **63** | calories from fat: **55** | total fat: **6.3g** | saturated fat: **5.8g** | cholesterol: **0mg** | FAT: | CARBS: | PROTEIN: |
| sodium: **23mg** | carbs: **1.7g** | dietary fiber: **0.5g** | net carbs: **1.2g** | sugars: **0.4g** | protein: **0.4g** | **90%** | **7%** | **3%** |

MACADAMIA NUT MILK

COCONUT-FREE • DAIRY-FREE • EGG-FREE • LOW-FODMAP • NIGHTSHADE-FREE • VEGAN • VEGETARIAN

MAKES 1 quart (950 ml) (4 servings)

PREP TIME: 5 minutes, plus 12 hours to soak nuts

COOK TIME: –

It's so important to use raw nuts for this recipe (and any nut milk recipe). Please don't think that the roasted, salted ones will make good milk. I've made this mistake before and cried over the loss of all those nuts.

If you want a thicker milk, just cut out a bit of the water. If I'm planning on using this milk for coffees, I remove 1 cup (240 ml) of the water to make it thicker. Then each serving is ¾ cup (180 ml) rather than 1 cup (240 ml).

See "About the optional add-ins" in the Cashew Milk recipe on page 342 for milk-making strategies regarding the optional add-ins.

1 cup (160 g) raw macadamia nuts

4 cups (950 ml) water

⅛ teaspoon finely ground Himalayan salt

¼ cup (25 g) unflavored MCT oil powder (optional)

1½ teaspoons vanilla extract (optional)

1. Place the macadamia nuts in a 12-ounce (350-ml) or larger sealable container. Cover with water. Seal and place in the fridge for 12 hours.

2. After 12 hours, strain and rinse the nuts, then place in a blender or food processor along with the 4 cups (950 ml) of fresh water and the salt. Blend or pulse on high for 1 to 2 minutes, until all the nuts are completely pulverized.

3. To strain the milk, set a fine-mesh strainer in or drape a piece of cheesecloth over a bowl that holds at least 48 ounces (1.4 L). Slowly pour the nut mixture through the strainer or cheesecloth, allowing the milk to drip into the bowl. If you're using a strainer, press on the pulverized nuts with a spoon to release the excess liquid. If using cheesecloth, pick up the sides of the cloth and wring out the excess liquid.

4. If you do not wish to include the optional add-ins, skip to Step 5. If using the optional add-ins, pour the strained nut milk back into the blender or food processor, then add the MCT oil powder and/or vanilla and blend or pulse on low for 10 seconds, just until incorporated.

5. Transfer the milk to a 1-quart (950-ml) or larger airtight container.

STORE IT: *Keep in the fridge for up to 4 days or in the freezer for up to 1 month.*

THAW IT: *Remove from the freezer and allow to thaw on the counter until at least 50% defrosted, then place in the fridge until ready to use.*

Per 1-cup/240-ml serving, without MCT oil powder:

calories: **56**	calories from fat: **40**	total fat: **5.3g**	saturated fat: **1.2g**	cholesterol: **0mg**		FAT:	CARBS:	PROTEIN:
sodium: **95mg**	carbs: **1.2g**	dietary fiber: **0g**	net carbs: **1.2g**	sugars: **0g**	protein: **0.9g**	**85%**	**9%**	**6%**

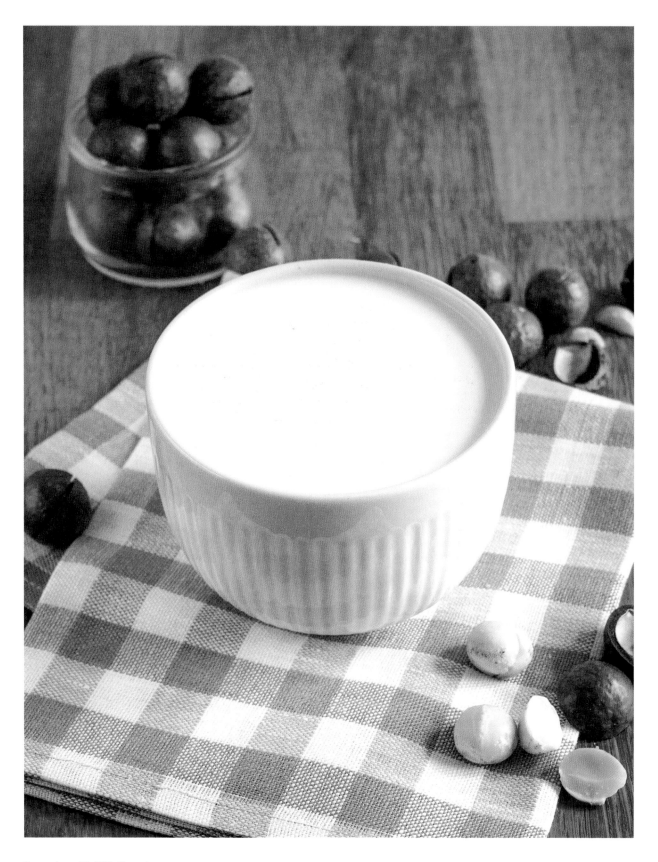

Per serving, with MCT oil powder:

calories: **74** | calories from fat: **55** | total fat: **7g** | saturated fat: **2.9g** | cholesterol: **0mg**

sodium: **95mg** | carbs: **1.7g** | dietary fiber: **0g** | net carbs: **1.7g** | sugars: **0g** | protein: **1.1g**

FAT:	CARBS:	PROTEIN:
85%	**9%**	**6%**

WATERMELON COOLER

COCONUT-FREE • DAIRY-FREE • EGG-FREE • LOW-FODMAP • NIGHTSHADE-FREE • NUT-FREE • VEGAN • VEGETARIAN

OPTION: AIP

MAKES four 4-ounce (120-ml) servings

PREP TIME: 5 minutes

COOK TIME: –

My sister and I could drink these until we turned into watermelons! During a recent trip home, we ordered a version of this drink while out for dinner with the rest of the family. It was so tasty, but loaded with sugar. We asked for no agave syrup, but I'm sure the watermelon juice they used contained sugar, too. So, I promised my sis I'd remake the recipe and put it in my next book. Here ya go, Christina! Just for you.

4½ ounces (128 g) fresh watermelon cubes, divided

12 mint leaves, divided

8 ice cubes, divided

4 ounces (120 ml) vodka, divided

4 teaspoons lime juice, divided

1⅓ cups (315 ml) sparkling or still water, divided

1. Set out four 4-ounce (120-ml) or larger glasses. Take a quarter of the watermelon cubes and cut them into ¼-inch (6-mm) dice. Divide the diced watermelon among the glasses. To each glass, add 3 mint leaves, 2 ice cubes, 1 ounce (30 ml) of vodka, and 1 teaspoon of lime juice.

2. Place the remaining watermelon pieces in a bowl and mash with a fork until you've removed as much of the juice as possible. Divide the juice among the glasses, about 2 teaspoons per glass. Fill each glass with sparkling water and enjoy!

make it AIP:
Omit the alcohol.

Per serving:

| calories: **70** | calories from fat: **0** | total fat: **0g** | saturated fat: **0g** | cholesterol: **0mg** |
| sodium: **2mg** | carbs: **1.3g** | dietary fiber: **0g** | net carbs: **1.3g** | sugars: **0.6g** | protein: **0.1g** |

FAT:	CARBS:	PROTEIN:	ALCOHOL:
0%	7%	1%	92%

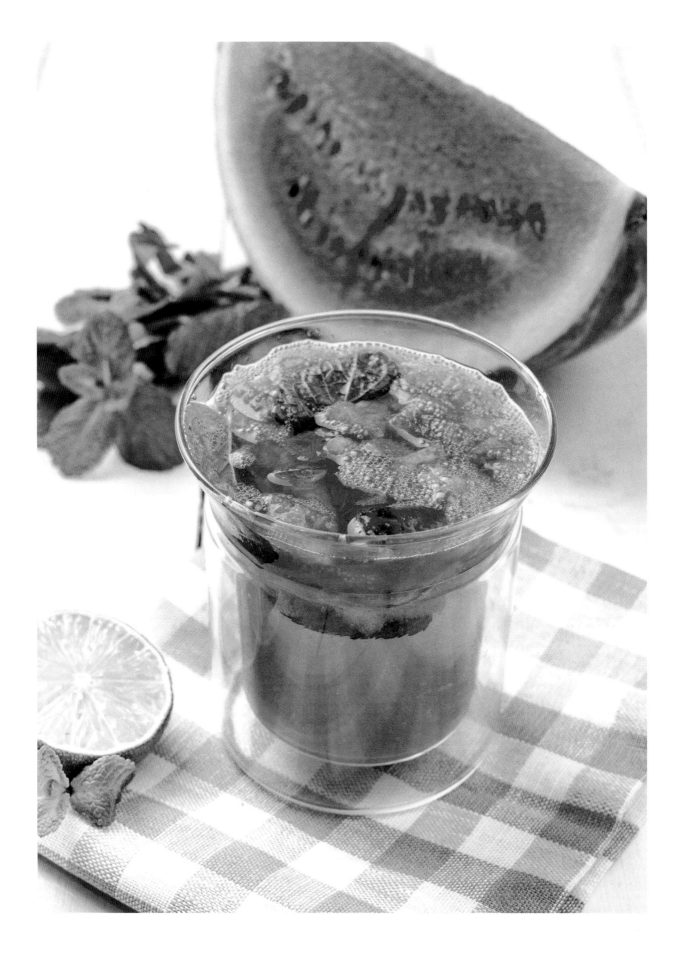

FROZEN MARGARITAS!

COCONUT-FREE • DAIRY-FREE • EGG-FREE • NIGHTSHADE-FREE • NUT-FREE • VEGAN • VEGETARIAN
OPTIONS: AIP • LOW-FODMAP

MAKES four 8-ounce (240-ml) servings

PREP TIME: 5 minutes

COOK TIME: –

I don't drink often, but when I do, it's almost always a margarita or two. What's not to love about the classic lime-infused drink? Well, except for all the sugar. Here's a sugar-free option that'll keep everyone happy. Plus, it has a salted rim if you're into that sort of thing.

FOR THE RIM (OPTIONAL):

2 tablespoons coarse sea salt

1 lime wedge

4 cups (520 g) ice (about 32 cubes)

½ cup (120 ml) lime juice

¼ cup (40 g) confectioners'-style erythritol, or 6 drops liquid stevia

4 ounces (120 ml) tequila

4 lime wedges, for garnish (optional)

1. Have on hand four 8-ounce (240-ml) or larger glasses.

2. To rim the glasses with salt, place the salt on a small plate or saucer. Moisten the rims of the glasses with the lime wedge. Holding the glass at an angle, carefully rotate the rim of each glass in the salt, coating the outer lip in the salt.

3. Place the ice, lime juice, sweetener, and tequila in a blender and blend on high for 30 seconds or until slushy.

4. Divide the margarita mixture among the 4 glasses. Garnish each with a lime wedge, if desired. Best enjoyed immediately.

make it AIP:
Omit the alcohol and use stevia or enjoy unsweetened.

make it LOW-FODMAP:
It is unclear whether tequila is low-FODMAP, as it has not been tested. Logically, it should be, but be cautious. You can prepare this drink with vodka instead of tequila if you're concerned.

Per serving, with salted rim:

					FAT:	CARBS:	PROTEIN:	ALCOHOL:
calories: **77**	calories from fat: **1**	total fat: **0.1g**	saturated fat: **0g**	cholesterol: **0mg**	**1%**	**11%**	**1%**	**87%**
sodium: **3501mg**	carbs: **2.1g**	dietary fiber: **0.1g**	net carbs: **2g**	sugars: **0.4g**	protein: **0.1g**			

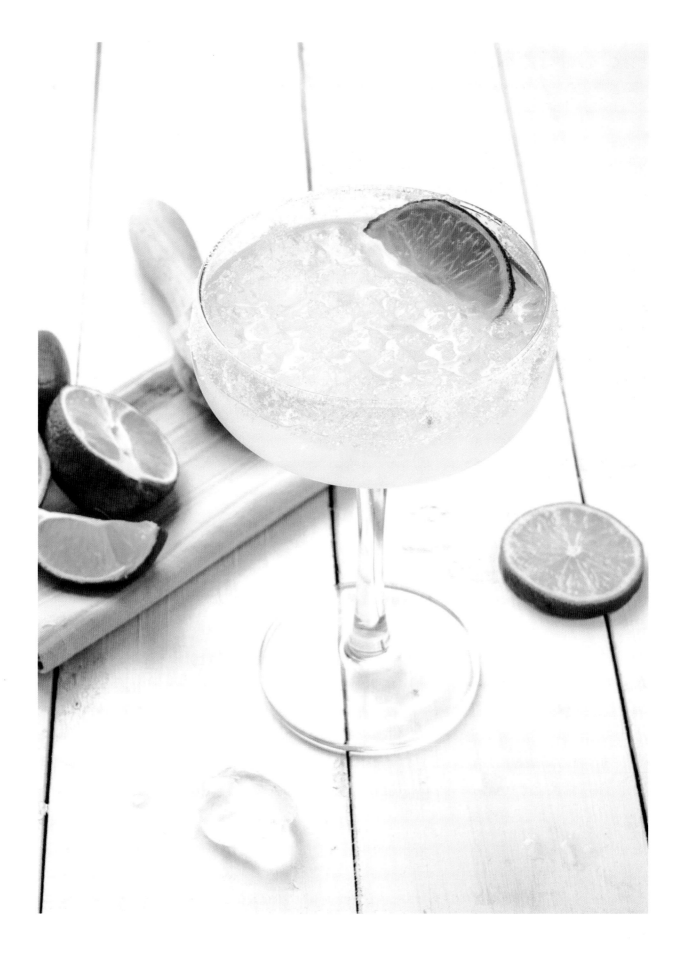

KETO FIZZ

AIP • DAIRY-FREE • EGG-FREE • LOW-FODMAP • NIGHTSHADE-FREE • NUT-FREE • VEGAN • VEGETARIAN

MAKES one 16-ounce (475-ml) serving

PREP TIME: 1 minute

COOK TIME: –

I wish I could say that I developed this recipe after careful attention and planning, but it wasn't like that. We were long overdue for a grocery run, so we were out of everything, including drinking water. That's when I found some carbonated water at the bottom of the pantry and some coconut milk in the freezer. Out of desperation, I defrosted the coconut milk, then combined it with the carbonated water. There's really nothing much else to it, other than to say that the flavor of this fizz is similar to a milkshake sans the blast of sugar and sugar high afterward.

⅓ cup (80 ml) full-fat coconut milk

2 or 3 drops liquid stevia (optional)

12 ounces (355 ml) sparkling water, chilled

Place the coconut milk in a tall 16-ounce (475-ml) or larger glass. Add the stevia, if using, and stir until combined. Pour in the sparkling water. Best enjoyed immediately.

Per serving:

calories: **116** | calories from fat: **108** | total fat: **12g** | saturated fat: **10g** | cholesterol: **0mg**
sodium: **25mg** | carbs: **1g** | dietary fiber: **0g** | net carbs: **1g** | sugars: **1g** | protein: **1g**

FAT:	CARBS:	PROTEIN:
93%	**3%**	**4%**

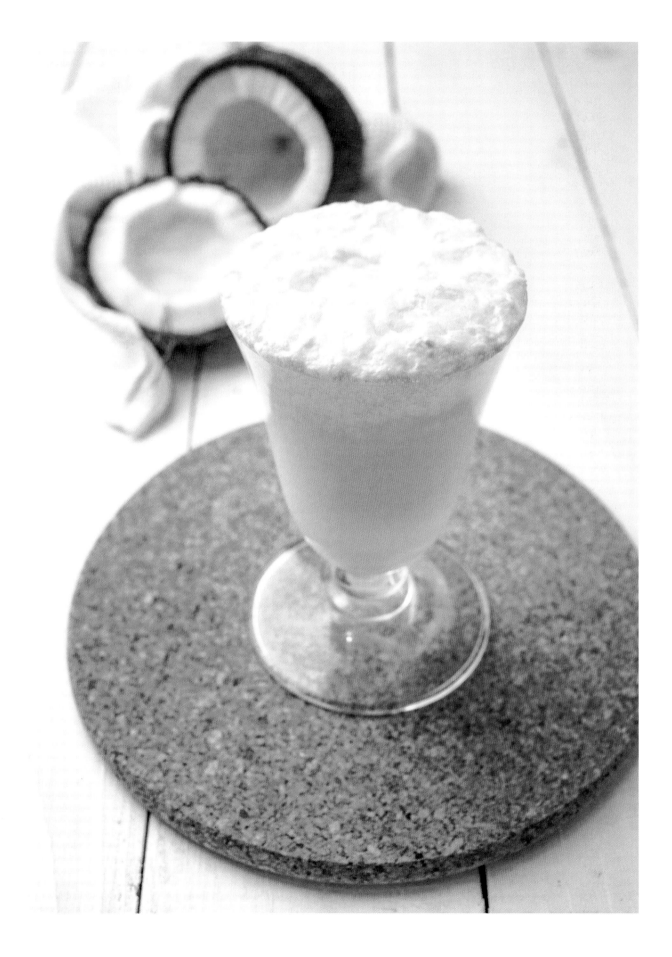

STRAWBERRY MILKSHAKE

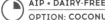 AIP • DAIRY-FREE • EGG-FREE • LOW-FODMAP • NIGHTSHADE-FREE • NUT-FREE • VEGAN • VEGETARIAN
OPTION: COCONUT-FREE

MAKES two 8-ounce (240-ml) servings

PREP TIME: 5 minutes

COOK TIME: –

This recipe calls for full-fat coconut milk frozen into cubes. Why not use frozen strawberries to thicken the shake? You could, but the consistency wouldn't be as thick and creamy. Frozen coconut milk gives shakes and smoothies a luxurious texture, almost like ice cream. I always have a tray of frozen coconut milk on hand for shakes and smoothies like this one. The cubes not only cool down the drink but also add a bunch of extra fat! This can be a helpful alternative to relying on more costly fats like MCT oil when making smoothies.

The easiest way to make the frozen coconut milk cubes is to measure out the coconut milk and then pour it into an ice cube tray. But if that's too much work for you, just swap the frozen coconut milk with chilled coconut milk and replace the fresh strawberries with frozen.

This milkshake doubles as a wicked ice pop mixture if you have any leftovers you can't finish!

6 ounces (170 g) strawberries, hulled (fresh or frozen and defrosted)

⅔ cup (160 ml) water

½ cup (120 ml) full-fat coconut milk, frozen into cubes

½ teaspoon vanilla extract

1. Place all the ingredients in a blender or food processor. Blend on high for 40 to 50 seconds, until all the coconut milk cubes have been broken up and the texture of the shake is smooth.

2. Divide between two 8-ounce (240-ml) or larger glasses. Best enjoyed immediately.

make it COCONUT-FREE:
Use heavy cream instead of coconut milk.

STORE IT: *If there are leftovers or you need to make the shake ahead of time, store it in an airtight container in the fridge for up to 3 days. When ready to enjoy, give it a little shake. Alternatively, pour the leftovers into ice pop molds and freeze.*

Per serving:

calories: **121** | calories from fat: **88** | total fat: **9.8g** | saturated fat: **0g** | cholesterol: **0mg** | sodium: **1mg** | carbs: **7.2g** | dietary fiber: **1.7g** | net carbs: **5.5g** | sugars: **4.3g** | protein: **1.1g**

FAT:	CARBS:	PROTEIN:
73%	**23%**	**4%**

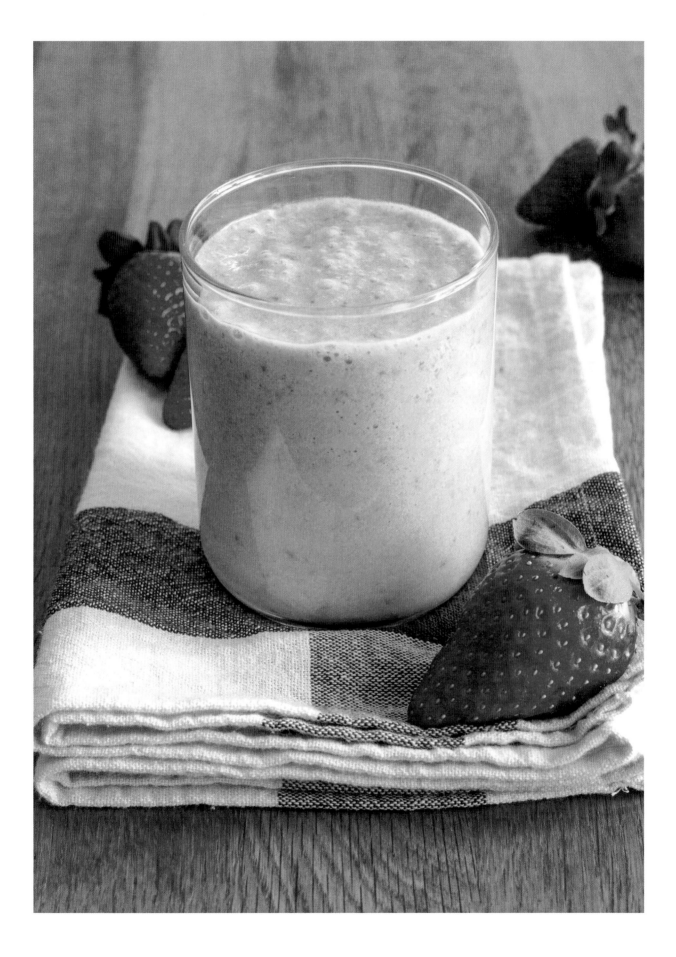

MATCHA MILKSHAKE

EGG-FREE • NIGHTSHADE-FREE • VEGETARIAN
OPTIONS: COCONUT-FREE • DAIRY-FREE • NUT-FREE • VEGAN

MAKES one 8-ounce
(240-ml) serving

PREP TIME: 5 minutes

COOK TIME: –

This milkshake is a special treat that is simple to make and quite tasty if you love matcha! Any low-carb ice cream will do the trick here. If you want a dairy-free version, So Delicious makes a keto-friendly coconut milk ice cream that's sweetened with erythritol. In fact, I'm enjoying a pint right now as I'm writing this. If you can eat dairy, there are many low-carb ice cream options for you, including Halo Top.

For the milk, any type—from dairy milk to almond milk—will work. Homemade Cashew Milk (page 342), Coconut Milk (page 344), and Macadamia Nut Milk (page 346), or store-bought versions of these, are all good options.

To lower the carb count, use chilled full-fat coconut milk in place of the ice cream.

½ cup (120 ml) milk (nondairy or regular)

2 teaspoons matcha powder

4 scoops low-carb ice cream (dairy-free or regular) (about 4½ oz/128 g)

1. Place the milk and matcha in an 8-ounce (240-ml) or larger airtight container. A pint-sized mason jar works fabulously.

2. Whisk the ingredients until the matcha is fully incorporated into the milk.

3. Add the ice cream, seal, and shake for 20 to 30 seconds.

4. Remove the lid and insert a straw. Best enjoyed immediately.

make it **COCONUT-FREE:**
Use a nut milk or dairy milk and a nut- or dairy-based ice cream.

make it **DAIRY-FREE/VEGAN:**
Use a nondairy milk and a dairy-free ice cream.

make it **NUT-FREE:**
Use a coconut- or dairy-based ice cream.

STORE IT: *If there are leftovers or you need to make the shake ahead of time, store it in an airtight container in the fridge for up to 3 days. When ready to enjoy, give it a little shake. Alternatively, pour the leftovers into ice pop molds and freeze.*

Per serving, made with full-fat coconut milk and erythritol-sweetened coconut milk ice cream:

			FAT:	CARBS:	PROTEIN:
calories: **193**	calories from fat: **126**	total fat: **14g**	saturated fat: **12.5g**	cholesterol: **0mg**	
sodium: **185mg**	carbs: **33g**	dietary fiber: **17.5g**	net carbs: **15.5g**	sugars: **2.5g**	protein: **1.5g**

FAT: **48%** CARBS: **50%** PROTEIN: **2%**

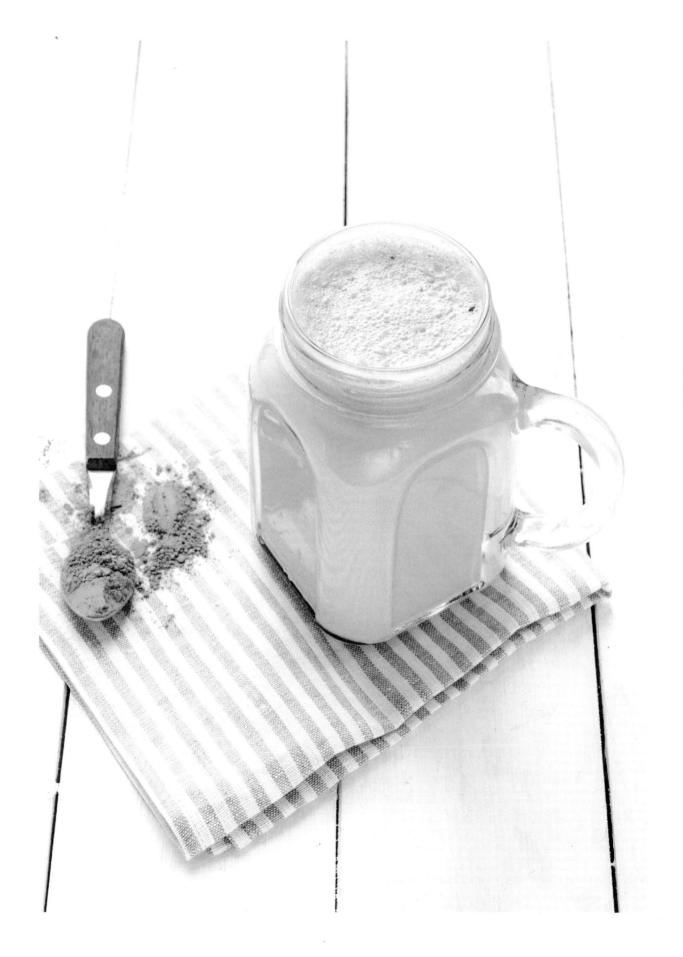

THE ULTRA GREEN

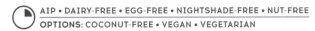
AIP • DAIRY-FREE • EGG-FREE • NIGHTSHADE-FREE • NUT-FREE
OPTIONS: COCONUT-FREE • VEGAN • VEGETARIAN

MAKES two 10-ounce (300-ml) servings

PREP TIME: 5 minutes

COOK TIME: –

If you love the taste of vegetables and can't get enough greenery into your body, this drink is for you. If you're not a huge fan of the color green or you can't have a salad without oodles of dressing, then it's probably best to pass on this one—hardcore veggie lovers only!

I freeze the zucchini and avocado pieces before making this smoothie because it adds chill without having to rely on ice. Also, it's more economical to purchase produce when it's on sale, chop it up, and use it in various recipes over the months to come. You don't have to freeze them for this recipe, but I highly recommend trying it at least once.

1 cup (240 ml) nondairy milk

¾ cup (110 g) chopped zucchini, frozen

½ medium Hass avocado, peeled, pitted, cubed, and frozen (about 2 oz/ 55 g of flesh)

1 handful of fresh spinach (about 1 oz/ 30 g)

2 tablespoons collagen peptides or protein powder

1 tablespoon coconut oil or unflavored MCT oil powder

¾ teaspoon matcha powder

1. Place all the ingredients in a blender or food processor. Blend until smooth, 30 to 40 seconds.

2. Divide between two 10-ounce (300-ml) or larger glasses. Best enjoyed immediately.

make it COCONUT-FREE:
Opt for a nondairy milk not made from coconut, like almond or hazelnut milk, and use MCT oil powder instead of coconut oil.

make it VEGAN:
Do not use collagen. Opt for a plant-based protein powder.

make it VEGETARIAN:
Do not use collagen. Opt for a plant- or egg-based protein powder.

STORE IT: *If there are leftovers or you need to make the drink ahead of time, store it in an airtight container in the fridge for up to 3 days. When ready to enjoy, give it a little shake. Alternatively, pour the leftovers into ice pop molds and freeze.*

Per serving, made with full-fat coconut milk, collagen, and coconut oil:

							FAT:	CARBS:	PROTEIN:
calories: **200**	calories from fat: **129**	total fat: **14.3g**	saturated fat: **9g**	cholesterol: **0mg**			**64%**	**15%**	**21%**
sodium: **131mg**	carbs: **7.3g**	dietary fiber: **3.3g**	net carbs: **4g**	sugars: **2.7g**	protein: **10.6g**				

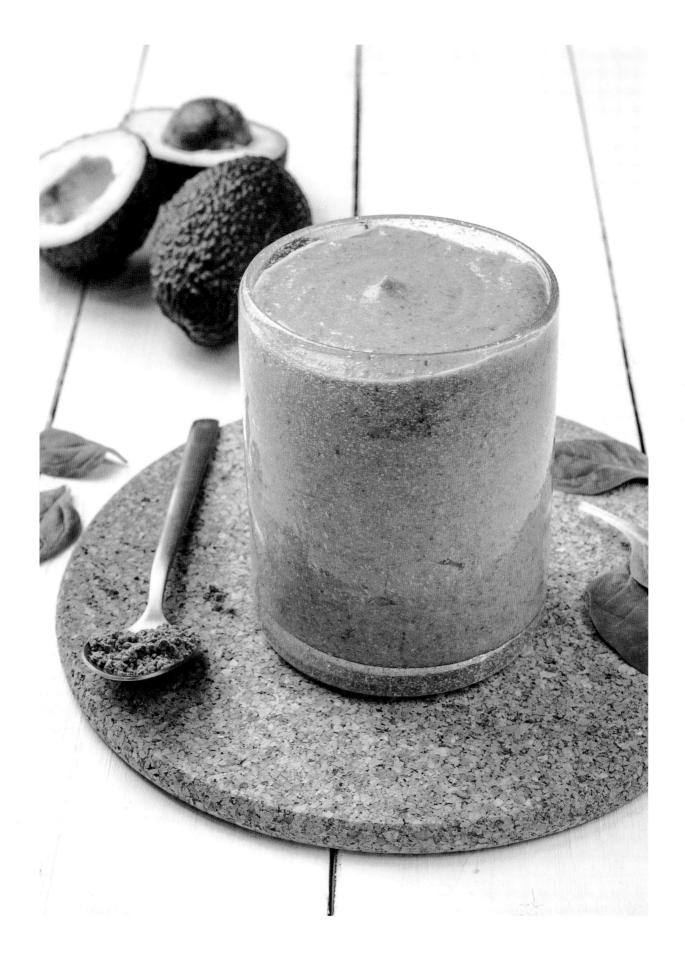

CHILLED CHAI

EGG-FREE • LOW-FODMAP • NIGHTSHADE-FREE

OPTIONS: AIP • COCONUT-FREE • DAIRY-FREE • NUT-FREE • VEGAN • VEGETARIAN

MAKES one 16-ounce (475-ml) serving

PREP TIME: 10 minutes

COOK TIME: –

If you can have dairy, go for dairy milk here. Otherwise, I enjoy making this drink with lite or full-fat coconut milk. It also works fabulously with Cashew Milk (page 342).

1 chai tea bag (decaf or regular)

1 cup (240 ml) boiling water

2 tablespoons unflavored MCT oil powder

2 tablespoons collagen peptides or protein powder

1½ teaspoons erythritol, or 2 drops liquid stevia (optional)

6 ice cubes

½ cup (120 ml) milk (nondairy or regular)

1. Set the tea bag in a large mug and pour the boiling water over it. Allow to steep for 10 to 15 minutes.

2. Meanwhile, place the MCT oil powder, collagen, and sweetener, if using, in a blender or food processor.

3. Once the tea has steeped, remove the bag and pour the tea into the blender or food processor. Blend on high for 20 to 30 seconds, just until incorporated. Alternatively, you can add the ingredients to the mug with the tea and whisk with a fork until fully incorporated.

4. Place the ice cubes in a tall 20-ounce (600-ml) glass. Pour the tea mixture into the glass, then pour the milk over the top.

> **STORE IT:** *Store covered in the fridge for up to 3 days. When ready to enjoy, give it a little shake.*

make it AIP:
Use coconut milk and stevia or enjoy unsweetened.

make it COCONUT-FREE:
Use a nut milk or dairy milk.

make it DAIRY-FREE:
Use a nondairy milk.

make it NUT-FREE:
Use coconut milk or dairy milk.

make it VEGAN:
Do not use collagen. Opt for a plant-based protein powder. Use a nondairy milk.

make it VEGETARIAN:
Do not use collagen. Opt for a plant- or egg-based protein powder.

Per serving, made with collagen and lite coconut milk:

calories: **217** | calories from fat: **126** | total fat: **14g** | saturated fat: **0g** | cholesterol: **0mg**
sodium: **58mg** | carbs: **3.5g** | dietary fiber: **2g** | net carbs: **1.5g** | sugars: **0g** | protein: **12g**

FAT:	CARBS:	PROTEIN:
58%	6%	36%

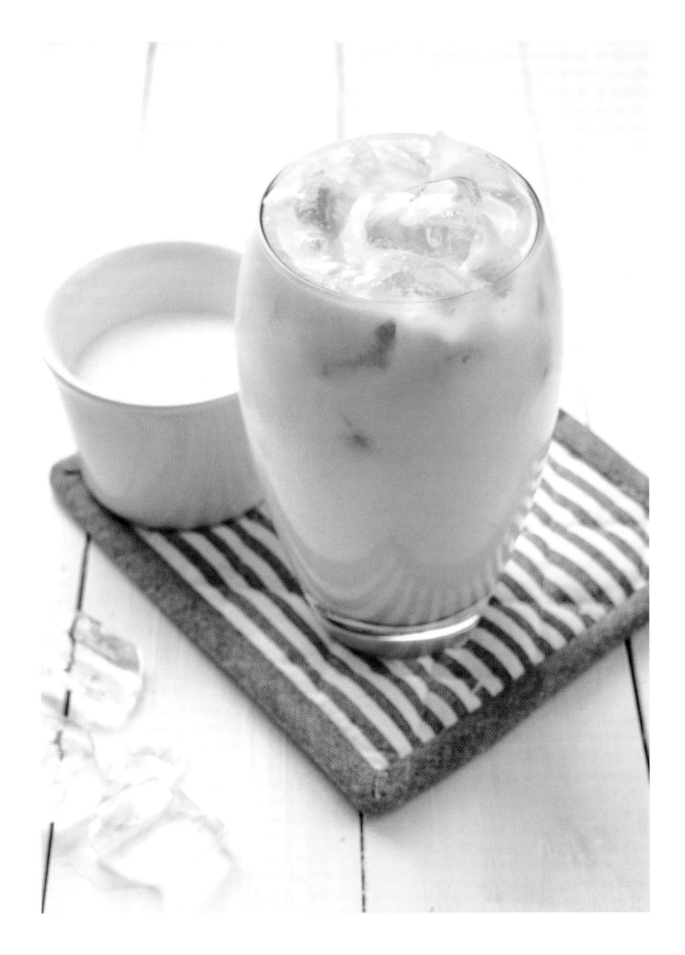

VANILLA SHAKE

LOW-FODMAP • NIGHTSHADE-FREE

OPTIONS: COCONUT-FREE • DAIRY-FREE • NUT-FREE • VEGETARIAN

MAKES one 8-ounce (240-ml) serving

PREP TIME: 2 minutes

COOK TIME: –

You can have so much fun with this recipe after you get accustomed to making it. Swap out the almond butter for any nut butter under the sun, and play around with seed butters, too! Swap out the water for brewed coffee, steeped and chilled tea (green tea is awesome here), or nondairy milk.

The collagen is optional, but I'll never say no to growing healthy hair, skin, and nails. If you don't do collagen, you can substitute your favorite protein powder, as you can in most of the recipes in this book. The adjustment will change the nutritional details a bit, but it's better that you make this shake out of your favorite ingredients than avoid it altogether. It's a simple concept that you will use over and over again.

If you have a concern about consuming raw egg yolk, you could purchase pasteurized eggs or simply leave the egg yolk out of your shake.

4 ice cubes

½ cup (120 ml) water

2 tablespoons collagen peptides or protein powder (optional)

1 tablespoon coconut oil, unflavored MCT oil powder, or ghee

1 tablespoon smooth unsweetened almond butter

1 large egg yolk

1 teaspoon erythritol, or 1 drop liquid stevia

½ teaspoon vanilla extract

1. Place all the ingredients in a blender or food processor and blend on high for 30 seconds or until the ice is pulverized.

2. Transfer to an 8-ounce (240-ml) or larger glass. Best enjoyed immediately.

make it COCONUT-FREE:
Use MCT oil powder or ghee.

make it DAIRY-FREE:
Do not use ghee.

make it NUT-FREE:
Use a seed butter.

make it VEGETARIAN:
Do not use collagen. Opt for a plant- or egg-based protein powder.

STORE IT: *If there are leftovers or you need to make the shake ahead of time, store it in an airtight container in the fridge for up to 3 days. When ready to enjoy, give it a little shake. Alternatively, pour the leftovers into ice pop molds and freeze.*

Per serving, made with coconut oil, without collagen/protein powder:

						FAT:	CARBS:	PROTEIN:
calories: **283**	calories from fat: **244**	total fat: **27.1g**	saturated fat: **14.1g**	cholesterol: **210mg**		**86%**	**5%**	**9%**
sodium: **9mg**	carbs: **3.9g**	dietary fiber: **1.6g**	net carbs: **2.3g**	sugars: **1.1g**	protein: **6.1g**			

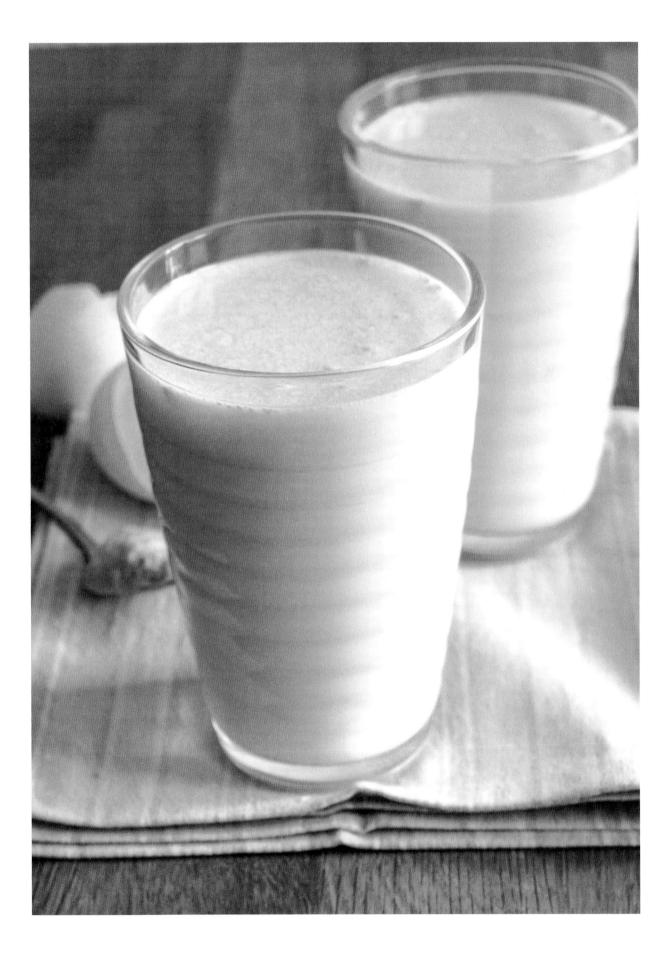

RECIPE QUICK REFERENCE

✓ meets this criteria | O option | *(see page 53 for details)*

RECIPE	PAGE	SIZE	❄	🍲	👤	⏱	AIP	COCONUT-FREE	DAIRY-FREE	EGG-FREE	LOW-FODMAP	NIGHTSHADE-FREE	NUT-FREE	VEGAN	VEGETARIAN
Quick 'n' Easy Barbecue Sauce	70	SMALL	✓	✓	✓	✓		O	✓	✓			✓	✓	✓
Thai Dressing	72	SMALL		✓	✓	✓			✓	✓		O	O	✓	✓
Chive & Onion Cream Cheese	74	SMALL		✓	✓	✓		O	✓	✓			✓	✓	✓
Ranch Dressing	76	SMALL		✓	✓	✓			✓	O		✓	✓	O	✓
Honey Mustard Dressing & Marinade	78	SMALL	✓	✓	✓	✓	✓	✓	✓	✓		✓	✓		✓
Green Speckled Dressing	80	SMALL		✓	✓	✓		O	✓	O	O	✓	✓	O	✓
Bacon Dressing	82	SMALL	✓	✓	✓	✓	O	✓	✓	✓	✓	✓	✓		
Avocado Lime Dressing	84	SMALL		✓	✓	✓	✓	✓	✓	✓		✓	✓	✓	✓
Lemon Turmeric Dressing & Marinade	86	SMALL	✓	✓	✓	✓	✓	✓	✓	✓		✓	✓	✓	✓
Basil Vinaigrette & Marinade	88	SMALL		✓	✓	✓	O	✓	✓	✓	O	✓	✓	O	✓
Poppy Seed Dressing	90	SMALL	✓	✓	✓	✓			✓	✓	O	✓	✓		✓
Teriyaki Sauce & Marinade	92	SMALL	✓	✓	✓	✓		O	✓	✓		✓	✓	✓	✓
Creamy Italian Dressing	94	SMALL		✓	✓	✓		✓	✓	O	O	O	✓	O	✓
Chocolate Sauce	96	SMALL	✓	✓	✓	✓	O	✓	✓	✓		✓	✓	✓	✓
Herby Vinaigrette & Marinade	98	SMALL		✓	✓	✓	O	✓	✓	✓	O	✓	✓	✓	✓
Ready-in-Seconds Hollandaise Sauce	100	SMALL		✓	✓	✓		O	O		✓	O	✓		
Egg-Free Mayonnaise	102	SMALL		✓	✓	✓		✓	✓	✓		✓	✓	✓	✓
Mayonnaise	104	SMALL		✓	✓	✓		✓	✓			✓	✓		✓
Chocoholic Granola	108	SMALL	✓	✓	✓			O	✓	✓	O	✓		✓	✓
Avocado Breakfast Muffins	110	SMALL		✓	✓	✓		O	✓				✓		✓
Herb Chicken Sausages with Braised Bok Choy	112	SMALL	✓	✓	✓	✓	O	O	O	✓	O	O			
Buffalo Chicken Breakfast Muffins	114	SMALL		✓	✓	✓		O	O		O	O	✓		
Prosciutto Biscuits	116	SMALL	✓	✓	✓	✓			✓		✓	✓	✓		
Salmon Bacon Rolls with Dipping Sauce	118	MEDIUM		✓	✓	✓	O	✓	✓	O	O	O	✓		
Hey Girl	120	MEDIUM		✓		✓	O	O	✓	O		✓	✓	O	O
Pumpkin Spice Latte Overnight "Oats"	122	MEDIUM		✓				O	✓	✓	✓	✓	O	O	✓
Rocket Fuel Hot Chocolate	124	MEDIUM		✓		✓	O	✓	✓	✓		✓	✓	O	O
Full Meal Deal	126	MEDIUM		✓	✓	✓			O			O	✓		✓
Liver Sausages & Onions	128	MEDIUM	✓	✓	✓		O	✓	O	✓		✓	✓		
Cross-Country Scrambler	130	MEDIUM		✓				✓	✓		✓		✓		
Eggs Benedict	132	MEDIUM			✓	✓		O	O			✓	✓	O	
Mug Biscuit	134	MEDIUM	✓	✓		✓			O			✓	✓		✓
Keto Breakfast Pudding	136	MEDIUM		✓		✓		✓	✓	O		✓	✓	O	O
Pepper Sausage Fry	138	MEDIUM	✓	✓	✓	✓	O	O	✓	✓	O	O			
Indian Masala Omelet	140	MEDIUM		✓				✓	O				✓		✓
Sticky Wrapped Eggs	142	MEDIUM		✓	✓			O	✓		✓	O			
All Day Any Day Hash	144	LARGE	✓	✓	✓			O	O	✓			✓		
Something Different Breakfast Sammy	146	LARGE				✓		✓	✓	O		O	✓	O	O
Super Breakfast Combo	148	LARGE	✓			✓	O	O	✓	✓	O	✓	O	O	O
Coffee Shake	150	LARGE		✓		✓		O	O	✓	O	✓	✓	O	✓
Chili Lime Chicken Bowls	154	SMALL	✓	✓	✓			✓	✓	✓			✓		
German No-Tato Salad	156	SMALL		✓	✓	✓		✓	✓	O	O	✓	✓		
Salmon Salad Cups	158	MEDIUM		✓	✓		O	✓	✓	O	✓	✓	✓		
Steak Fry Cups	160	MEDIUM	✓	✓	✓			O	✓				✓		
Broccoli Ginger Soup	162	MEDIUM	✓	✓	✓	✓	O		✓				✓		
Antipasto Salad	164	MEDIUM		✓	✓			✓	✓				✓		
Sauerkraut Soup	166	MEDIUM	✓	✓	✓	✓	O	✓	✓	✓		✓	✓		

RECIPE	PAGE	SIZE	❄	🍱	👤	⏱	AIP	COCONUT-FREE	DAIRY-FREE	EGG-FREE	LOW-FODMAP	NIGHTSHADE-FREE	NUT-FREE	VEGAN	VEGETARIAN
Easy Chopped Salad	168	MEDIUM		✓		✓	○	✓	✓	✓		○	✓	✓	✓
Cajun Shrimp Salad	170	MEDIUM		✓	✓	✓		✓	✓	✓			✓		
Speckled Salad	172	MEDIUM		✓		✓	○	✓	✓	✓	○	✓	✓	✓	✓
Keto Lasagna Casserole	174	LARGE	✓	✓	✓			○	○				○		
Kale Salad with Spicy Lime-Tahini Dressing	176	LARGE		✓	✓	✓		✓	✓	✓			✓	✓	✓
Zucchini Pasta Salad	178	LARGE		✓	✓	✓		✓	✓	○	✓		○	○	✓
Coconut Red Curry Soup	180	LARGE	✓	✓	✓	✓	○	✓	✓	✓			✓		
Chimichurri Steak Bunwiches	182	LARGE	✓	✓	✓	✓		✓	✓			○	✓		
Mexican Chicken Soup	184	LARGE	✓	✓	✓	✓		○	○	✓			✓		
Sammies with Basil Mayo	186	LARGE		✓		✓		✓	✓	○		✓	✓		
Cream Cheese Meat Bagels	188	LARGE	✓	✓	✓			○	○		○	○	✓		
BLT-Stuffed Avocados	190	LARGE				✓	○	✓	✓	✓			✓		
Broccoli Tabbouleh with Greek Chicken Thighs	192	LARGE	✓	✓	✓	✓	○	✓	✓	✓			✓		
Paprika Chicken Sandwiches	194	HUGE		✓	✓	✓		○	✓	○			○		
Crispy Thighs & Mash	198	MEDIUM	✓	✓	✓			○	○	✓			✓		
Noodles & Glazed Salmon	200	MEDIUM	✓	✓	✓	✓		○	○	✓	○	○	○		
Scallops & Mozza Broccoli Mash	202	MEDIUM	✓	✓	✓			○	○	✓			✓		
BBQ Beef & Slaw	204	MEDIUM	✓	✓	✓			○	✓	✓			✓		
Cream of Mushroom–Stuffed Chicken	206	MEDIUM	✓	✓	✓			○	○	✓			✓		
Crispy Pork with Lemon-Thyme Cauli Rice	208	MEDIUM	✓	✓	✓			○	○	✓			✓		
One-Pot Porky Kale	210	MEDIUM	✓	✓	✓			○	○	○			○		
Salmon & Kale	212	MEDIUM	✓	✓	✓			○	✓	✓			○		
Creamy Spinach Zucchini Boats	214	MEDIUM		✓	✓				✓	○			○		
My Favorite Creamy Pesto Chicken	216	MEDIUM	✓	✓	✓	✓		○	○	✓	○	○	○		
Chicken Laksa	218	MEDIUM	✓	✓	✓	✓		○	✓	✓			○		
Super Cheesy Salmon Zoodles	220	MEDIUM	✓	✓				○	○	✓	○	○	○		
Epic Cauliflower Nacho Plate	222	MEDIUM		✓				○	○	○					
Shhh Sliders	224	MEDIUM	✓	✓	✓	✓		✓	✓			○	○		
Shrimp Curry	226	MEDIUM	✓	✓	✓			○	✓	✓			✓		
Cabbage & Sausage with Bacon	228	LARGE	✓	✓	✓		○	✓	✓	✓			○	✓	
Secret Stuffed Peppers	230	LARGE	✓	✓	✓		○	✓	○	✓	○	○	✓		
Shrimp Fry	232	LARGE	✓	✓		✓	○	○	✓	✓	○	○	✓		
Roasted Broccoli & Meat Sauce	234	LARGE	✓	✓	✓			✓	✓	✓	○		✓		
Cheesy Meatballs & Noodles	236	LARGE	✓	✓	✓	✓	○	○	○	✓			✓		
Zucchini Lasagna	238	LARGE	✓	✓	✓			○	○				✓		
Mexican Meatzza	240	LARGE		✓	✓			○	○				○		
Noodle Bake	242	LARGE		✓	✓		○	○	○	✓		○	✓		
Bacon-Wrapped Stuffed Chicken	244	LARGE	✓	✓	✓		○	✓	✓	✓		✓	✓		
One-Pot Stuffin'	246	LARGE	✓	✓	✓		○	○	✓	✓		✓	○		
Southern Pulled Pork "Spaghetti"	248	LARGE		✓	✓			✓	✓	✓			✓		
Sweet Beef Curry	250	LARGE	✓	✓	✓			○	✓	✓		○	✓		
Open-Faced Tacos	252	HUGE	✓	✓	✓	✓		○	○	✓	○		✓		
Breaded Shrimp Salad	254	HUGE		✓	✓	✓		○	✓				✓		
Shredded Mojo Pork with Avocado Salad	256	HUGE	✓	✓	✓			✓	✓	✓			✓		
Crunchy Jicama Fries	260	SMALL			✓		○	✓	✓	○		○	✓	○	✓
Sautéed Asparagus with Lemon-Tahini Sauce	262	SMALL		✓	✓	✓		✓	✓	✓		✓	✓	✓	✓
Liver Bites	264	SMALL	✓	✓	✓		○	✓	✓	✓		✓	✓		

RECIPE QUICK REFERENCE *(continued)*

✓ **meets this criteria** | ○ **option** | *(see page 53 for details)*

RECIPE	PAGE	SIZE	❄	◷	👥	⏱	AIP	COCONUT-FREE	DAIRY-FREE	EGG-FREE	LOW-FODMAP	NIGHTSHADE-FREE	NUT-FREE	VEGAN	VEGETARIAN
Wedge Dippers	266	SMALL		✓	✓	✓	○	○	✓	○		✓	✓	○	✓
Mac Fatties	268	SMALL	✓		✓				✓	✓	○	○		✓	✓
Cauliflower Patties	270	SMALL	✓	✓	✓	✓		○	○			✓		○	✓
Tapenade	272	SMALL		✓	✓	✓		✓	✓	✓			✓	○	○
Hummus Celery Boats	274	SMALL		✓	✓			✓	✓	✓	○	○		✓	✓
Fried Cabbage Wedges	276	SMALL		✓	✓	✓	✓	○	✓	✓	○	✓	✓	○	✓
Salami Chips with Buffalo Chicken Dip	278	SMALL		✓	✓	✓	○	✓	✓	✓	○	○	✓		
Dairy-Free (But Just as Good) Queso	280	MEDIUM		✓	✓			○	✓	✓				○	○
Toasted Rosemary Nuts	282	MEDIUM	✓	✓	✓	✓		○	○	✓	✓	○		○	✓
Chimichurri	284	MEDIUM		✓	✓	✓	○	✓	✓	✓	○		✓	○	○
Breaded Mushroom Nuggets	286	MEDIUM		✓				✓	✓			○			
Cucumber Salmon Coins	288	MEDIUM		✓		✓		✓	✓	○	○	✓	✓		
Radish Chips & Pesto	290	MEDIUM		✓				✓	✓	✓		✓		✓	✓
BLT Dip	292	MEDIUM		✓	✓			✓	✓	○					
Tuna Cucumber Boats	294	LARGE		✓		✓		✓	✓	○	○	✓	✓		
Zucchini Cakes with Lemon Aioli	296	LARGE		✓				✓				✓	✓		
Keto Diet Snack Plate	298	LARGE		✓		✓		✓	✓			✓	✓		
Bacon-Wrapped Avocado Fries	300	LARGE			✓	✓	✓	✓	✓	✓		✓	✓		
Ketone Gummies	304	SMALL		✓	✓		✓	✓	✓	✓	✓	✓	✓		
Strawberry Shortcake Coconut Ice	306	SMALL		✓	✓	✓	○	○	✓	✓	✓	✓	✓	✓	✓
Grandma's Meringues	308	SMALL		✓	✓			○	✓		✓	✓	✓		✓
Haystack Cookies	310	SMALL	✓	✓	✓			○	✓	✓	✓	✓	✓	○	✓
Cheesecake Balls	312	SMALL	✓	✓	✓			○	○	✓	✓	✓	✓		○
Cinnamon Bombs	314	SMALL	✓		✓	✓	○	○	○	✓	✓	✓	○	○	✓
Superpower Fat Bombs	316	SMALL	✓		✓	✓		○	○	✓	✓	✓	✓	○	○
Jelly Cups	318	SMALL			✓		○	○	○	✓	✓	✓	○		
Fudge Bombs	320	SMALL	✓		✓	✓		○	○	✓	✓	✓	○	○	✓
Brownie Cake	322	SMALL	✓	✓	✓			○	○			✓			✓
Cinnamon Sugar Muffins	324	SMALL	✓	✓	✓			○	○		○	✓			✓
Edana's Macadamia Crack Bars	326	MEDIUM	✓	✓	✓			○	○		✓	✓			✓
N'oatmeal Bars	328	MEDIUM	✓	✓	✓			✓	✓	✓		✓	✓	✓	✓
Blueberry Crumble with Cream Topping	330	MEDIUM	✓	✓	✓	✓		○	○			✓		○	✓
Chocolate Soft-Serve Ice Cream	332	MEDIUM		✓	✓		○	✓	✓			✓	○	○	○
Keto Arnold Palmer	336	SMALL		✓		✓	○	✓	✓	✓	✓	✓	✓	✓	✓
Turmeric Keto Lemonade	338	SMALL		✓		✓	○	✓	✓	✓	✓	✓	✓	✓	✓
Egg Cream	340	SMALL		✓				○	○	✓	✓	✓	○	○	✓
Cashew Milk	342	SMALL	✓	✓	✓			✓	✓	✓		✓		✓	✓
Coconut Milk	344	SMALL	✓	✓	✓	✓	✓		✓	✓		✓	✓	✓	✓
Macadamia Nut Milk	346	SMALL	✓	✓	✓			✓	✓	✓		✓		✓	✓
Watermelon Cooler	348	SMALL			✓	✓	○	✓	✓	✓	✓	✓	✓	✓	✓
Frozen Margaritas!	350	SMALL			✓	✓	○	✓	✓	✓	○	✓	✓	✓	✓
Keto Fizz	352	SMALL			✓	✓	✓		✓	✓	✓	✓	✓	✓	✓
Strawberry Milkshake	354	SMALL	✓		✓	✓	✓	○	✓	✓	✓	✓	✓	✓	✓
Matcha Milkshake	356	SMALL	✓		✓			○	○	✓		✓	○	○	✓
The Ultra Green	358	SMALL	✓	✓		✓	✓	○	✓	✓		✓	✓	○	○
Chilled Chai	360	SMALL		✓		✓	○	○	✓	✓		✓		○	○
Vanilla Shake	362	SMALL	✓	✓		✓		○	○		✓	✓	○		○

RECIPE INDEX

SAUCES AND SPREADS

BREAKFAST

144

146

148

150

All Day Any Day Hash

Something Different Breakfast Sammy

Super Breakfast Combo

Coffee Shake

LUNCH

154

156

Chili Lime Chicken Bowls

German No-Tato Salad

158

160

162

164

166

168

170

Salmon Salad Cups

Steak Fry Cups

Broccoli Ginger Soup

Antipasto Salad

Sauerkraut Soup

Easy Chopped Salad

Cajun Shrimp Salad

172

Speckled Salad

174

176

178

180

182

184

186

Keto Lasagna Casserole

Kale Salad with Spicy Lime-Tahini Dressing

Zucchini Pasta Salad

Coconut Red Curry Soup

Chimichurri Steak Bunwiches

Mexican Chicken Soup

Sammies with Basil Mayo

188

190

192

Cream Cheese Meat Bagels

BLT-Stuffed Avocados

Broccoli Tabbouleh with Greek Chicken Thighs

194

Paprika Chicken
Sandwiches

DINNER

198

Crispy Thighs &
Mash

200

Noodles & Glazed
Salmon

202

Scallops & Mozza
Broccoli Mash

204

BBQ Beef & Slaw

206

Cream of Mushroom–
Stuffed Chicken

208

Crispy Pork with
Lemon-Thyme
Cauli Rice

210

One-Pot Porky Kale

212

Salmon & Kale

214

Creamy Spinach
Zucchini Boats

216

My Favorite Creamy
Pesto Chicken

218

Chicken Laksa

220

Super Cheesy
Salmon Zoodles

222

Epic Cauliflower
Nacho Plate

224

Shhh Sliders

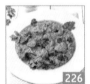
226

Shrimp Curry

228

Cabbage & Sausage
with Bacon

230

Secret Stuffed
Peppers

232

Shrimp Fry

234

Roasted Broccoli &
Meat Sauce

236

Cheesy Meatballs &
Noodles

238

Zucchini Lasagna

240

Mexican Meatzza

242

Noodle Bake

244

Bacon-Wrapped
Stuffed Chicken

246

One-Pot Stuffin'

248

Southern Pulled
Pork "Spaghetti"

250

Sweet Beef Curry

252

254

256

Open-Faced Tacos

Breaded Shrimp
Salad

Shredded
Mojo Pork with
Avocado Salad

SAVORY SNACKS

260

262

264

266

268

270

272

Crunchy
Jicama Fries

Sautéed Asparagus
with Lemon-Tahini
Sauce

Liver Bites

Wedge Dippers

Mac Fatties

Cauliflower Patties

Tapenade

274

276

278

Hummus
Celery Boats

Fried Cabbage
Wedges

Salami Chips
with Buffalo
Chicken Dip

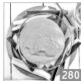
280

282

284

286

288

290

292

Dairy-Free (But Just
as Good) Queso

Toasted
Rosemary Nuts

Chimichurri

Breaded Mushroom
Nuggets

Cucumber
Salmon Coins

Radish Chips &
Pesto

BLT Dip

294

296

298

300

Tuna Cucumber
Boats

Zucchini Cakes
with Lemon Aioli

Keto Diet
Snack Plate

Bacon-Wrapped
Avocado Fries

SWEET SNACKS

 304
Ketone Gummies

 306
Strawberry Shortcake
Coconut Ice

 308
Grandma's
Meringues

 310
Haystack Cookies

 312
Cheesecake Balls

 314
Cinnamon Bombs

 316
Superpower
Fat Bombs

 318
Jelly Cups

 320
Fudge Bombs

 322
Brownie Cake

 324
Cinnamon Sugar
Muffins

 326
Edana's Macadamia
Crack Bars

 328
N'oatmeal Bars

 330
Blueberry Crumble
with
Cream Topping

 332
Chocolate Soft-
Serve Ice Cream

EXTRA SIPS

 336
Keto Arnold Palmer

 338
Turmeric Keto
Lemonade

 340
Egg Cream

 342
Cashew Milk

 344
Coconut Milk

 346
Macadamia Nut
Milk

 348
Watermelon Cooler

 350
Frozen Margaritas!

 352
Keto Fizz

 354
Strawberry
Milkshake

 356
Matcha Milkshake

 358
The Ultra Green

 360
Chilled Chai

 362
Vanilla Shake

GENERAL INDEX